Topics in
Structural Heart Disease

Emerging Concepts in Cardiology

Topics in
Structural Heart Disease

Craig T. Basson, MD, PhD

Gladys and Roland Harriman Professor of Medicine
Director, Cardiovascular Research
Division of Cardiology
Department of Medicine
Weill Medical College of Cornell University
New York Presbyterian Hospital
New York, New York

Bruce B. Lerman, MD

H. Altschul Master Professor of Medicine
Chief, Division of Cardiology
Department of Medicine
Weill Medical College of Cornell University
New York Presbyterian Hospital
New York, New York

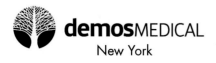
demosMEDICAL
New York

Acquisitions Editor: Richard Winters
Cover Design: Joe Tenerelli
Compositor: NewGen North America
Printer: King Printing

Visit our website at www.demosmedpub.com

Library of Congress Cataloging-in-Publication Data

Topics in structural heart disease / [edited by] Craig T. Basson, Bruce B. Lerman.
   p.; cm.
   Includes bibliographical references and index.
   ISBN 978–1–933864–59–4
  1. Heart—Diseases. 2. Heart—Diseases—Diagnosis. I. Basson, Craig T.
II. Lerman, Bruce B.
  [DNLM: 1. Cardiovascular Diseases—diagnosis. WG 141 S927 2010]
  RC682.S795 2010
  616.1'2—dc22   2009034460

Medicine is an ever-changing science. Research and clinical experience are continually expanding our knowledge, in particular our understanding of proper treatment and drug therapy. The authors, editors, and publisher have made every effort to ensure that all information in this book is in accordance with the state of knowledge at the time of production of the book.

Nevertheless, the authors, editors, and publisher are not responsible for errors or omissions or for any consequences from application of the information in this book and make no warranty, express or implied, with respect to the contents of the publication. Every reader should examine carefully the package inserts accompanying each drug and should carefully check whether the dosage schedules mentioned therein or the contraindications stated by the manufacturer differ from the statements made in this book. Such examination is particularly important with drugs that are either rarely used or have been newly released on the market.

Special discounts on bulk quantities of Demos Medical Publishing books are available to corporations, professional associations, pharmaceutical companies, health care organizations, and other qualifying groups. For details, please contact:

Special Sales Department
Demos Medical Publishing
11 W. 42nd Street, 15th Floor
New York, NY 10036
Phone: 800–532–8663 or 212–683–0072
Fax: 212–941–7842
E-mail: rsantana@demosmedpub.com

Made in the United States of America
09 10 11 12 13   5 4 3 2 1

Contents

Preface   ix
Contributors   xi

1   Computed Tomography Evaluation of Coronary
    Artery Disease   1
    Fay Y. Lin and James K. Min

2   Magnetic Resonance Imaging for Assessment
    of the Postmyocardial Infarction Heart   19
    Sidney Glasofer and Jonathan W. Weinsaft

3   Exercise Electrocardiography: The Diagnostic
    and Prognostic Value of Heart Rate   37
    *Paul Kligfield, Joy M. Gelbman, and
    Peter M. Okin*

4   ECG Left Ventricular Hypertrophy:
    Detection and Prognosis   51
    Seth R. Bender and Peter M. Okin

5   Diabetes   69
    Richard B. Devereux and Giovanni de Simone

6   The Noninvasive Vascular Laboratory: Physiologic
    Testing and Vascular Ultrasonography for the
    Assessment of Peripheral Arterial Disease   89
    George Bell and Ingrid Hriljac

7   Cardiac and Aortic Causes of Stroke   117
    Maria G. Karas and Jorge R. Kizer

8   Cardiovascular Manifestations of
    Systemic Lupus Erythematosus   141
    Mary J. Roman

9   Tetralogy of Fallot in the Adult Congenital
    Heart Disease Patient   153
    Kirsten O. Healy and Gina LaRocca

Index   169

Preface

Despite recent advances in the management of cardiovascular diseases, these conditions continue to wreak havoc in our society. Cardiovascular disease remains the leading cause of death in the United States, and more than 2,000 Americans die every day from heart disease. One in five deaths involve coronary heart disease and one in eight involve heart failure. Recent studies have reported different rates of testing and treatment utilization by physicians in various geographic locations, and quality of care analyses continue to highlight the need to educate and to encourage physicians to implement the most modern therapeutic strategies.

The Emerging Topics in Cardiology series is devoted to describing state-of-the-art approaches to common problems in cardiovascular disease that will be of use to internists and cardiologists. The discussions are rooted in the most current literature available and dovetail with available American Heart Association/American College of Cardiology guidelines. Reflections, opinions, and editorializations that may temper the rote application of these guidelines and that may project future advances and changes in practice are offered by Cornell cardiologists who are subspecialists in the topics explored.

In this first volume, *Topics in Structural Heart Disease*, our colleagues tackle a variety of disorders that reflect acquired and congenital structural cardiovascular pathologies. Etiologies, diagnostic modalities, and therapies are all considered. Examination of the effects of diabetes and systemic lupus erythematosis on the structure and function of the heart and blood vessels provides an opportunity to explore the impact of inflammatory and immune processes on the cardiovascular system; we address how these processes affect diagnosis, prognosis, and treatment. Diagnostic evaluations of structural cardiovascular disease that lead to prognostication and appropriate management require a variety of complex imaging and other noninvasive modalities. Technologies continue to evolve at a rapid pace and cardiology has seen marked advances. Therefore, chapters address, wholly or in part, contemporary application of echocardiography, computed tomography, magnetic resonance imaging, and vascular ultrasound to care for patients with cardiac and vascular disease. Imaging modalities are also critical to the assessment of individuals with congenital as well as acquired heart disease, and the evaluation of the patient with Tetralogy of Fallot is a key paradigm for how we can approach the increasingly prevalent issue of adults with congenital structural heart disease. To consider how physicians might best determine the functional significance of structural disorders that lead to ischemic and/or hypertrophic heart disease, this volume describes the refined application of exercise testing and electrocardiography. Finally, we consider how knowledge regarding these cardiovascular pathologies and diagnostic modalities can be utilized along with modern advances in biomarker risk factors to improve diagnosis and prognosis in our patients with stroke.

The editors are grateful to our colleagues at Cornell Cardiology who have invested their time, energy, and insights into this series. We hope that practicing physicians will find this volume and this series a unique tool in their daily practice as they care for patients with heart disease. Future volumes will address additional topics in heart disease, and it is our intent to provide a resource of cutting edge consultation that improves cardiovascular health for all.

Craig T. Basson, MD, PhD
Bruce B. Lerman, MD

Contributors

George Bell, MD
Fellow in Medicine
Division of Cardiology
Department of Medicine
Weill Medical College of Cornell University
New York Presbyterian Hospital
New York, New York

Seth R. Bender, MD
Fellow in Medicine
Division of Cardiology
Department of Medicine
Weill Medical College of Cornell University
New York Presbyterian Hospital
New York, New York

Giovanni de Simone, MD
Department of Clinical and Experimental Medicine
Federico II University Hospital
Naples, Italy

Richard B. Devereux, MD
Professor of Medicine
Director, Echocardiography Laboratory
Division of Cardiology
Department of Medicine
Weill Medical College of Cornell University
New York Presbyterian Hospital
New York, New York

Joy M. Gelbman, MD
Assistant Professor of Medicine
Division of Cardiology
Department of Medicine
Weill Medical College of Cornell University
New York Presbyterian Hospital
New York, New York

Sidney Glasofer, MD
Fellow in Medicine
Division of Cardiology
Department of Medicine
Weill Medical College of Cornell University
New York Presbyterian Hospital
New York, New York

Kirsten O. Healy, MD
Fellow in Medicine
Division of Cardiology
Department of Medicine
Weill Medical College of Cornell University
New York Presbyterian Hospital
New York, New York

Ingrid Hriljac, MD
Assistant Professor of Medicine
Division of Cardiology
Department of Medicine
Weill Medical College of Cornell University
New York Presbyterian Hospital
New York, New York

Maria G. Karas, MD
Fellow in Medicine
Division of Cardiology
Department of Medicine
Weill Medical College of Cornell University
New York Presbyterian Hospital
New York, New York

Jorge R. Kizer, MD, MSc
Associate Professor of Medicine
Division of Cardiology
Department of Medicine
Weill Medical College of Cornell University
New York Presbyterian Hospital
New York, New York

Paul Kligfield, MD
Professor of Medicine
Director, Cardiac Graphics Laboratory
Division of Cardiology
Department of Medicine
Weill Medical College of Cornell University
New York Presbyterian Hospital
New York, New York

Gina LaRocca, MD
Assistant Professor of Medicine
Division of Cardiology
Department of Medicine
Weill Medical College of Cornell University
New York Presbyterian Hospital
New York, New York

Fay Y. Lin, MD
Assistant Professor of Medicine
Division of Cardiology
Department of Medicine
Weill Medical College of Cornell University
New York Presbyterian Hospital
New York, New York

James K. Min, MD
Assistant Professor of Medicine
Division of Cardiology
Department of Medicine
Weill Medical College of Cornell University
New York Presbyterian Hospital
New York, New York

Peter M. Okin, MD
Professor of Medicine
Director of Clinical Affairs
Division of Cardiology
Department of Medicine
Weill Medical College of Cornell University
New York Presbyterian Hospital
New York, New York

Mary J. Roman, MD
Professor of Medicine
Associate Director, Echocardiography Laboratory
Division of Cardiology
Department of Medicine
Weill Medical College of Cornell University
New York Presbyterian Hospital
New York, New York

Jonathan W. Weinsaft, MD
Assistant Professor of Medicine
Director, Cardiac MRI
Division of Cardiology
Department of Medicine
Weill Medical College of Cornell University
New York Presbyterian Hospital
New York, New York

Topics in
Structural Heart Disease

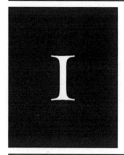

Computed Tomography Evaluation of Coronary Artery Disease

FAY Y. LIN
JAMES K. MIN

OUTLINE

CCTA Technology   1

Practice of CCTA   2

Usefulness of a Noninvasive
Imaging Test   5

Prognostic Value of CCTA   13

Cost Considerations   14

Radiation Considerations   15

Current Indications and Appropriateness
Criteria for CCTA   15

Future Directions of CCTA   16

References   16

In the last several decades, the paradigm for evaluation of individuals with suspected coronary artery disease (CAD) has employed a combination of clinical assessment and noninvasive functional-based imaging methods for diagnosis, risk stratification, and net reclassification. These functional imaging modalities—most commonly performed by myocardial perfusion single-photon emission computed tomography (MPS) and, to a lesser extent, stress echocardiography, positron emission tomography (PET), and magnetic resonance imaging (MRI)—are aimed at identification of obstructive coronary stenoses by detection of regional differences in coronary flow reserve or left ventricular wall motion.

Recently, coronary computed tomographic angiography (CCTA) has emerged as a promising, noninvasive anatomic method for direct visualization of atherosclerotic plaque within coronary arteries. Developments in computed tomography (CT) technology—driven primarily by improvements in temporal and spatial resolution and volume coverage—now permit routine evaluation of the coronary arteries and cardiovascular structures with exquisite clarity and accuracy. The purpose of this chapter is to review the principles of anatomic coronary artery evaluation by CCTA, and to describe the scientific evidence to date regarding its diagnostic accuracy, prognostic risk potential, and cost effectiveness.

■ CCTA TECHNOLOGY

Coronary artery evaluation by CT has been traditionally difficult to achieve. The constant and often unpredictable motion of the coronary arteries requires imaging techniques with high temporal resolution, while the small diameter of the coronary arteries demands high spatial resolution. Furthermore, as CT image acquisition requires breathhold to prevent significant respiratory motion artifact, adequate z-axis coverage (i.e., in the craniocaudal direction) is necessary to limit examination times to that achievable by most patients. The recent introduction of 64-detector row CT scanners now permits adequate volume coverage that, when coupled with submillimeter spatial resolution and subsecond temporal resolution, results in virtually artifact-free cardiac and coronary artery imaging.

Since their introduction in 2005, 64-detector row CT scanners have become the benchmark standard for CCTA performance. Performance of CCTA by these

CT scanners has historically relied on half-scan integral reconstruction, whereby data sampled during one-half of the CT x-ray source rotation (i.e., 180°) is used to reconstruct a transaxial image. By this method, the temporal resolution of CCTA ranges between 160 and 220 msec. Data are collected by multidetector rows equipped with in-plane spatial resolutions that range between 0.5 and 0.8 mm. During each rotation of the CT x-ray source, approximately 2 cm of z-axis coverage are achieved. The combination of these characteristics enables image acquisition of the heart in approximately 5–10 seconds.

As the temporal resolution of traditional 64-detector row CT scanners is limited, individuals undergoing CCTA traditionally require heart rates below 65 beats per minute (bpm) in order to achieve optimal image quality. Numerous technological advances have been introduced in order to permit CT image acquisition at higher heart rates. One solution available on every 64-detector row CT scanner is termed multisegment reconstruction. By this technique, data are sampled at time intervals shorter than that required for half-scan reconstruction (e.g., 90°) and combined over several consecutive cardiac cycles. This method can double or even quadruple the temporal resolution of CCTA, but requires interpolation of data from multiple cardiac cycles with very little beat-to-beat variation. As this technique has not been uniformly successful in improving image quality or diagnostic accuracy, other solutions have been advanced.

An additional potential solution has been to increase the z-axis coverage of the CT scanners. This is made possible by increasing the numbers of detector rows from 64 to 128, then to 256, and now to 320. A 320-detector row CT enables image acquisition of the entire heart in one single rotation of the CT x-ray source, although the spatial and temporal resolutions remain unchanged. The advantages of the increased numbers of detector rows is reduced susceptibility to cardiac arrhythmias and a potentially lower radiation dose.

An alternative method at improving temporal resolution has been to increase the numbers of x-ray sources on the CT scanner. Traditional 64-detector row CT scanners here entailed a single x-ray source with a single detector array directly opposite the source. In contrast, a recently introduced dual-source CT scanner combines two x-ray sources with two sets of detector arrays at 90° from each other within a single gantry. This scanner enables image acquisition with 90° rotation (as opposed to 180° rotation), and improves temporal resolution to 83 msec. Recent studies examining the use of dual-source CCTA have been promising, indicating improved image quality at higher heart rates (1).

Despite improved volume coverage and enhanced temporal resolution, CT acquisition of the heart has been limited by spatial resolutions of 0.5 to 0.8 mm, or approximately 2 to 4 times less than that of invasive coronary angiography. Recently, a new-generation CT scanner has been introduced with a 0.2-mm resolution, which results in improved coronary artery lumen diameter visualization and potentially enhanced detection of atherosclerotic plaque.

■ PRACTICE OF CCTA

For typical CCTA, patients are evaluated for resting heart rate. If heart rates greater than 65 bpm are present, heart-rate lowering medications—most commonly oral or intravenous beta blockers—are administered. For angiographic visualization, iodinated contrast is injected to increase the relative density of the vascular lumen to the vessel wall in a manner similar to invasive coronary angiography. The initiation of scan acquisition is timed for the arrival of maximal coronary opacification within the coronary arteries. Axial or helical CT images are acquired during a single breathhold—which is variably dependent upon the rotational speed of the x-ray source, the area of coverage by the multidetector array, and the speed at which the patient passes through the scanner (defined as pitch). Data at identical points in the cardiac cycle from multiple heartbeats are matched, and coverage of the coronary artery bed generally requires 4 to 8 gantry rotations, over separate RR intervals, with a 64-slice scanner. Computer processing then enables image reconstruction of data, resulting in a 3-dimensional isotropic voxel data set for each specified interval within a cardiac cycle. Isotropic voxel data represent an advantage of CT over other imaging modalities, in that equally precise spatial resolution exists in the x-, y-, and z-planes. Each voxel within the array displays a shade of gray depending on the average attenuation of the tissue within the voxel; dense objects, such as bone and calcium, are coded lighter in color, while objects with lower attenuation, such as air, are coded darker.

Although CT data are acquired in the transaxial plane, CT images may also be viewed in reformatted slices that occur in any plane in space due to the isotropic nature of the acquired voxels (Figure 1.1). In this regard, a curved lumen of a coronary artery that traverses through multiple planes may be projected simultaneously as a single plane by simple postprocessing techniques, or visualized en face in a manner analogous to intravascular ultrasound (Figure 1.2). Coronary artery stents and bypass grafts may be evaluated in a manner similar to native coronary arteries (Figure 1.3). Noncoronary cardiac anatomy may also be visualized in 3-dimensions (Figure 1.4). For coronary arteries that exhibit motion artifact, clarity may be achieved by viewing coronary arteries at different points in the cardiac cycle depending upon the most quiescent phase for that particular artery.

The current capabilities of CT present both limitations and advantages to the visual interpretation of CCTA (2). First, at the current limit of spatial resolution, the voxel coverage of a small coronary artery does not permit quantification of luminal stenosis to the level of precision of invasive coronary angiography, with a spatial resolution of approximately 0.15 to 0.2 mm. However, coronary artery luminal diameters and cross-sectional areas may be semi-quantified, and intraluminal coronary stenosis is generally quantified as a percentage range—for example, 0%, 1–25%, 25–50%, 50–75%, and 75–100%. Second, at the current limit of temporal resolution, patients must have slow and regular heart rates that are less than 60 bpm in order to preclude significant cardiac motion artifact, and must be able to maintain effective breathholds of at least 5 to 10 seconds to avoid respiratory motion artifact. Patients with atrial fibrillation or other sources of beat-to-beat variability will have scans of considerably worse—and often uninterpretable—image quality for the coronary arteries. Third, as with all other imaging studies, dense objects such as hardware, stents, or calcification may introduce significant artifacts. Fourth, the radiation dose required for a conventional CCTA throughout the entire cardiac cycle is estimated at 10–15 mSv; by way of comparison, invasive angiography generally results in approximately 5–7 mSv of radiation, while myocardial perfusion stress testing requires 15–30 mSv of radiation, depending on the choice of radioisotope. Recent CCTA radiation dose reduction techniques, such as prospectively ECG-triggered CCTA, 100 kV tube voltage image, and ECG tube current modulation can substantially reduce radiation doses to the 2–3 mSV range—which is comparable to the level of annual background radiation exposure—without compromise in diagnostic image quality for the coronary arteries.

In contrast to invasive angiography or functional stress testing, which aim primarily to identify patients with obstructive coronary artery stenosis, CCTA offers a means of anatomic evaluation of the coronary arteries

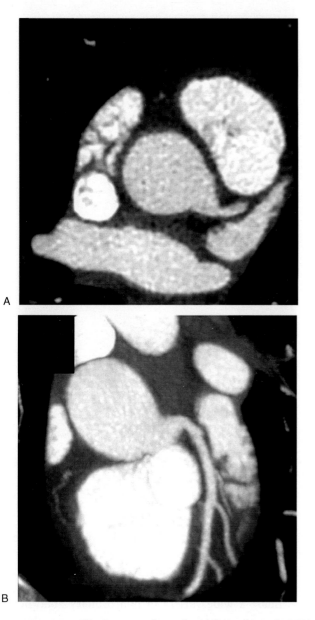

FIGURE 1.1 (A) Contrast-enhanced, ECG-gated axial CCTA image of left main artery. (B) Reformatted view of left anterior descending artery.

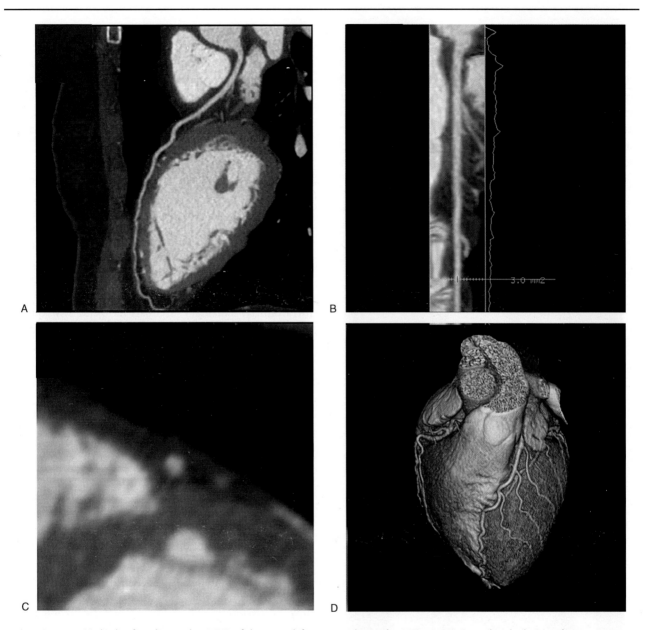

FIGURE 1.2 Methods of evaluation by CCTA of the same left anterior descending artery. (A) Curved multiplanar reformat. (B) Linear center-line reformat with automated calculation of cross-sectional area. (C) Cross-sectional view. (D) Three-dimensional reconstruction.

that not only estimates luminal diameter stenosis, but also provides information regarding coronary atherosclerosis composition and remodeling (Figure 1.5). Indeed, at present, CCTA is the only noninvasive test that provides data similar to intravascular ultrasound or optical coherence tomography to visualize coronary arteries beyond simple lumenography. Further, CCTA is able to demonstrate all anatomy within a 3-dimensional

acquisition throughout a cardiac cycle; thus, it is ideal for evaluations of relative anatomy, such as coronary artery anomalies, pulmonary veins, and coronary vein morphology (Figure 1.6). In fact, CCTA may be used to evaluate a wide variety of noncoronary abnormalities, including aortic disease, left atrial anatomy, shunts, masses, left ventricular hypertrophy, infarcts, wall motion abnormalities, and valvular, pericardial, and congenital

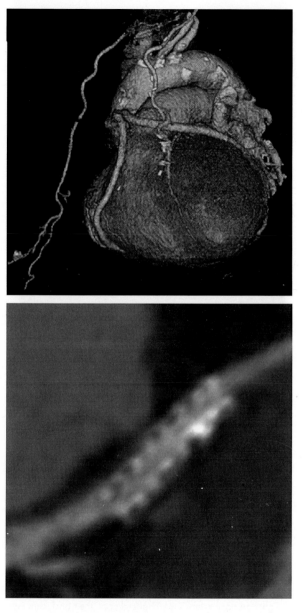

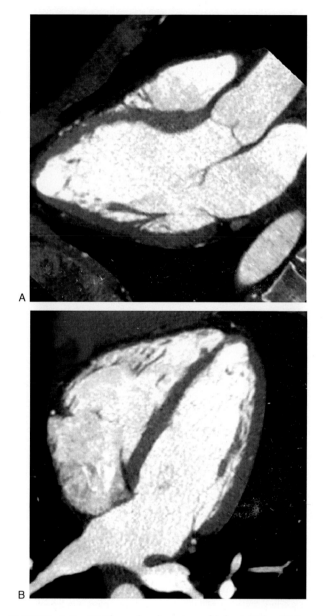

FIGURE 1.3 (A) Three-dimensional reconstruction of coronary artery bypass graft in a left anterior oblique view. There is a patent left internal mammary artery graft to the left anterior descending artery. There is a patent saphenous venous Y-graft to the obtuse marginal and posterior descending arteries. The right internal mammary artery is uninvolved. (B) Coronary stent with mild in-stent restenosis in curved multiplanar reformat.

FIGURE 1.4 (A) Three-chamber view of left ventricle. (B) Four-chamber view.

heart disease, as well as noncardiac causes of chest pain such as hiatal hernias (Figure 1.7). Quantitative evaluation of ventricular mass, volumes, and function may also be accurately performed (Figure 1.8).

■ USEFULNESS OF A NONINVASIVE IMAGING TEST

The primary use of CCTA is for the evaluation of coronary arteries in individuals with suspected CAD; thus, a brief discussion of the utility of diagnostic testing for CAD in general is warranted.

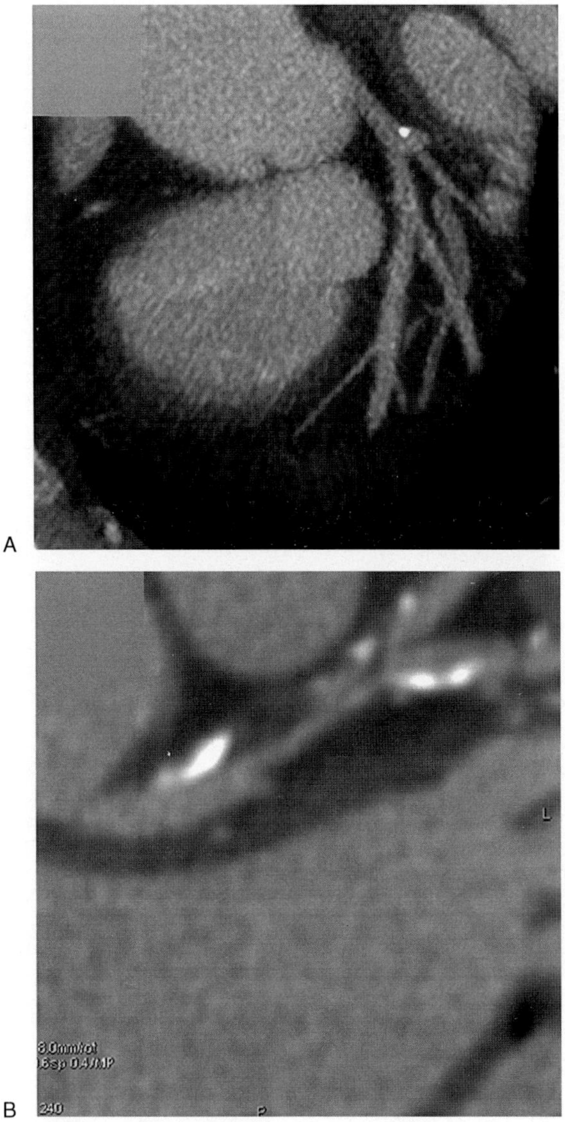

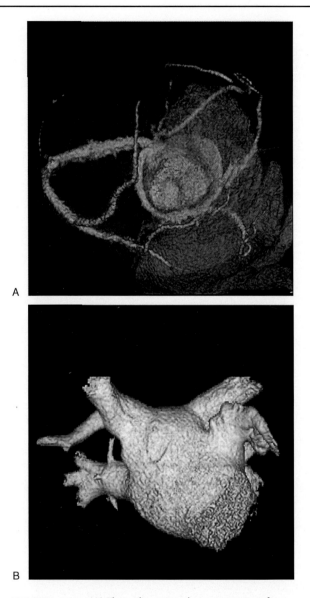

FIGURE 1.5 (A) Very mild focal calcified plaque in the left main coronary artery and very mild diffuse noncalcified plaque in the left anterior descending artery. (B) Obstructive left main coronary artery with diffuse mixed plaque. Both positive and negative remodeling are seen.

FIGURE 1.6 (A) Three-dimensional reconstruction of an anomalous right coronary artery superimposed upon the translucent myocardium in a left anterior oblique caudal projection. The single coronary artery originates in the right aortic cusp and trifurcates into the right coronary artery, the left circumflex artery posterior to the aortic root, and the left anterior descending artery anterior to the pulmonary artery. (B) Three-dimensional model of the left atrium in an anteroposterior view, demonstrating the relative position of the pulmonary veins, left atrial appendage, and mitral valve. In this patient, the indentation of the fossa ovalis is also visualized medially.

The discriminatory power of a noninvasive diagnostic test can be generally characterized by its performance against a gold standard—such as invasive coronary angiography—for diagnosis of obstructive CAD or for prediction of a future adverse CAD event. Sensitivity, specificity, and the area under the receiver-operating curve (AUC) are useful statistical measures that describe the accuracy of finding true positives, true negatives, and simultaneous maximization of both in any population;

an ideal test would have a sensitivity and specificity of 100%, and an AUC of 1. From sensitivity and specificity measures, positive and negative predictive values or likelihood ratios can be calculated. In contrast to sensitivity

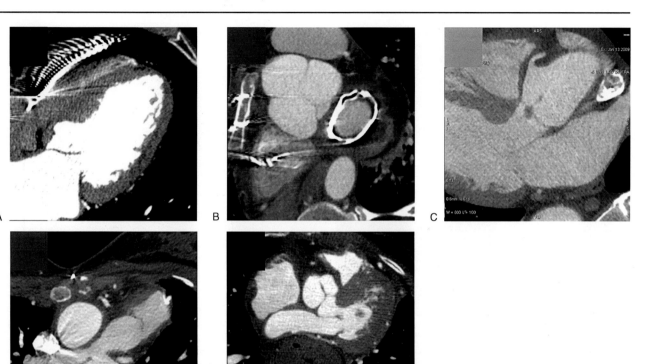

FIGURE 1.7 (A) Hypoattenuation of the anterolateral wall consistent with a subendocardial infarct. An automated implanted cardiac defibrillator lead is also seen in the right ventricle with streak artifact. (B) Aortic root aneurysm measuring 5.0 cm and a mitral annuloplasty ring visualized en face. A pacemaker is also visible in the right ventricle. (C) Mildly dilated aortic root with an aortic valve fibroelastoma. (D) Tetralogy of Fallot with bilateral branch pulmonary artery stenosis. Calcification is seen anterior to the right ventricular outflow tract at the site of prior repair. (E) Large hiatal hernia visible in axial images at the level of the aortic root. The left atrium is distorted posteriorly by the stomach.

and specificity, these metrics are highly dependent upon the prevalence of disease within a tested population, and are generally more relevant to guiding individual patient care. In short, the posttest likelihood of disease is dependent not only upon the diagnostic performance of a test, but also on the pretest likelihood of disease.

The classic assessment of pretest likelihood of CAD employs the Diamond-Forrester model of Bayesian analysis. The major branch point of this algorithm for individuals depends upon age, gender, and the presence and quality of symptoms. This algorithm, aimed at predicting the likelihood of anatomic obstructive CAD, has been widely employed for use in cardiac imaging and testing (Figure 1.9) (3). For a noninvasive diagnostic test of moderate discriminatory diagnostic value, patients with intermediate pretest probabilities of disease obtain the greatest degree of clinically significant risk reclassification, while those with high or low pretest probabilities are more likely to be falsely risk reclassified. As the discriminatory

value of the test improves, fewer patients would be misclassified and the pretest probability range for which useful risk reclassification can be achieved would widen. The discriminatory prognostic power of a test depends similarly upon disease distribution, with additional variation beyond diagnosis by natural history, disease treatment, and behavior of physicians and patients.

Cardiac imaging physicians have characterized numerous test characteristics of traditional modalities for prognosis above and beyond angiographic definitions of CAD for both symptomatic assessment and asymptomatic screening. As a relatively young technology, CCTA is only beginning to define the significance of its test findings.

Diagnostic Accuracy of CCTA to Detect and Exclude Obstructive Coronary Artery Stenosis

The cornerstone of any new diagnostic technology is the assessment of its diagnostic accuracy; in the case of

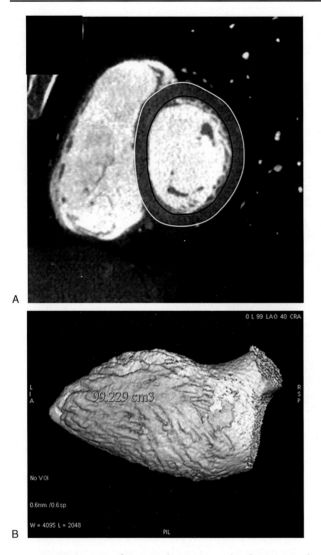

A

B

FIGURE 1.8 (A) Left ventricular mass and volumes may be calculated using Simpson's rule of disks or (B) three-dimensional reconstructions.

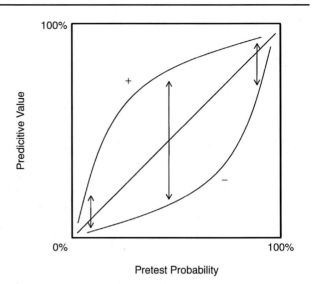

FIGURE 1.9 Discriminative properties of a diagnostic test at different levels of pretest probability or disease prevalence. Testing in intermediate-probability patients yields greater reclassification for positive predictive value (+) and negative predictive value (–) than testing in high- or low-probability patients.

CCTA, it is the identification of obstructive coronary artery stenosis. A recent meta-analysis of 12 studies using 64- or more detector row CCTA demonstrated good performance for the identification of >50% stenosis: sensitivity 97% (95% confidence interval [CI] 95–98%), specificity 90% (95% CI 86–93%), positive predictive value 93% (95% CI 91–96%), and negative predictive value 96% (95% CI 92–98%) (4). This high diagnostic performance—in particular, the high negative predictive value to exclude obstructive CAD—suggests a potential role for CCTA in low- to intermediate-risk patients in whom exclusion of

disease would identify individuals in whom no further testing or therapy would be warranted. Critics of CCTA contend, however, that despite meta-analytic data, prior studies of CCTA have relied upon single centers and retrospective study designs that were limited by workup bias, thus missing patients who may have otherwise been found to be false negatives. This limitation is not unique to CCTA, and has been observed for studies of exercise treadmill testing, echocardiography, and myocardial perfusion scintigraphy.

In response, two recent prospective multicenter studies—ACCURACY and CORE 64—have evaluated the diagnostic test performance of CCTA free of workup bias in patients with differing disease prevalences. The Assessment by Coronary Computed Tomographic Angiography of Individuals Undergoing Invasive Coronary Angiography, or ACCURACY trial, was a U.S.-based study that enrolled patients at 16 centers already referred for elective coronary angiography for CCTA prior to ICA (5). Of the 230 subjects, only 72 (24.8%) and 32 (13.9%) were found to have >50% or >70% stenosis. The diagnostic sensitivities, specificities, and positive and negative predictive values to detect a >50% or >70% stenosis were 95%, 83%, 64%, and 99%, respectively, and 94%, 83%, 48%, and 99%

respectively. The AUC for identification of patients with >50% or >70% stenosis was 0.96 and 0.95, respectively. This study definitively established the high diagnostic accuracy for both detection and exclusion of obstructive coronary artery stenosis at both the 50% and 70% thresholds.

Sensitivity and specificity of CCTA in ACCURACY (95% and 83%, respectively) compares favorably to other noninvasive imaging cardiac tests including exercise echocardiography (86% versus 81%, respectively) and exercise MPS (87% and 73%, respectively); furthermore, negative predictive values of CCTA are superior to all other modalities (6). Of note, the ACCURACY trial is the only study to date to report diagnostic test performance of CCTA in a symptomatic population with a low-intermediate prevalence of CAD—which has been the population in which it is proposed to be most useful according to the most recent CCTA American College of Cardiology Appropriateness Criteria (7). This accounts for the lower positive predictive value in comparison to earlier studies, which tested patients with more advanced disease than would be considered inappropriate under current guidelines.

In contrast, the 291 patients enrolled in the multicenter CORE 64 study possessed high pretest likelihood of CAD and, indeed, were found to have a 56% prevalence of >50% intraluminal stenosis, despite exclusion for elevated coronary artery calcium >600 Agatston units (8). As may be expected with the higher likelihood of disease, the negative predictive value of CCTA was lower, at 83%. However, it is notable that the AUC, which describes the discriminatory power of diagnostic testing across a range of cutoffs, was very high for angiographic disease at 0.91; by comparison, the AUC of a gold standard diagnostic test such as angiography itself would be 1.0, while the AUC for MPS ranges from 0.72 to 0.79, and stress perfusion MRI from 0.84 to 0.86 (9). In addition, the AUC for prediction of later revascularization was very similar between CCTA and invasive angiography (0.84 versus 0.81). These data suggest that in the appropriate patient population, CCTA may be potentially useful for triage of patients to a medical or invasive treatment strategy.

Diagnostic Accuracy of CCTA Intraluminal Stenosis to Detect Perfusion Defects

Several landmark studies using nuclear perfusion methods have documented the inverse relationship between hyperemic myocardial blood flow and degree of coronary artery stenosis. In this regard, many recent studies have aimed to determine the relationship of CCTA-identified obstructive CAD to myocardial perfusion scintigraphy-identified ischemia. Bax et al. described a cohort of 114 patients with intermediate likelihood of CAD undergoing myocardial perfusion scanning and CCTA. Of those with no visualized plaque by CCTA, 90% had a normal perfusion scan. Of those with any CAD by CCTA—whether obstructive or nonobstructive—55% had a normal perfusion scan (10). Among those with >50% stenosis by CCTA, 50% had a normal perfusion scan. It is notable that among a subset that was subsequently sent to invasive angiography, agreement between invasive angiography and CCTA was high at 90%, while agreement between invasive angiography and myocardial perfusion scintigraphy was much lower at 64%.

Gaemperli and colleagues furthered these findings by the examination of 78 patients undergoing 64-slice CCTA, myocardial perfusion scintigraphy, and invasive angiography (11). Invasive angiograms were evaluated by quantitative coronary angiography (QCA). In this cohort, obstructive coronary artery stenosis was identified in 46 patients (59%). They found a sensitivity, specificity, negative and positive predictive value of 95%, 53%, 94%, and 58% respectively. However, these discordances between CCTA obstructive plaque and MPS-identified ischemia were also observed with QCA, with similar AUC (0.88 [0.80–0.96] for CCTA, 0.87 [0.79–0.94] for QCA) and with identical probabilities of ischemic detection by CCTA and QCA diameter stenoses.

From these data, investigators have argued that MPS and CCTA may provide discrete and potentially complementary information related to CAD—that is, detection of myocardial ischemia and detection of coronary atherosclerosis.

Diagnostic Accuracy of CCTA for Acute Coronary Syndrome

Recently, the ROMICAT investigators reported their findings from an observational, double-blinded cohort study of 368 patients presenting to the emergency department with acute chest pain. Patients with initial negative troponin and ECGs received 64-slice CCTA, and were followed for the diagnosis of acute coronary syndrome (ACS) during the index hospitalization and major adverse cardiovascular events for a 6-month follow-up period (12). Of these patients, 8% developed ACS during the hospitalization and 0% had any cardiac events; of the ACS patients, 7 out of 31 had nonobstructive plaque by CCTA, but none had no plaque at all. Using the triage criterion of either any plaque or >50% stenosis, the sensitivities were 100% and 77%, the specificities were 54% and 87%, the NPVs were 100% and 98%, and the PPVs were 17% and 35%, respectively. In this patient population, the absence of any coronary artery disease on CCTA would have allowed for early safe discharge for 50% of the patients, and the AUC for the presence of stenosis was 0.82, as compared to the AUC for the TIMI risk score of 0.63. However, the low positive predictive value of CCTA underscores the findings that a 50% threshold for intraluminal coronary artery stenosis is an imperfect metric for the identification of ACS.

Diagnostic Accuracy of CCTA for the Evaluation of Coronary Artery Bypass Graft Patency

Given that most coronary artery bypass grafts are larger than native coronary arteries and are not directly located on the epicardial surface of the heart (and thus are not subject to cardiac motion artifact), there has been a keen interest in the evaluation of coronary artery bypass grafts by CCTA. While these characteristics are seemingly attractive, the imaging of bypass grafts by CCTA is nevertheless complex and not without limitations. Indeed, among internal mammary artery grafts, which tend toward smaller sizes than saphenous vein grafts, a multitude of surgical staples and clips may accompany the mammary grafts and cause significant partial volume and beam hardening artifacts. Nevertheless, prior studies that evaluated the diagnostic performance of CCTA for the detection of occlusion or stenosis have been promising. A recent meta-analysis of 15 studies evaluating the performance of 16- and 64-detector row CT scanners observed a sensitivity, specificity, positive predictive value, and negative predictive value of 98%, 97%, 93%, and 99%, respectively (13).

In many cases the detection or exclusion of bypass graft patency is sufficient. However, there is often a clinical need to evaluate not only the patency of the bypass grafts, but also the native coronary arteries as well—in particular, the distal run-off vessels. In these circumstances, native coronary artery evaluation is rendered more difficult by several factors, including surgical clips that result in artifact, severe calcific coronary

atherosclerosis, and small vessel luminal diameter. In addition, imaging of internal mammary artery grafts requires widening of the z-axis coverage—with a concomitant increase in scan time—thereby increasing the chance for patient motion, cardiac motion, and contrast mistiming. From these observations, routine bypass graft imaging for limited assessment of graft patency can produce excellent results, while comprehensive evaluation of graft patency and native coronary circulation is much more difficult.

Diagnostic Accuracy of CCTA for the Evaluation of Coronary Artery Stents

Similar to the evaluation of coronary artery vessels with significant calcifications, the examination of coronary artery stents remains a challenge for current generation CCTA. Both calcium and metal are prone to significant CT artifacts—including partial volume and beam hardening artifacts—that often limit the visualization of coronary artery lumen. Unlike bypass graft patency, the diagnostic performance of coronary artery stent evaluation by CCTA is less robust, with reported sensitivity, specificity, positive likelihood ratio, and negative likelihood ratio of 84%, 91%, 12.2, and 0.23, respectively, in a recent meta-analysis of 15 studies using 16- or 64-detector row CT scanners (14). Furthermore, most prior studies have evaluated patient cohorts in which the prevalence of significant in-stent restenosis was low, thereby limiting the potential generalizability of the accrued data.

Certain observations have arisen from these prior studies and indicate circumstances in which stent imaging by CCTA may be more successful. Stents with larger diameters—that is, 3.5 mm or greater—that are located in the proximal portions of vessels tend toward higher diagnostic accuracy. In addition, not all stents are equally assessable by CCTA. For example, the magnesium and cobalt alloys that make up many of the drug-eluting stents tend to be easier to visualize than certain bare metal stents that are composed of tantalum.

Newer generation CT scanners with improved spatial resolution and beam hardening correction algorithms will enable more accurate assessment of in-stent restenosis. However, until then, coronary artery stent imaging is not routinely encouraged by most experts, and if performed, should be limited to larger stents composed of metal alloys with favorable characteristics for visualization by CCTA.

Beyond Obstructive Versus Nonobstructive Stenosis for Identification of Individuals with Ischemia

Although CCTA diagnostic accuracy has been assessed using traditional invasive angiography thresholds (e.g., 50% or 70% intraluminal diameter stenosis) for definition of obstructive CAD, simple "lumenography" with binary classification of disease oversimplifies the risk of individual patients. Invasive quantification of fractional flow reserve (FFR) has led to novel insights into the "functional" significance of angiographic lesions— that is, the ability of a coronary artery stenosis to limit epicardial coronary artery blood flow. De Bruyne et al. compared coronary pressures and FFR in normal arteries to those with diffuse atherosclerosis that were nonobstructive by angiography (15). Those with diffuse nonobstructive disease demonstrated significantly greater pressure gradients between the aorta and distal coronary artery with hyperemia (10 ± 8 mm Hg versus 3 ± 3 mm Hg) and significantly lower FFR (0.89 ± 0.08 versus 0.97 ± 0.02), indicating higher resistance to flow. In fact, among 8% of the diffusely diseased vessels, the FFR was <0.75, generally considered the threshold for inducible ischemia.

Thus, several recent CCTA studies have examined other plaque characteristics beyond intraluminal stenosis severity—such as location, distribution, composition, and overall plaque burden—as potentially useful metrics for prediction of individuals in whom coronary artery plaque is identified and myocardial ischemia risk may be heightened. Lin et al. studied 163 patients undergoing MPS and 64-detector row CCTA (16). In addition to classification of patients as having or not having obstructive CAD, coronary artery plaque was also graded by a segments-at-risk score as well as a plaque composition score. The segments-at-risk score, which preferentially weighted proximally located plaque, comprised a measure of coronary plaque burden accounting for proximity in location. Plaque composition scores indicated numbers of coronary segments exhibiting noncalcified, calcified, or mixed plaque types. In this analysis, CCTA measures of obstructive versus nonobstructive plaque did not identify individuals with mildly abnormal (summed stress score >4) or moderate-to-severely abnormal (summed stress score >8) MPS. Nevertheless, measures of overall coronary plaque burden considering plaque proximity within the coronary artery tree identified individuals with mildly abnormal

MPS (OR 2.78, 95% CI 1.01–7.68, $P = 0.05$) as well as moderate-to-severely abnormal MPS (2.65, 95% CI 0.91–7.77, $P = 0.07$). Furthermore, increasing numbers of segments exhibiting mixed plaque similarly identified individuals with moderate-to-severely abnormal MPS (odds ratio [OR] 3.95, 95% CI 1.39–11.2, $P = 0.01$). These findings indicate that measures of overall plaque burden, location, and composition may enhance detection of individuals with coronary artery stenoses that cause myocardial ischemia.

The same group extended these findings in a recent study of 165 individuals with suspected CAD who underwent exercise treadmill testing (17). Using a Duke CAD index based upon the angiographically-derived Duke coronary artery jeopardy score accounting for plaque severity and location in the left main or proximal left anterior descending artery, CCTA identified patients with increasing severity exercise-induced ST-segment depression as well as decreasing Duke treadmill score. Notably, increasing gradations of CAD by CCTA from none to nonobstructive to obstructive stenosis predicted shorter overall Bruce treadmill protocol exercise times.

These collective findings suggest that a more comprehensive assessment of coronary artery plaque may result in enhanced prediction of individuals with concurrent CCTA-evident CAD and myocardial ischemia.

Beyond Obstructive Versus Nonobstructive Stenosis for Risk Stratification

Notwithstanding the diagnostic benefit derived from identification of obstructive CAD or flow-limiting ischemia, most myocardial infarctions occur in individuals with low-grade nonobstructive stenoses. Lessons learned from intravascular ultrasound demonstrate the importance of plaque composition and remodeling on incident adverse cardiac events. Ehara and colleagues examined the frequency and number of calcium deposits by intracoronary vascular ultrasound (IVUS) among 178 patients with acute myocardial infarction, unstable angina, and stable angina pectoris (18). In individuals presenting with acute myocardial infarction, the number of calcium deposits within a 90° arc per patient were significantly higher than in those presenting with stable angina pectoris. Conversely, individuals presenting with stable angina pectoris were significantly more likely to exhibit longer lengths of calcified plaque (P <0.0001). When plaque was graded as having no calcification, spotty calcification, intermediate calcification, or extensive calcification, individuals presenting with acute myocardial infarction or unstable angina pectoris were more likely to exhibit spotty calcifications or no calcification, as compared to extensive calcifications in individuals with stable angina pectoris ($P < 0.0001$). A further IVUS study of 73 patients presenting with acute myocardial infarction examining coronary arterial remodeling in relation to plaque composition revealed positive remodeling to be more common than negative remodeling (55% versus 25%).

These IVUS results point out a divergence between risk stratification and diagnosis of chronic chest pain on the per-plaque level. Indeed, patients presenting with stable angina pectoris possess culprit plaques that tend toward arterial segments with negative remodeling and greater extent and lengths of calcified plaque. Plaques associated with acute coronary syndromes tend to be located within artery segments that exhibit more positive remodeling and are associated with primarily noncalcified plaques, typically with spotty calcifications. On a per-patient basis, patients with angiographically obstructive CAD may be at elevated risk for ACS not only because of their stenotic lesions, but also because of the numerous nonobstructive lesions also present in the coronary tree; however, those with angiographically nonobstructive CAD may have a level of risk that varies depending on the burden, extent, and composition of their nonobstructive disease. The ability of CCTA to visualize low-grade plaques outside the lumen promises to expand these insights to a wider patient population than would be otherwise eligible for IVUS or FFR.

Can CCTA Offer a Noninvasive Method of Plaque Characterization?

In light of these prior IVUS findings, many prior studies have attempted to use CCTA to measure adverse plaque characteristics. These studies have focused upon noninvasive characterization of plaque volume, composition, and remodeling in a diverse range of individuals.

Plaque Volume

Leber et al. compared CCTA and IVUS in 58 vessels in 37 patients for the presence and quantification of any plaque (19). CCTA demonstrated high specificity for the detection of any plaque, successfully excluding plaque in 484 of 525 (92%) vessel segments. Plaques not detected by CCTA were thinner (0.9 ± 0.3 mm versus 1.5 ± 0.3 mm, $P < 0.05$), located in smaller vessels (3.6 ± 1.1 mm

versus 4.5 ± 1.2 mm, $P < 0.05$), and comprised less percent of plaque cross-sectional area ($22 \pm 5\%$ versus $42 \pm 16\%$, $P < 0.05$).

Plaque Composition

Leber et al. also examined the ability of CCTA to identify different plaque compositions in comparison to IVUS among 36 vessels in 19 patients (19). Each vessel, divided into 3-mm sections, was assessed for plaque type by both modalities. Calcified and "mixed" plaques were correctly identified by CCTA compared to IVUS in 41 of 43 (95%) cases, while noncalcified plaques were correctly identified in 54 of 65 (83%) cases. Overall plaque volume per vessel by CCTA compared favorably to IVUS-measured plaque ($r^2 = 0.69$, $P < 0.01$), with a general underestimation of mixed and noncalcified plaque volumes ($P = 0.03$), and a trend toward overestimation of calcified plaques. For plaques with "lipid" cores and for plaques with spotty calcifications, CCTA identified 7 of 10 (70%) and 27 of 30 (90%) of lesions correctly.

Plaque Remodeling

Hoffman et al. measured a remodeling index (vessel cross-sectional area/reference segment cross-sectional area) in coronary artery plaques from 44 patients undergoing CCTA and ICA who were examined for a remodeling index in comparison to IVUS measurements (20). Both vessel area (0.82) and remodeling index (0.77) by CCTA correlated well with IVUS. Positive remodeling by CCTA, confirmed by IVUS, was more common in nonstenotic arteries as compared to stenotic arteries.

Plaque Characteristics in Stable and Unstable Coronary Syndromes

Motoyama et al. recently evaluated plaque composition and remodeling in 38 patients with ACS and 33 patients with stable angina pectoris (21). Using either 16- or 64-detector row CCTA, positive remodeling (87% versus 12%, $P < 0.0001$), noncalcified plaques (79% versus 9%, $P < 0.0001$), and spotty calcifications (63% versus 21%, $P = 0.0005$) were noted to significantly more frequent in ACS culprit lesions as compared to lesions in stable angina patients. In contrast, extensive calcification was noted more often (55% versus 22%, $P = 0.004$) in individuals with stable angina as compared to ACS. Indeed, when examining a criterion of positive remodeling or noncalcified plaque or spotty calcifications within a coronary artery lesion, the sensitivity for detection as well as the negative predictive value for exclusion of the ACS culprit lesions was 100%.

Hoffman et al. also compared 14 patients with ACS to 9 patients with stable angina by CCTA (22). In patients with ACS, plaque area (17.5 ± 5.9 mm² versus 13.5 ± 10.7 mm²), positive remodeling (1.4 ± 0.3 versus 1.2 ± 0.3), and noncalcified plaque (100% versus 77%) were more often noted. In contrast, calcified plaque was more commonly observed in patients with stable angina (85%) compared to ACS patients (71%). These studies bear out in CCTA the lessons learned from IVUS: plaques that cause stable angina are distinct from those causing myocardial infarction, and "hot" plaques are not necessarily negatively remodeled, stenotic plaques—hence the lack of specificity of the 50% intraluminal stenosis criterion, and the high specificity of the presence of any plaque for exclusion of ACS in the ROMICAT study.

■ PROGNOSTIC VALUE OF CCTA

Anatomic evaluation by invasive coronary angiography is among the oldest mainstays of cardiovascular testing for incremental prognostic value above clinical evaluation, and risk stratification with ICA has been well characterized with measures such as the Duke coronary artery jeopardy score according to the severity, extent, and location of CAD (23). Anatomic evaluation by CCTA, with analogous measures of plaque severity and burden, has the potential to perform comparably and, perhaps superiorly, to invasive angiography for prognosis. By comprehensive visualization of both intraluminal and extraluminal plaque, CCTA may provide finer gradations of risk stratification than what is currently available, particularly among patients with greater degrees of positive than negative remodeling, and mixed noncalcified and calcified plaque. Given these findings, much interest has focused upon assessing the prognostic value of CCTA. Measures of risk stratification by CCTA can be measured by different clinical event states (e.g., death versus MACE) as well as in conjunction with or apart from other noninvasive testing strategies.

Prognostic Value of CCTA for All-Cause Mortality

A recent study reported the 15-month survival of 1,127 low-intermediate risk symptomatic patients with suspected CAD undergoing CCTA as their primary imaging modality (24). In patients with no evident plaque in any coronary artery, in the left main artery, or in the proximal left anterior descending artery, the negative predictive values for death by all causes in a 15-month follow-up period were 99.7%, 97.8%, and 98.4%, respectively. Indeed, among the 333 patients with no evident coronary artery plaque by CCTA, death rates were significantly lower (0.3% versus 4.8%, hazard ratio [HR] 0.12, 95% CI 0.02–0.89, $P = 0.04$) than in the remaining population studied. In addition, CCTA measures of CAD severity, extent, location, and distribution significantly predicted the risk of all-cause death. Moderate (≥50–69%) and severe (≥70%) luminal diameter stenoses by CCTA were associated with higher mortality risk compared with less obstructive plaques, and risk of death rose with numbers of major epicardial vessels affected.

Using a modified Duke coronary artery jeopardy score, CCTA effectively stratified grades of risk for all-cause death by increasing coronary artery plaque severity, location, distribution, and extent, with the highest mortality observed in patients with moderate or severe CCTA-identified plaque of the left main artery. Increasing risk was conferred by: (a) 2 segments with moderate plaque or 1 segment with severe plaque ($P = 0.013$); (b) 3 segments with moderate plaque, 2 segments with severe plaque, or severe plaque in the proximal LAD ($P = 0.002$); (c) 3 segments with severe plaque or 2 segments with severe plaque that included the proximal LAD ($P = 0.001$); and (d) moderate or severe left main artery plaque ($P < 0.001$), with a 15% 1.5-year mortality.

Prognostic Value of CCTA Plaque Severity for Adverse Events

CCTA has also been evaluated for its ability to stratify risk for incident major adverse cardiac events (MACE). In a recent 16-month study of 100 patients with suspected or known CAD, 16- and 64-detector row CCTA measures of nonobstructive ($P = 0.04$) and obstructive ($P < 0.01$) plaque, especially of the left main or left anterior descending artery ($P < 0.001$), successfully identified individuals at higher risk of death, nonfatal myocardial infarction, unstable angina requiring hospitalization, and/or target vessel revascularization (25). Among 1,000 asymptomatic patients who underwent CCTA as part of a general health evaluation, those with no plaque had no MACEs over an average observation of 17 months, while 15 of the 215 individuals with any plaque had unstable angina or revascularization (26). In both of these unblinded studies, events were primarily driven by revascularization. However, the pooled data from 5 studies assessing prognosis of CCTA demonstrate a substantial difference in annualized cardiovascular death or MI rates in individuals with obstructive (n = 79/543; 14%) versus nonobstructive (8/1371; 0.6%) plaque.

Prognostic Value of Plaque Composition by CCTA

A recent analysis of 810 patients with nonobstructive CAD of mild or moderate stenosis severity (25–75%) by CCTA focused on the role of low-density plaques (Hounsfield unit density <68 HU). Over 35 months of follow-up, low density plaques with higher lipoid or fibrous content conferred a significantly higher risk of MACE (HR 4.60, 95% CI 1.08–5.92). These findings underline the risks presented by plaques that would not have been visualized otherwise by calcium scoring or ischemia testing, and raise the possibility of the value of plaque characterization above and beyond severity of intraluminal obstruction to identify at-risk individuals as candidates for aggressive medical therapy.

Warranty Period of Normal CCTA

While from the aforementioned studies, it appears that the absence of any plaque by CCTA predicts a low risk of later death or MACEs over the intermediate term, long-term outcomes for individuals undergoing 64-detector row CCTA is not yet available (given its recent introduction in 2005). However, older generation scanners such as electron beam computed tomographic angiography (EBCTA) have a longer accumulated experience for study. In a recent analysis by Ostrom et al., 2,538 patients with suspected CAD but without known prior CAD who had undergone EBCTA were followed for an average of 6.5 years, with 86 deaths observed (27). Patients with no visualized plaques had an excellent survival of 98.3%, while those with any diagnosed CAD had a 3-fold greater mortality with a survival of 95.3%. The extent and severity of plaque predicted all-cause mortality in a graded fashion by the extent and severity of disease, with significantly elevated hazards seen not only for 3-vessel (HR 2.59, 95% CI 1.99–3.68), 2-vessel (HR 2.31, 95% CI 1.86–2.89), and 1-vessel obstructive disease (HR 1.82, 95% CI 1.45–2.3), but also for 3-vessel nonobstructive disease (HR 1.74, 95% CI 1.49–2.05), nearly equal to the risks of single-vessel obstructive disease. Angiographic disease by EBCTA significantly improved incremental prognostic power compared with traditional risk factor assessment alone (AUC 0.83 versus 0.69, P = 0.0001). In the future, 64-slice CCTA, with its attendant superior diagnostic performance, should perform as well as or better than EBCTA for long-term prognosis.

Prognostic Value of Noncoronary Findings by CCTA

While CCTA has been evaluated for its diagnostic accuracy for cardiac structure and function—including ventricular and atrial volume measures, valvular regurgitation and stenosis, and aortic atherosclerosis—prognostic valuations of these measures have not yet been comprehensively performed. Indeed, only recently have age- and gender-specific normative reference values for the heart and great vessels by CCTA been developed. Nevertheless, prior studies using nongated chest CT highlight the potential additive prognostic value of noncoronary findings.

In a recent 5-year follow-up of 361 patients with stable angina pectoris undergoing multidetector CT, presence of aortic calcifications conferred significantly higher risk for cardiovascular events (HR 4.65, 95% CI 1.19–18.26, P = 0.028) (28). Similarly, in an analysis of 1,155 subjects free of known CAD, CT measures of intrathoracic and pericardial fat were significantly correlated with higher triglycerides (P < 0.0001), hypertension (P < 0.0001), impaired fasting glucose (P < 0.001), diabetes mellitus (P < 0.009), and metabolic syndrome (P < 0.00001) (29). These and other prognostically valuable findings, such as left-ventricular function, volumes, and mass, as well as left-atrial volume and size, may add predictive value beyond coronary arteries regarding comprehensive risk of incident MACE.

■ COST CONSIDERATIONS

Enthusiasm for adoption of CCTA must be tempered within a modern-day, cost-conscious medical environment. A recent study evaluated the downstream clinical and cost outcomes in individuals undergoing CCTA by way of Medicare category III transaction codes (30). Within an insurance database encompassing greater than 10 million lives, 142,535 adult individuals were identified as having undergone CCTA or myocardial perfusion scintigraphy (MPS) during a 3-month period with no prior history of CAD. Patients undergoing CCTA ($n = 1,938$) were compared to matched MPS ($n = 7,752$) patients for 9-month CAD-related health expenditures and clinical outcomes. At the 9-month follow-up, no differences were noted for CCTA or MPS individuals for rates of hospitalizations (4.2% versus 4.1%, P = not significant [NS]), CAD-related outpatient visits (17.4% versus 13.3%, P = NS), myocardial infarction (0.4% versus 0.6%, P = NS), and new-onset angina (3.0% versus 3.5%, P = NS). Despite the lack of differences in clinical outcomes, adjusted CAD-related costs were 33% lower for individuals undergoing CCTA by an average of $467 (95% CI, $99–984, $P < 0.001$).

Goldstein et al. performed a randomized controlled trial comparing a strategy incorporating CCTA to triage for discharge in minimal disease, stress-testing for intermediate lesions or nondiagnostic scans, and ICA for stenosis >70% among 197 patients (31). Both the CCTA and the MPS standard of care strategies were completely safe with 0% adverse events over 6 months, with reduced diagnostic time (3.4 h versus 15.0 h, $P < 0.001$) and lowered costs ($1,586 versus $1,872, $P < 0.001$) for CCTA in comparison to MPS. Together, these findings suggest that, for appropriate patients, use of CCTA as a strategy for evaluation is as clinically effective as MPS while reducing healthcare costs.

■ RADIATION CONSIDERATIONS

The higher spatial and temporal resolution of CCTA requires greater overlap of scan coverage and therefore higher doses of radiation than chest CT. Risks of radiation from CT have been estimated, although never confirmed. Einstein and colleagues applied estimates of lifetime attributable risk (LAR) of cancer incidence associated with radiation exposure to estimate the LARs of different cancers with different CCTA protocols (32). Simulations resulted in radiation estimates of lifetime cancer risks which varied from 1 in 143 for a 20-year-old woman to 1 in 3,261 for an 80-year-old man. Myocardial perfusion scintigraphy, the most

prevalent alternate noninvasive imaging modality, has similar overall estimated doses of radiation to CCTA depending upon the isotope and protocol, but with different patterns of tissue specific exposure; however, a similar LAR estimation procedure has yet to be performed (33). This important work highlights the importance of careful patient selection and of weighing risks and benefits of diagnostic imaging by all modalities, and deserves confirmation in long-term follow-up studies.

Prospective ECG gating, which dose modulates radiation to reduce exposure during portions of the cardiac cycle with maximal motion and limited value for coronary artery evaluation, is quickly becoming the standard of safety for 64-slice CCTA. Maruyama et al. recently evaluated 229 patients undergoing CCTA with either prospective or retrospective ECG gating (34). Of those patients, 56 were not eligible for prospective gating because of elevated heart rates, ≥65 bpm. Of the remainder, prospective gating reduced radiation dose by 79% to 4.3 ± 1.4 mSv, compared with retrospective gating with doses of 21.1 ± 6.7 mSv, without reducing the number of evaluable segments (95.5 versus 96.6%, $P = 0.14$), sensitivity (96.4 versus 97.0%, $P = 0.84$) or specificity (98.5 versus 97.6%, $P = 0.12$). At our center, all CCTAs are performed with prospective ECG gating unless evaluation of cardiac function is specifically requested or patients are unable to obtain heart rates of less than 65 bpm.

■ CURRENT INDICATIONS AND APPROPRIATENESS CRITERIA FOR CCTA

The first and most recent appropriateness guidelines for CCTA date from 2006, prior to publication of a large portion of the data reviewed in this chapter (7). As such, CCTA is deemed appropriate primarily for structural evaluation of coronary artery and congenital anomalies, as well as preprocedural planning for cardiac surgery or ablation. For patients with chest pain, CCTA is restricted to the following three groups:

- Evaluation of chest pain syndromes with intermediate pretest probability of CAD *and* either ECG uninterpretable *or* unable to exercise
- Evaluation of acute chest pain with intermediate pretest probability of CAD *and* no ECG changes and serial enzymes negative

• Evaluation of chest pain syndrome after an uninterpretable or equivocal stress test (by exercise, perfusion, or stress echo)

The Mayo Clinic recently applied appropriateness criteria retrospectively to CCTAs performed in a single center over 6 months in 2007, with 28% found to be appropriate and 17% inappropriate (35). Of the inappropriate scans, almost two-thirds could be attributed to two indications: Asymptomatic patients with a low pretest probability of CAD, or symptomatic chest pain patients with moderate to severe ischemia on a stress test. Moreover, 45% of the scans were unclassifiable by the current criteria.

These results highlight the need to expand guideline definitions to address the currently unclassifiable patients, and current efforts are underway to update the CCTA appropriate use guidelines. The study also demonstrates overuse of CCTA within the two described indications, but also points to the need for guideline revisions to incorporate new data. The pace of new evidence in the field of CCTA, and the new treatment paradigm subsequent to the COURAGE trial favoring initial medical management of nonsurgical ischemic disease, call for an update of current appropriateness guidelines. Indeed, the 2006 AHA scientific statement for cardiac CT and the 2007 acute coronary syndrome guidelines indicate that "it may be reasonable to measure atherosclerosis burden using electron-beam or multidetector CT in clinically selected intermediate-CAD-risk individuals (e.g., those with a 10 to 20% Framingham 10-year risk estimate) to refine clinical risk predication and to select patients for aggressive target values for lipid-lowering therapies" as a Class IIb recommendation, and notes the evidence for assessment of the low- to intermediate-risk chest pain patient from the initial results of the ROMICAT trial (6,36).

■ FUTURE DIRECTIONS OF CCTA

Advancements in technology are accelerating rapidly. Dual-source CT demonstrates improvements in temporal resolution and decreased artifact. For instance, 256- and 320-slice scanners decrease the duration of breathhold and allow single-heartbeat imaging in patients with erratic heart rates. Both offer advantages

for the development of perfusion imaging. Improvements in detectors and data reconstruction algorithms also promise improvements in spatial resolution with new high-definition CT scanners.

Many exciting clinical applications of cardiac CT are in development, both for coronary and noncoronary cardiac evaluation. Automated plaque quantification promises to bring greater objectivity and refinement of risk stratification to the current categorical evaluation of CCTA intraluminal stenosis, positive remodeling, plaque composition, and plaque volume. Infarction and perfusion imaging may be possible simultaneous to coronary anatomic evaluation. CCTA is proving useful for preprocedural planning, from pulmonary and coronary vein anatomy, to prior to electrophysiologic intervention to visualization for cardiothoracic surgery in reoperations or complex congenital heart disease. Finally, no technological improvement is meaningful without evaluation of the impact on patient outcomes and societal costs. Randomized controlled trials are needed to assess the value of CCTA in the evaluation of symptomatic low- to intermediate-risk patients with suspected CAD.

■ REFERENCES

1. Brodoefel H, Burgstahler C, Tsiflikas I, et al. Dual-source CT: effect of heart rate, heart rate variability, and calcification on image quality and diagnostic accuracy. *Radiology* 2008; 247(2):346–55.
2. Roberts WT, Bax JJ, Davies LC. Cardiac CT and CT coronary angiography: technology and application. *Heart* 2008 94(6):781–92.
3. Diamond GA, Forrester JS. Probability of CAD. *Circulation* 1982; 65(3):641–2.
4. Vanhoenacker PK, Heijenbrok-Kal MH, Van Heste R, et al. Diagnostic performance of multidetector CT angiography for assessment of coronary artery disease: meta-analysis. *Radiology* 2007; 244(2):419–28.
5. Budoff MJ, Dowe D, Jollis JG, et al. Diagnostic performance of 64-multidetector row coronary computed tomographic angiography for evaluation of coronary artery stenosis in individuals without known coronary artery disease: results from the prospective multicenter ACCURACY (Assessment by Coronary Computed Tomographic Angiography of Individuals Undergoing Invasive Coronary Angiography) trial. *J Am Coll Cardiol* 2008; 52(21):1724–32.
6. Fraker TD, Jr., Fihn SD, et al. 2007 chronic angina focused update of the ACC/AHA 2002 guidelines for the management of patients with chronic stable angina: a report of the American College of Cardiology/American Heart Association

Task Force on Practice Guidelines Writing Group to develop the focused update of the 2002 guidelines for the management of patients with chronic stable angina. *J Am Coll Cardiol* 2007; 50(23):2264–74.

7. Hendel RC, Patel MR, Kramer CM. ACCF/ACR/SCCT/SCMR/ASNC/NASCI/SCAI/SIR 2006 appropriateness criteria for cardiac computed tomography and cardiac magnetic resonance imaging. A report of the American College of Cardiology Foundation Quality Strategic Directions Committee Appropriateness Criteria Working Group. *J Am Coll Radiol* 2006; 3(10):751–71.

8. Miller JM, Rochitte CE, Dewey M, et al. Diagnostic performance of coronary angiography by 64-row CT. *N Engl J Med* 2008; 359(22):2324–36.

9. Sakuma H, Suzawa N, Ichikawa Y, Makino K, Hirano T, Kitagawa K, Takeda K. Diagnostic accuracy of stress first-pass contrast-enhanced myocardial perfusion MRI compared with stress myocardial perfusion scintigraphy. *AJR Am J Roentgenol* 2005; 185(1):95–102.

10. Schuijf JD, Wijns W, Jukema JW, et al. Relationship between noninvasive coronary angiography with multi-slice computed tomography and myocardial perfusion imaging. *J Am Coll Cardiol* 2006; 48(12):2508–14.

11. Gaemperli O, Schepis T, Valenta I, et al. Functionally relevant coronary artery disease: comparison of 64-section CT angiography with myocardial perfusion SPECT. *Radiology* 2008; 248(2):414–23.

12. Hoffmann U, Nagurney JT, Moselewski F, et al. Coronary multidetector computed tomography in the assessment of patients with acute chest pain. *Circulation* 2006; 114(21):2251–60.

13. Hamon M, Lepage O, Malagutti P, Riddell JW, Morello R, Agostini D. Diagnostic performance of 16- and 64-section spiral CT for coronary artery bypass graft assessment: meta-analysis. *Radiology* 2008; 247(3):679–86.

14. Cademartiri F, Schuijf JD, Pugliese F, et al. Usefulness of 64-slice multislice computed tomography coronary angiography to assess in-stent restenosis. *J Am Coll Cardiol* 2007; 49(22):2204–10.

15. De Bruyne B, Hersbach F, Pijls NH, et al. Abnormal epicardial coronary resistance in patients with diffuse atherosclerosis but "Normal" coronary angiography. *Circulation* 2001; 104(20):2401–6.

16. Lin F, Shaw LJ, Berman DS, et al. Multidetector computed tomography coronary artery plaque predictors of stress-induced myocardial ischemia by SPECT. *Atherosclerosis* 2008; 197(2):700–9.

17. Lin FY, Saba S, Weinsaft JW, et al. Relation of plaque characteristics defined by coronary computed tomographic angiography to ST-segment depression and impaired functional capacity during exercise treadmill testing in patients with low to intermediate risk of coronary artery disease. *Am J Cardiol* 2008; 103(1):50–8.

18. Ehara S, Kobayashi Y, Yoshiyama M, et al. Spotty calcification typifies the culprit plaque in patients with acute myocardial infarction: an intravascular ultrasound study. *Circulation* 2004; 110(22):3424–9.

19. Leber AW, Knez A, Becker A, et al. Accuracy of multidetector spiral computed tomography in identifying and differentiating the composition of coronary atherosclerotic plaques: a comparative study with intracoronary ultrasound. *J Am Coll Cardiol* 2004; 43(7):1241–7.

20. Achenbach S, Ropers D, Hoffmann U, et al. Assessment of coronary remodeling in stenotic and nonstenotic coronary atherosclerotic lesions by multidetector spiral computed tomography. *J Am Coll Cardiol* 2004; 43(5):842–7.

21. Motoyama S, Kondo T, Sarai M, et al. Multislice computed tomographic characteristics of coronary lesions in acute coronary syndromes. *J Am Coll Cardiol* 2007; 50(4):319–26.

22. Hoffmann U, Moselewski F, Nieman K, et al. Noninvasive assessment of plaque morphology and composition in culprit and stable lesions in acute coronary syndrome and stable lesions in stable angina by multidetector computed tomography. *J Am Coll Cardiol* 2006; 47(8):1655–62.

23. Califf RM, Phillips HR, 3rd, Hindman MC, et al. Prognostic value of a coronary artery jeopardy score. *J Am Coll Cardiol* 1985; 5(5):1055–63.

24. Min JK, Shaw LJ, Devereux RB, et al. Prognostic value of multidetector coronary computed tomographic angiography for prediction of all-cause mortality. *J Am Coll Cardiol* 2007; 50(12):1161–70.

25. Pundziute G, Schuijf JD, Jukema JW, et al. Prognostic value of multislice computed tomography coronary angiography in patients with known or suspected coronary artery disease. *J Am Coll Cardiol* 2007; 49(1):62–70.

26. Choi EK, Choi SI, Rivera JJ, et al. Coronary computed tomography angiography as a screening tool for the detection of occult coronary artery disease in asymptomatic individuals. *J Am Coll Cardiol* 2008; 52(5):357–65.

27. Ostrom MP, Gopal A, Ahmadi N, et al. Mortality incidence and the severity of coronary atherosclerosis assessed by computed tomography angiography. *J Am Coll Cardiol* 2008; 52(16):1335–43.

28. Eisen A, Tenenbaum A, Koren-Morag N, et al. Calcification of the thoracic aorta as detected by spiral computed tomography among stable angina pectoris patients: association with cardiovascular events and death. *Circulation* 2008; 118(13):1328–34.

29. Rosito GA, Massaro JM, Hoffmann U, et al. Pericardial fat, visceral abdominal fat, cardiovascular disease risk factors, and vascular calcification in a community-based sample: the Framingham Heart Study. *Circulation* 2008; 117(5):605–13.

30. Min JK, Kang N, Shaw LJ, et al. Costs and clinical outcomes after coronary multidetector CT angiography in patients without known coronary artery disease: comparison to myocardial perfusion SPECT. *Radiology* 2008; 249(1):62–70.

31. Goldstein JA, Gallagher MJ, O'Neill WW, Ross MA, O'Neil BJ, Raff GL. A randomized controlled trial of multi-slice coronary computed tomography for evaluation of acute chest pain. *J Am Coll Cardiol* 2007; 49(8):863–71.

32. Einstein AJ, Henzlova MJ, Rajagopalan S. Estimating risk of cancer associated with radiation exposure from 64-slice computed tomography coronary angiography. *JAMA* 2007; 298(3):317–23.

33. Einstein AJ, Moser KW, Thompson RC, Cerqueira MD, Henzlova MJ. Radiation dose to patients from cardiac diagnostic imaging. *Circulation* 2007; 116(11):1290–305.

34. Maruyama T, Takada M, Hasuike T, Yoshikawa A, Namimatsu E, Yoshizumi T. Radiation dose reduction and coronary assessability of prospective electrocardiogram-gated computed tomography coronary angiography: comparison with retrospective electrocardiogram-gated helical scan. *J Am Coll Cardiol* 2008; 52(18):1450–5.

35. Miller J. RSNA Scientific Sessions 2008.

36. Anderson JL, Adams CD, Antman EM, et al. ACC/AHA 2007 guidelines for the management of patients with unstable angina/ non ST-elevation myocardial infarction: a report of the American College of Cardiology/American Heart Association Task Force on Practice Guidelines (Writing Committee to Revise the 2002 Guidelines for the Management of Patients With Unstable Angina/Non ST-Elevation Myocardial Infarction): developed in collaboration with the American College of Emergency Physicians, the Society for Cardiovascular Angiography and Interventions, and the Society of Thoracic Surgeons: endorsed by the American Association of Cardiovascular and Pulmonary Rehabilitation and the Society for Academic Emergency Medicine. *Circulation* 2007; 116(7):e148–304.

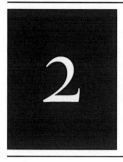

Magnetic Resonance Imaging for Assessment of the Postmyocardial Infarction Heart

SIDNEY GLASOFER

JONATHAN W. WEINSAFT

OUTLINE

Imaging Principles   19

Conventional Cardiac Imaging   20

Tissue Characterization   23

Emerging Concepts   27

Conclusions   31

References   31

In patients that have sustained myocardial infarctions, cardiac imaging is commonly used to guide therapy and assess prognosis. Cardiac magnetic resonance (CMR) is well suited for clinical use in the postinfarct period as it provides high-resolution tomographic imaging without exposure to ionizing radiation. Additionally, CMR provides multifaceted imaging applications that can be tailored to address pertinent clinical issues. CMR provides highly reproducible imaging of cardiac function and chamber dimensions, enabling accurate assessment of the postmyocardial infarction heart without the need for geometric assumptions. CMR can also measure cardiovascular flow, enabling quantification of secondary complications of infarction such as ventricular septal defects and valvular regurgitation. In addition to these standard techniques, CMR provides unique information concerning myocardial tissue characterization. Through the technique of delayed enhancement imaging, CMR can directly differentiate between infarcted and viable myocardium, characterizing myocardial tissue in a manner that closely correlates with ex-vivo pathology findings. Thus, within a single integrated examination, cardiac function, anatomy, flow, and tissue composition can be reliably assessed.

This chapter provides an overview of CMR for imaging of the postmyocardial infarction heart. First, it provides a general review of CMR imaging principles. Then it discusses the utilization of CMR as a tool to define cardiac function, anatomy, flow, and perfusion. Next, the utility of CMR tissue-characterization imaging for management of the postmyocardial infarction patient is detailed. Finally, emerging literature is reviewed in relation to broader applications of CMR, including tissue-based arrhythmic risk stratification, prognostic assessment, and thrombus detection following myocardial infarction.

■ IMAGING PRINCIPLES

CMR produces images through detection of signals produced by hydrogen protons. Hydrogen protons in the body are aligned by exposure to a uniform magnetic field, the strength of which is typically expressed in units of Tesla (typically 1.5 or 3.0 Tesla for cardiac imaging). Hydrogen protons, which uniformly rotate ("precess") in response to a static field, are exposed to additional radiofrequency pulses of variable strength and timing intervals. By varying the strength and distribution of magnetic gradients in relation to transient excitation pulses, CMR pulse sequences can be used to localize protons to different locations and characterize anatomy. High temporal resolution pulse sequences can be used to characterize function. Magnetic field (gradient) strength can also be tailored to characterize blood flow. Thus, by varying the timing and strength of field gradients and excitation pulses, CMR can characterize cardiovascular anatomy, function, and flow.

CMR can also provide unique information concerning tissue composition of structures within the body. On a fundamental level, CMR tissue characterization is attributable to the fact that the distribution of hydrogen protons varies in relation to tissue substrate. Differences in composition affect the manner in which tissue will be excited and relax in response to radiofrequency excitation pulses. For example, when exposed to a fixed magnetic field strength (Tesla) and a transient excitation pulse, magnitude and strength of both longitudinal and transverse magnetization will differ based on tissue properties. Longitudinal magnetization is commonly referred to as "T1" and transverse magnetization as "T2" properties. CMR pulse sequences can be tailored to exaggerate differences in T1 and T2 characteristics, therefore differentiating structures from one another based on tissue substrate rather than anatomic appearance. Gadolinium-based contrast agents, which produce T1 shortening, can be administered during CMR to discern differences in tissue characteristics. Ultimately, by combining anatomic, functional, and tissue-characterization imaging, CMR can provide important information regarding diagnosis and management of the postmyocardial infarction heart.

■ CONVENTIONAL CARDIAC IMAGING

Anatomy and Function

Myocardial infarction can produce alterations in left ventricular chamber geometry, wall thickness, and contractile function. Ejection fraction and chamber size are well-established prognostic indices in the postinfarct patient (1,2). Left ventricular mass has also been shown to predict outcome (3) and assess therapeutic response following acute coronary syndromes (4). Additionally, myocardial infarction can produce secondary mechanical complications such as free wall myocardial rupture, ventricular septal defects, papillary muscle rupture, and pericardial inflammation. Thus, imaging of both cardiac anatomy and function is important for the postmyocardial infarction heart.

Imaging Concepts

CMR provides high-resolution assessment of cardiac anatomy. For static imaging of cardiac structures, CMR typically employs pulse sequences that are tailored to display cardiac structures while suppressing signal from blood. This technique, commonly referred to as "black blood" imaging, is performed by applying a nonselective inversion pulse outside of the plane of reference while applying a second (reinversion) pulse within the imaging plane. This causes inflowing blood to be nulled (black) while preserving signal from fixed structures such as myocardium or pericardium (Figure 2.1A).

For combined functional and anatomic assessment, cine imaging is typically performed. Steady-state free precession (SSFP) is the pulse sequence that is most commonly used for this purpose (Figure 2.1B). SSFP provides excellent endocardial cavity definition, with quality independent of body habitus or imaging plane. Typical imaging parameters can produce in-plane spatial resolution of 1.0 mm by 1.3 mm with slice thickness of 6 to 8 mm. Using conventional breathhold imaging, each cine image typically requires a 6 to 12 second breathhold. Parallel imaging can be employed to reduce breathhold times. Real-time and navigator techniques have also been employed to obtain functional imaging without any breathhold requirement.

CMR quantification of left ventricular parameters is typically based on analysis of contiguous short-axis images. This enables 3-dimensional volumetric assessment based on planimetry of endocardial contours during systole and diastole. Epicardial contours can also be traced for quantification of left ventricular mass, calculated as total myocardial volume multiplied by specific gravity (1.05 g/cm³). Using this method, ejection fraction, mass, and stroke volume can be quantified using volumetric data without the need for geometric assumptions.

In clinical practice, cine-CMR assessment of regional wall motion is typically based on visual analysis. If quantitative assessment is necessary, myocardial tagging methods can also be used for assessment of regional contractility. Myocardial tagging is a method whereby saturation pre-pulses are applied to the myocardium, producing a grid-like pattern that is deformed as a function of regional contractility. Tagging sequences have been used to assess precise changes in regional myocardial contractility and LV remodeling following myocardial infarction (5–7).

CMR can be used to assess secondary complications of myocardial infarction. Pericardial thickening and effusion are well demonstrated on both cine-CMR and static anatomic imaging using black blood or other techniques. In addition to simple anatomical assessment,

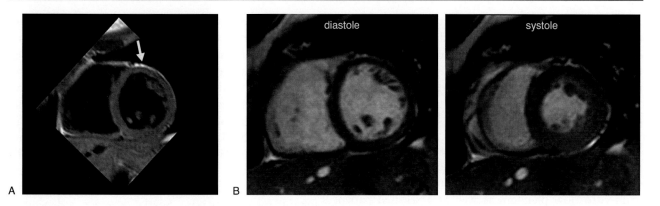

FIGURE 2.1 CMR anatomic and functional imaging. These images demonstrate two common imaging techniques for assessment of cardiac anatomy and function. (A) An example of black blood spin echo imaging. Note that myocardium can be discerned from epicardial fat (*yellow arrow*), which appears bright on T1-weighted images. (B) An example of steady-state free precession (SSFP) imaging. Because SSFP provides high temporal resolution imaging, it enables highly reproducible assessment of cardiac function and chamber size (systolic and diastolic frames shown).

cine-CMR can provide important functional information concerning free wall invagination and/or ventricular interdependence, which can be seen in the context of pericardial tamponade and constriction, respectively.

Clinical Applications

Cine-CMR has been used as an imaging standard for left ventricular geometry and function (8,9). Reproducibility comparisons to echocardiography have demonstrated favorable results for CMR (10). CMR temporal resolution (approximately 50 msec) is typically higher than other tomographic imaging methods such as computed tomography (CT) or single-photon emission computed tomography (SPECT). These capabilities enable CMR to detect subtle changes in left ventricular performance that can be important for assessment of the postmyocardial infarction heart. In experimental studies, cine-CMR has been used to assess serial changes in left ventricular function and remodeling following attempted gene and stem cell transfer (11–13). In the clinical setting, cine-CMR has been shown to be useful for assessment of postinfarction remodeling in relation to infarct size (14), revascularization strategies (15), exercise training (16), and pharmacologic therapy (4,17).

Cardiac Flow

Flow assessment is an important component of imaging in the postmyocardial infarction period. Myocardial infarction can be a direct cause of regurgitant flow as tissue necrosis can involve valvular structures. For example, because both the anterolateral and posteromedial papillary muscles are supplied by epicardial coronary arteries, coronary occlusion can directly impair mitral valve function. Indeed, papillary muscle infarction is an established cause of worsening mitral regurgitation in the postmyocardial infarction setting (18). Valvular regurgitation may also develop as a secondary consequence of myocardial infarction. Residual myocardial ischemia, adverse chamber remodeling, as well as elevated intracardiac filling pressures, can all contribute to valvular dysfunction. Mechanical complications of infarction such as ventricular septal defects can also impact flow within the postinfarct heart.

Imaging Concepts

CMR can employ several techniques for assessment of valvular function and blood flow. Valvular morphology is typically assessed on standard functional (SSFP) images. Because regurgitant flow is often nonlaminar, flow distortions disturb field homogeneity and are thereby apparent on functional SSFP imaging. This technique enables qualitative assessment of regurgitant severity. Functional imaging provides an added advantage of assessing anatomic and geometric factors that may contribute to valvular incompetence. These include chamber dilation, papillary muscle morphology, or regional contractile dysfunction.

CMR can also quantify cardiac flow through use of dedicated "phase velocity encoded" pulse sequences, which enable quantification of forward and regurgitant volumes, as well as flow velocity. Phase velocity encoded imaging is designed to detect changes in proton alignment (phase shift) as blood traverses a known magnetic field gradient. Bipolar gradients are applied to establish parameters for the proportional relationship between blood velocity and phase, which can then be used to quantify blood velocity and flow.

Clinical Applications

Phase velocity encoded imaging has been validated in both clinical and experimental settings. Chatzimavroudis et al. compared transaortic phase contrast imaging both to in-vitro flow phantom as well as a selected patient population, demonstrating high correlations ($r = 0.99$) in both settings (19). Hundley et al. compared left ventricular stroke volume by phase contrast to invasive hemodynamic measurements (20). In this study, mean differences were 3 ± 9 mL and -3 ± 11 mL as compared to Fick and thermodilution methods, respectively. Phase contrast imaging has been shown to correlate well with echocardiography for assessment of mitral (21) and aortic regurgitation (22). This technique has also been validated for quantification of atrial septal defects (23) and can be used for assessment of ventricular septal defects, which are established mechanical complications of myocardial infarction. Because CMR is not limited by acquisition plane, phase contrast imaging can be broadly applied for assessment of valvular flow, septal defects, and global left ventricular performance of the postinfarct heart.

Myocardial Perfusion

Myocardial infarction most often results from atherosclerotic plaque rupture with secondary coronary vascular occlusion. For patients that present early following the onset of ST-elevation infarction, prompt revascularization of the infarct-related vessel is critical for restoration of coronary blood flow and salvage of viable myocardium (24). However, initial revascularization strategies may often be delayed or incomplete following ST-elevation myocardial infarction, causing detection of residual myocardial ischemia to be important for guiding therapy (24). Additionally, for low-risk patients that present with non-ST elevation myocardial infarction, functional imaging for detection of ischemia is often used as a primary test to guide therapy (25).

Imaging Concepts

CMR can assess stress-induced myocardial ischemia. Both vasodilator as well as inotropic stress protocols have been used for this purpose. CMR vasodilator protocols typically encompass perfusion imaging during rest and pharmacologic (adenosine) stress. A gadolinium-based contrast agent (typically 0.1 mm/kg) is infused as a bolus during stress and rest conditions. As gadolinium produces T1 shortening, regions of normal perfusion take up gadolinium and appear bright whereas ischemic regions are hypoperfused and appear dark. Perfusion images are acquired during first pass of gadolinium, which typically occurs within 10 to 20 seconds of contrast administration. Thus, high temporal resolution imaging is required for this for this purpose. Spatial coverage is dependent on both heart rate as well as gradient performance, with three to six short-axis slices typically acquired.

CMR perfusion imaging has been performed using standard gradient echo (GRE), gradient echo-echo planar hybrid, and steady state free precession (SSFP) pulse sequences (26–31). Interpretation is commonly based on visual qualitative assessment (28,30,31), although quantitative calculations based on regional signal-intensity time curves have also been used for this purpose (32). Figure 2.2 provides a representative stress CMR image that demonstrates regional hypoperfusion within the inferior wall and inferoseptum (Fig. 2.2A); invasive angiography was consistent with CMR findings, demonstrating occlusion of the right coronary artery (Fig. 2.2B).

Clinical Applications

Stress-perfusion CMR is well validated as an accurate technique for the identification of coronary obstruction. Among a broad population in whom x-ray coronary angiography was performed independent of stress CMR findings, Klem et al. reported that sensitivity of stress CMR was 89%, and specificity was 87% (31). In a recent meta-analysis of 24 studies (1,516 patients), sensitivity of stress-perfusion CMR was 91% (CI 85–94%) and specificity was 81% (CI 77–85%) (33).

Stress perfusion CMR has performed well when compared to other modalities. In a multicenter dose ranging study, Schwitter et al. reported that diagnostic performance of stress CMR at the optimal gadolinium dose (0.1 mmol/kg) was similar to that of SPECT for diagnosis of angiography-evidenced coronary obstruction (AUC 0.86 ± 0.06 versus 0.75 ± 0.09, $P = 0.12$) (34). When comparing this CMR subgroup to the overall SPECT population, the investigators reported that stress CMR performed better than SPECT (AUC 0.67 ± 0.05, $P = 0.01$). While the reasons for the improved

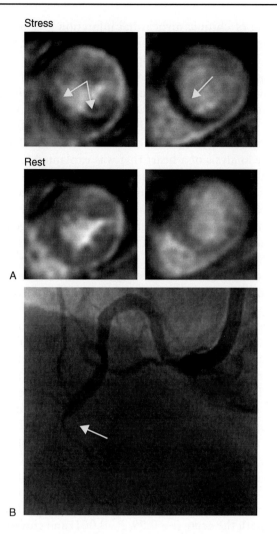

Stress

Rest

A

B

FIGURE 2.2 CMR perfusion imaging. (A) A representative example of stress (*upper panel*) and rest (*lower panel*) CMR perfusion imaging. Of note, stress CMR demonstrates a dense perfusion deficit involving the mid-distal inferior wall and septum (*yellow arrows*) whereas rest CMR demonstrates normal perfusion. (B) Invasive x-ray angiography, which was consistent with CMR, demonstrating obstruction of the mid right coronary artery (*yellow arrow*).

performance of CMR are not established, this may be partially attributable to the higher spatial resolution as compared to SPECT. Indeed, the importance of spatial resolution in relation to heart size has been demonstrated using stress CMR alone. Among a cohort of women referred for stress CMR, Klem et al. reported that diagnostic performance varied in relation to heart size, with impaired detection of coronary disease in patients with lower myocardial mass and smaller chamber volumes (35). As the spatial resolution of stress

CMR is higher than that of SPECT, one would expect improved diagnostic performance of CMR among patients with smaller left ventricular size.

■ TISSUE CHARACTERIZATION

Viable myocardium is defined by the presence of living myocytes whereas cellular necrosis is a hallmark of myocardial infarction. Thus, on a tissue substrate level, distinction between viable and infarcted myocardium is one that is independent of contractile function or response to inotropic stimuli. Additionally, from a clinical standpoint, the disconnect between viability and contractile function is well established, as viable myocardium may be hypocontractile in the setting of chronic hypoperfusion or acute ischemia (36–40).

Delayed Enhancement CMR

CMR can assess viability based on myocardial tissue characteristics rather than contractile function. Infarcted and viable myocardium can be distinguished from one another using the technique of delayed enhancement (DE-) CMR. With this technique, areas of infarcted myocardium appear bright ("hyperenhanced") whereas viable myocardium appears dark (Fig. 2.3). Imaging is performed 10 to 30 minutes following the infusion of gadolinium (0.10–0.20 mmol/kg), with postcontrast inversion times adjusted throughout this period in order to null viable myocardium. DE-CMR is often performed using a segmented gradient echo sequence (41,42). Single-shot and navigator-based techniques have also been applied for this purpose (43,44).

Pathophysiologic Basis

DE-CMR has been shown to provide a near exact correlation with histopathology-evidenced size of infarcted and viable myocardium (41,42,45). Infarct size is highly reproducible in both the acute and chronic infarct setting (46,47). As DE-CMR provides high spatial resolution imaging, infarcts that involve as little as one thousandth of total left ventricular myocardial mass can be detected (48). Infarcts of this size are undetectable by techniques that assess myocardial perfusion or contractile function (45,49).

While the cellular mechanisms for myocardial hyperenhancement have not been fully elucidated, the physiologic processes responsible for this phenomenon are believed to relate to myocyte cellular alterations that produce an increase in local gadolinium concentration within areas of infarcted myocardium. In both the acute and chronic infarct setting, hyperenhancement is believed to result from an absence of viable myocytes to exclude distribution of gadolinium. Increases in gadolinium volume of distribution decrease T1 recovery time, producing hyperenhancement on DE-CMR. The concept that hyperenhancement results from myocardial tissue changes as a consequence of cellular necrosis is supported by experimental data. In animal studies, local concentrations of gadolinium-based contrast agents are increased in areas of acute myocardial infarction (50,51). Whole body data suggests that in normal myocardial regions, gadolinium is excluded from the myocyte intracellular space by intact sarcolemmal membranes (52,53). When acute cell death occurs, the integrity of the sarcolemmal membrane is disrupted, thereby providing a mechanism for extravasation of gadolinium and resultant hyperenhancement. The loss of sarcolemmal membrane integrity is thought to be very closely related to cell death (54–56), and the concept that hyperenhancement is related to cell death explains the near exact relationship of hyperenhencement to myocyte necrosis (Fig. 2.3).

Relative increases in extracellular collagen content is also believed to contribute to hyperenhancement in the setting of chronic myocardial infarction (57,58). On a tissue level, the interstitial space between collagen fibers may be greater than the space between densely packed living myocytes that is characteristic of viable myocardium. Due to this expanded volume of distribution, an increase in concentration of gadolinium in chronically infarcted versus viable myocardium is observed. Histopathology data support this proposed mechanism. In the analysis of a heart that was explanted following CMR, Moon et al. (59) demonstrated that myocardial areas with hyperenhancement on DE-CMR exhibited increased collagen content on histopathology, with a linear relationship between the degree of collagen content and the percentage of hyperenhanced pixels.

Multiple studies have demonstrated that hyperenhancement on DE-CMR is a specific marker of myocardial necrosis that closely correlates with infarct size and morphology (41,45,60–62). These concepts were established by Kim et al. (41) in a study of dogs subjected to transient coronary occlusion (to produce transient myocardial ischemia) or permanent coronary ligation (to produce irreversible myocardial injury). In-vivo cine and DE-CMR were performed at various time points (one day, three days, eight weeks) following coronary manipulation. Following sacrifice, ex-vivo DE-CMR was performed on the animals, and histopathology analysis and TTC staining were subsequently performed for determination of infarct size. In animals subjected to coronary ligation, there was a near exact correlation between DE-CMR and histopathology evidenced infarct size both the acute ($r = 0.99$, $P < 0.001$) and chronic ($r = 0.97$, $P < 0.001$) infarct settings. DE-CMR also provided accurate assessment of infarct morphology, closely replicating histopathology-evidenced infarct shape and contours. On the other hand, in animals subjected to transient coronary occlusion, affected coronary territories did not demonstrate either hyperenhancement or histopathology evidenced infarct despite transient impairment in myocardial contractility.

DE-CMR is capable of distinguishing between infarcted and reversibly injured myocardium. This was demonstrated by Fieno et al. (60), who studied a series of dogs subjected to coronary occlusion with or without reperfusion. In animals with reperfused infarcts, coronary re-occlusion was performed prior to sacrifice and fluorescent microparticles were then injected into the heart to identify areas of jeopardized but viable myocardium at risk of infarction. In-vivo DE-CMR was performed at serial time points (1 day to 8 weeks), prior

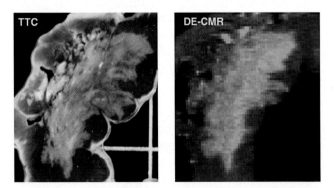

FIGURE 2.3 CMR infarct imaging. Comparison of ex-vivo delayed enhancement CMR (A) with acute myocyte necrosis defined by histopathology (B). Note that the size and shape of the infarcted region (yellowish-white region) defined histologically by triphenyltetrazolium (TTC) stain is nearly exactly matched by the size and shape of the hyperenhanced (bright) region of DE-CMR. (Adapted from Kim RJ, Fieno DS, Parrish TB, et al. Relationship of MRI delayed contrast enhancement to irreversible injury, infarct age, and contractile function. *Circulation.* 1999;100:1992–2002, with permission.)

to animal sacrifice with ex-vivo DE-CMR and subsequent histopathology analysis (TTC stain) performed for quantification of infarcted and viable myocardium. In-vivo and ex-vivo DE-CMR provided near identical findings for quantification of infarct size ($r = 0.99$) with close agreement between histopathology and DE-CMR evidenced infarct size (lowest $r = 0.95$, largest bias 1.7% of total left ventricular area). Furthermore, this study also demonstrated that hyperenhancement is not present in areas of reversible ischemic injury.

Studies comparing DE-CMR to other imaging techniques such as SPECT have shown that DE-CMR provides improved infarct detection. This was demonstrated by Wagner et al. (45), who performed both tests in a canine infarct model. Animals were sacrificed following DE-CMR and SPECT, with histopathology used as a gold standard measure of infarcted myocardium. Level of agreement between DE-CMR and SPECT varied according to transmural extent of infarction. Among segments in which the histologically demonstrated infarct size was greater than 75% of wall thickness, all showed demonstrated infarction by both DE-CMR and SPECT. Conversely, among segments identified by histopathology as having a subendocardial infarction, DE-CMR detected infarction in 92%, whereas SPECT demonstrated infarction in only 28% (Fig. 2.4). This may relate to differences in spatial resolution, which is greater for DE-CMR as compared to SPECT.

Beyond direct infarct detection, CMR also has been shown to provide important information regarding microvascular supply to infarcted territories. In the setting of acute myocardial infarction, microvascular supply can be compromised even if epicardial flow is restored (63,64). Both DE-CMR as well as perfusion techniques have been used to demonstrate microvascular obstruction (MVO). In order to study the relationship between perfusion CMR and histopathology-evidenced MVO, Wu et al. performed mechanical coronary occlusion and reperfusion in a series of closed-chest dogs (65). CMR was performed prior to animal sacrifice and histopathology (thoioflavin-S staining) was then used as a standard for MVO. For matched LV cross sections obtained 9 days following myocardial infarction, MVO measured 7.11 ± 3.68% of LV myocardium by first pass CMR, and 9.18 ± 4.34% by histopathology ($P < 0.05$). Other studies have used DE-CMR for MVO; since contrast uptake is necessary to produce hyperenhancement, absence of contrast within infarcted regions can also be used to demonstrate MVO. One advantage of DE-CMR

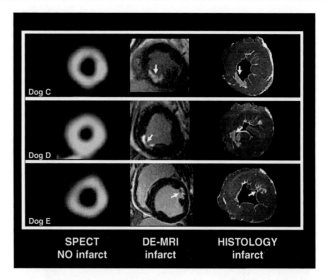

FIGURE 2.4 Improved infarct detection with DE-CMR. Short axis views from three dogs with subendocardial infarctions. Note that unlike SPECT images, the DE-MRI images readily demonstrate the infarcted regions. (Adapted from Wagner A, Mahrholdt H, Holly TA, et al.: Contrast-enhanced MRI and routine single-photon emission computed tomography (SPECT) perfusion imaging for identification of subendocardial myocardial infarcts: an imaging study. *Lancet.* 2003;361:374–379, with permission.)

over first pass perfusion is that it enables assessment of MVO in relation to overall infarct size. Figure 2.5 provides a representative example of DE-CMR-evidenced MVO, seen as an area of signal void (black) within the core of a region of hyperenhanced (bright) infarction.

Clinical Applications

Timely restoration of coronary blood flow has proven to be the cornerstone in the treatment of acute myocardial infarction as this is linked to salvage of viable myocardium, preservation of contractile function, and long-term improvement in survival (66–70). However, in some cases, prompt myocardial revascularization may be delayed or unsuccessful, resulting in variable degrees of infarct transmurality. Transmural extent of infarction (TEI) as measured by DE-CMR has been shown to be a powerful predictor of contractile response to revascularization and medical therapy.

Guidance of Revascularization

DE-CMR has been shown to predict functional improvement after reperfused acute myocardial infarction. This was demonstrated by Choi et al. in a study of consecutive

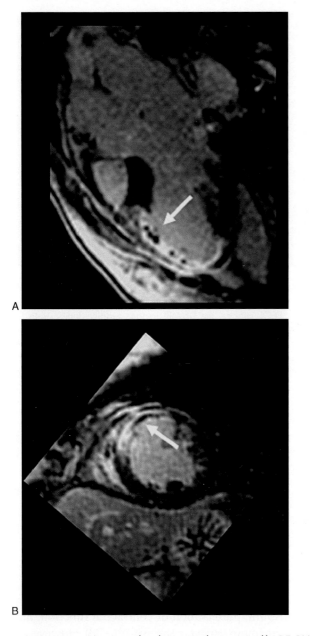

FIGURE 2.5 Microvascular obstruction demonstrated by DE-CMR. Representative 3-chamber (A) and short axis (B) DE-CMR demonstrating MVO (*yellow arrows*) within the left ventricular anterior wall and anteroseptum. In this patient example, DE-CMR was performed within 1 week following a myocardial infarction involving the left anterior descending artery. Note that a characteristic feature of DE-CMR evidenced MVO is localized absence of contrast uptake (black) that is completely surrounded by hyperenhanced myocardium (white).

12 weeks thereafter for assessment of functional recovery. Transmural extent of infarction (TEI) as measured by DE-CMR was highly predictive of improvement in wall motion following infarction (*P* <0.001). When quantified on a segmental basis, 77% (213/275) of segments without infarction showed improvement whereas 5% (3/64) of segments with 75 to 100% TEI showed improvement. In addition to prediction of segmental functional recovery, DE-CMR predicted improvement in global function: The presence of dysfunctional but viable myocardium (less than 25% TEI) was directly related to change in mean wall thickening score (*r* = 0.87, *P* <0.0001) and ejection fraction (*r* = 0.65, *P* = 0.002). Other studies in the acute infarct setting have yielded similar findings, providing confirmatory evidence that transmural extent of infarct on DE-CMR predicts functional improvement following acute myocardial infarction (72,73) and that the predictive value of DE-CMR is superior to that of functional imaging parameters such as ejection fraction (74).

In addition to infarct transmurality, DE-CMR simultaneously identifies the presence of microvascular obstruction within infarcted regions. This added data allows for more informed prediction of remodeling beyond direct measure of infarct size. In a study of patients with acute myocardial infarction, Gerber et al. found that MVO seen on DE-MRI predicted impairment in functional recovery as assessed at 7 months following AMI (75). Similarly, in a study of patients that underwent CMR following acute myocardial infarction (mean 6.1 ± 2.2 days), Hombach et al. demonstrated that DE-CMR-evidenced MVO, infarct size, and transmural extent of infarction each predicted subsequent adverse left ventricular remodeling as defined by > 20% increase in left ventricular end-diastolic volume on follow-up CMR (mean 225 ± 92 days post-AMI) (76). During clinical follow-up, presence of MVO (*P* = 0.04), increased left ventricular end-diastolic volume (*P* = 0.04), and impaired LVEF (*P* <0.01) were each found to be independent predictors of adverse clinical events as defined by death, myocardial infarction, heart failure related hospitalization, or follow-up coronary revascularization.

DE-CMR-evidenced MVO has been compared to other markers of infarct reperfusion. Nijveldt et al. compared CMR parameters to angiographic (TIMI) flow grade, myocardial blush grade, and ST segment resolution among 60 patients with acute myocardial infarction treated with primary stenting (64). In this study, the presence of MVO increased in association with transmural extent of infarction (*P* <0.001) and was significantly

patients who presented with their first myocardial infarction and were successfully revascularized (71). All patients underwent cine and DE-CMR within seven days of their infarction as well as follow-up cine CMR 8 to associated with incomplete ST segment resolution (P = 0.01). Among all parameters evaluated, MVO by DE-CMR was the strongest predictor of adverse remodeling, as evidenced by change in end-diastolic volume (β = 0.53, P = 0.001), end-systolic volume (β = 8.67, P = 0.001), and ejection fraction (β = 3.94, P = 0.006) at follow-up. Whereas this study found MVO to be a better predictor of functional recovery than infarct transmurality, others have yielded mixed results as to the relative predictive strength of MVO versus transmural extent of infarction (76–79). While debate remains as to whether MVO or transmural extent of infarction is the primary predictor of post myocardial remodeling, it is important to note that both variables are strongly associated with one another and can be simultaneously assessed by DE-CMR.

DE-CMR has been shown to provide improved prediction of regional response to revacularization when compared to other imaging modalities. Kitagawa et al. compared DE-CMR and thallium-201 SPECT imaging among a post myocardial infarction cohort (80). Cine-CMR was performed following the initial DE-CMR scan (mean 67 ± 17 days) for assessment of functional recovery. Viability assessment by both CMR and SPECT significantly correlated with improvement in regional wall thickening. However, the sensitivity, specificity, and accuracy of DE-CMR was superior to SPECT (98% versus 90%, P <0.01; 75% versus 54%, P <0.05; 92% versus 81%, P <0.001, respectively).

Guidance of Medical Therapy

Pharmacologic therapy is an important aspect of care for the post myocardial infarction patient. (24,25) DE-CMR has been shown to provide insight into clinical response to medical therapies. This was demonstrated by Bello et al. (81) in a study in which CMR was performed in patients with systolic heart failure (mean LVEF 26 ± 11%) prior to and six months after initiation of a beta-blocker regimen. All patients were already receiving a standard heart failure regimen, including ACE inhibitors or angiotensin receptor blockers, prior to initiation of beta-blockers. Similar to findings in patients undergoing coronary revascularization, an inverse relationship was found between transmural extent of infarction at baseline and likelihood of functional improvement after beta-blocker therapy. Contractility improved in 56% (674/1207) of segments with no hyperenhancement, but only 3% (8/232) of segments with over 75% hyperenhancement. On a per-patient basis, the percentage of left ventricular myocardium that was dysfunctional

but viable was directly related to improvement in ejection fraction (r = 0.57, P = 0.0003) and mean wall motion score (r = 0.70, P <0.001). This parameter was also directly related to improvement in left ventricular reverse remodeling, as measured by decrease in both end diastolic volume index (r = 0.45, P = 0.007) and end systolic volume index (r = 0.64, P = 0.007).

Assessment of Mechanical Complications

Mechanical complications of myocardial infarction often result from changes in myocardial tissue composition. Since DE-CMR provides unique information on myocardial tissue characteristics, it can provide insight into the etiology of infarct-related mechanical complications. For example, DE-CMR can detect papillary muscle infarction (76), a phenomenon that can contribute to worsening mitral regurgitation in the post infarct patient.

DE-CMR may also be used to differentiate between left ventricular aneurysm and pseudoaneurysm. This distinction is important as left ventricular pseudoaneurysm is often managed with surgical intervention (82), whereas aneurysmal dilation is typically managed conservatively. Diagnostic distinction between these phenomena can be challenging based on anatomical appearance alone. However, differentiation is may be aided based on tissue characterization. An aneurysm is composed of myocardium whereas a pseudo-aneurysm is composed of pericardium. Konen et al. tested the utility of DE-CMR among 22 patients with pathologically proven left ventricular aneurysm or pseudo-aneurysm (83). In this study, simple presence or absence of pericardial hyperenhancement had a sensitivity of 100% and specificity of 83% for diagnosis of pseudoaneurysm.

■ EMERGING CONCEPTS

While the utility of CMR for infarct characterization is well established, several recent investigations have demonstrated that tissue characterization imaging holds broader applications for the post myocardial infarction heart. Two specific applications hold particular importance with regard to risk assessment and clinical management. First, this section will explore the concept that DE-CMR can be used identify arrhythmogenic substrate in the post infarct heart, and thereby be used as a tool for prognostic assessment. Second, it will review data that suggest that DE-CMR tissue characterization may be useful to identify left ventricular thrombus and guide anticoagulant therapy following myocardial infarction.

DE-CMR for Post-MI Risk Stratification

Patients that have sustained myocardial infarctions are at increased risk for adverse arrhythmic events (84), which typically originate from ventricular foci. Myocardial scar provides a substrate for ventricular tachyarrhythmias (85–87). Data from animal studies indicates that both scar size (86,88) and morphology (88) influence arrhythmic risk. Imaging studies using modalities other than DE-CMR have also demonstrated scar to be a pro-arrhythmic substrate. For example, SPECT evidenced infarct size has been shown to be associated with risk of inducible ventricular tachycardia during electrophysiology study (EPS) (89,90), as well as death and recurrent ventricular tachyarrhythmias (91–93). DE-CMR evidenced hyperenhancement provides highly accurate assessment of both scar size and morphology, (41,60–62) with improved scar detection in comparison to other modalities such as SPECT (45). Thus, DE-CMR provides an important non-invasive tool for studying associations between scar characteristics and arrhythmic risk.

Current Evidence

The relationship between hyperenhancement and arrhythmogenic potential is supported by findings from several investigations. In a study of patients with coronary artery disease that underwent EPS based SCD risk stratification, Bello et al. (94) found that size (mass: 49 ± 5 gm versus 28 ± 5 gm, P <0.005) and surface area (172 ± 15 cm^2 versus 93 ± 14 cm^2, P <0.0005) of hyperenhanced myocardium was greater among patients with inducible sustained ventricular tachycardia in comparison to patients who were non-inducible. In this study, logistic regression and receiver operating characteristics (ROC) analysis demonstrated that risk stratification on the basis of hyperenhancement size or surface area provided improved prediction of inducible ventricular tachycardia versus ejection fraction alone. The relationship between hyperenhancement and arrhymogenic substrate has also been reported in patients with non-ischemic cardiomyopathy. Klem et al. (95) performed DE-CMR prior to EPS in a heterogeneous population of patients, 52% of whom had no evidence of coronary artery disease. Patients with inducible ventricular tachycardia had larger mean size of hyperenhanced myocardium (P <0.05) than non-inducible patients, with ROC analysis demonstrating

hyperenhancement size to be a better predictor of inducibility than ejection fraction (P <0.01). Absence of hyperenhancement identified a low-risk group as characterized by the fact that none of the patients without hyperenhancement (31% of study population) manifested inducible ventricular tachycardia during EPS. Studies have also reported that infarct morphology influences arrhythmogenic substrate. This was demonstrated by Nazarian et al. (96) in a study of patients with non-ischemic cardiomyopathy undergoing EPS. In this population, predominance of hyperenhancement involving 26 to 75% of wall thickness predicted inducible ventricular tachycardia (odds ratio 9.1, P = 0.02) even after adjustment for left ventricular ejection fraction.

Hyperenhancement on DE-CMR has been shown to predict clinical event risk in several populations. This was demonstrated in the acute myocardial infarction setting by Wu et al. (97), who performed CMR within one week of myocardial infarction and performed clinical follow-up thereafter. In multivariable analysis, adverse clinical outcomes (death, recurrent myocardial infarction, heart failure) were independently associated with infarct size by DE-CMR (HR 1.06 per % LV infarct, CI 1.00–1.11, P <0.05) even after controlling for ejection fraction (HR 0.96, HR 0.89–1.04, P = 0.39). DE-CMR has also been shown to predict outcomes in patients without clinically documented myocardial infarction. Kwong et al. (98) performed DE-CMR in a diverse cohort of patients without clinical history of myocardial infarction. In this study, presence of hyperenhancement was associated with increased cardiac mortality risk (hazard ratio 10.9, P <0.0001). Inclusion of hyperenhancement in multivariable models provided significant improvement to models comprised of clinical variables alone for prediction of mortality risk (model χ^2 improved from 5.97 to 23.78, P <0.0001). These findings are consistent with results reported by Kim et al. (99), who performed DE-CMR in a series of 185 patients without clinical history of myocardial infarction who were scheduled for invasive angiography. 27% of patients had myocardial infarction (hyperenhancement) detected by DE-CMR but unrecognized by either clinical history or ECG (Q wave) criteria. During clinical follow-up, DE-CMR evidenced but clinically unrecognized MI was an independent predictor of all-cause mortality (hazard ratio [HR] 11.4, 95% confidence interval [CI] 2.5-51.1) and cardiac mortality (HR 17.4, CI 2.2-137.4) even after controlling for New York Heart Association functional class and left ventricular ejection fraction.

Several studies have demonstrated that hyperenhancement pattern influences clinical risk. In a study of patients with established coronary artery disease, Yan et al. (100) found that presence of extensive peri-infarct regions of intermediate hyperenhancement (defined by hyperenhancement with signal intensity two to three standard deviations above normal) conferred increased mortality risk. Patients with above median volumes of peri-infarct regions were at highest risk for subsequent death (28% versus 13%, P <0.01). Even after adjustment for LVEF and age, size of peri-infarct regions was independently associated with all cause mortality (adjusted HR 1.42 per 10% increase, P = 0.005) as well as cardiovascular mortality (adjusted HR 1.49, P = 0.01). While Yan et al. studied a particularly high-risk cohort (20% mortality during 2.4 year median follow-up), findings from this study provide further support for a relationship between hyperenhancement and clinical risk.

Clinical Applications

Current evidence demonstrates that DE-CMR can be used to identify myocardial substrate for ventricular tachyarrhythmias. Presence and morphology of hyperenhancement has also been shown to stratify risk for mortality-related outcomes in selected patient groups. However, studies have yet to establish whether DE-CMR can be used as a screening test for arrhythmic risk-stratification of broad at-risk populations. Another related concern is whether DE-CMR can be used to better identify patients that will derive clinical benefit from preventative measures such as implantable cardiac defibrillators. These issues are currently under investigation by several groups and are likely to become an important focus of research.

DE-CMR for Post-MI Thrombus Assessment

Patients that sustain acute myocardial infarctions are at increased risk for thrombo-embolic events such as stroke (101). One presumed etiology of stroke following myocardial infarction is related to left ventricular thrombus, which provides a substrate for embolic events and a rationale for antithrombotic therapy (24). Echocardiography (echo) has been the predominant modality used to detect and guide therapeutic decisions regarding thrombus. Echo detects thrombus based on anatomical appearance. This approach is straightforward when thrombus is large or protuberant but can be challenging when thrombus in small in size or flat in

shape. Whereas thrombus may vary in shape and size, it is inherently defined by avascular tissue composition. DE-CMR can identify thrombus based on tissue characteristics and is emerging as a promising imaging tool for thrombus.

Thrombus Imaging

CMR can identify thrombus through both anatomic and tissue-specific imaging techniques, providing a unique imaging tool for comparison of different approaches for thrombus identification. Similar to echo, cine-CMR identifies thrombus on the basis of anatomical appearance. DE-CMR identifies thrombus based on tissue characteristics—as thrombus is inherently avascular, it is characterized by an absence of contrast uptake. By identifying thrombus based on tissue composition rather than anatomy, DE-CMR enables thrombus to be differentiated from surrounding myocardium irrespective of size or shape (Fig. 2.6).

CMR can also be used to identify structural risk factors for thrombus. For example, in prior population-based studies, thrombus has been associated with LV contractile dysfunction as well as chamber remodeling (102,103), which can both be assessed using cine-CMR. In addition, clinical studies in the post myocardial infarction setting have found thrombus to be associated with larger infarcts as measured by cardiac enzyme levels (104). DE-CMR directly images infarcted myocardium, thereby assessing an additional potential marker for thrombus. Thus, by providing both anatomical and tissue-characterization imaging, CMR offers comprehensive assessment of structural risk factors for thrombus.

Current Evidence

DE-CMR has been validated as an accurate technique for identification of left ventricular thrombus. Srichai et al. compared CMR findings to echo among a cohort of 361 patients that had a gold standard of pathological verification within 30 days of imaging (105). Sensitivity and specificity of CMR yielded a sensitivity of 88% and specificity of 99% in comparison to 23% and 96% for transthoracic echo. Similarly, in a study of patients with ischemic heart disease in whom both DE-CMR and echo were performed within a one day interval, Mollet et al. found that echo failed to identify 58% of thrombi visualized on DE-CMR (106).

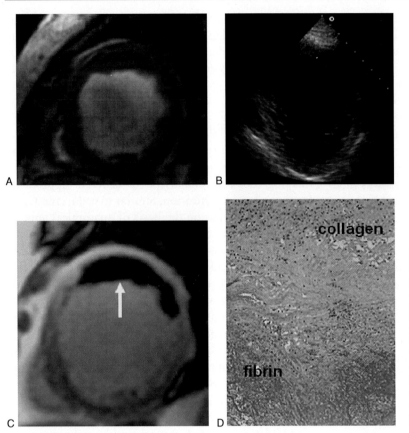

FIGURE 2.6 Thrombus tissue characterization by DE-CMR. Representative patient example demonstrating improved thrombus detection by DE-CMR. Anatomic imaging by echo (A,B) and cine-CMR (C) both show no evidence of left ventricular thrombus. DE-CMR tissue characterization imaging, obtained in matching imaging plane (mid LV short axis), demonstrates a mural thrombus (yellow arrow) adherent to the anterior wall (C). Histopathology (H & E stain, low power), obtained following surgical exploration, confirmed the presence of thrombus with organizing features including prominent collagen and fibrin content (D).

The clinical utility of DE-CMR for thrombus detection was also demonstrated by Weinsaft et al., who studied prevalence of thrombus among a cohort of 784 patients with systolic heart failure (107). DE-CMR was compared to cine-CMR in order to compare tissue characterization to anatomic imaging approaches to thrombus detection. Prevalence of thrombus was higher by DE-CMR as compared to cine-CMR (7.0% versus 4.7%, P <0.005), with cine-CMR less likely to detect small intracavitary or mural thrombus. Clinical follow-up supported DE-CMR an appropriate reference standard for thrombus as evidenced by the fact that patients with thrombus by DE-CMR had over a 7-fold higher rate of endpoints (CVA, TIA, or pathology verification of thrombus) than patients without thrombus (15.1% versus 2.1%, P <0.0001). In comparison, there was only a 3.0-fold higher rate of endpoints in patients with thrombus by cine-CMR (8.6% versus 2.8%, P = 0.06). Following this validation study, this group used DE-CMR as a reference standard to evaluate performance of both non-contrast and contrast echo among patients at clinical risk for thrombus due to chronic heart

failure or recent myocardial infarction (108). Consistent with prior studies that have compared DE-CMR to echo (105,106), Weinsaft et al. found that non-contrast echo was negative in over half of all patients with thrombus by tissue-characterization imaging. Echo contrast yielded nearly a 2-fold increase in sensitivity (61% versus 33%), as well as an improvement in overall accuracy (92% versus 82%) versus as compared to non-contrast echo (both P <0.05). However, 39% of thrombi detected by DE-CMR were not detected by contrast echo. Similar to prior cine-CMR comparisons, thrombus detected by DE-CMR but missed by echo was more likely to be mural in shape or, when apically located, small in size (both P <0.05).

DE-CMR has also been shown to identify substrate for thrombus. This was demonstrated by Weinsaft et al., who examined clinical and imaging parameters associated with thrombus among their initial heart failure population (107). Prevalence of thrombus was over 5-fold greater among patients with ischemic as compared to those with non-ischemic cardiomyopathy, despite similar ejection fraction in both groups. When DE-CMR was used to compare myocardial infarct size in each group, the investigators found that infarct size was threefold higher (P <0.0001) in patients with ischemic disease, paralleling the increased prevalence of thrombus. In multivariate analysis, transmural infarct size by DE-CMR was independently associated with thrombus, remaining significant even after controlling for clinical risk factors and ejection fraction. A relationship between infarct size and thrombus is consistent with prior clinical data that had suggested that patients with larger infarcts were at greatest risk for thrombus (104,109). However, the association between thrombus and infarct size had been commonly attributed to consequent systolic dysfunction or chamber remodeling, rather than an independent effect of infarct itself. While the mechanism relating infarcted myocardium to formation of thrombus is not fully understood, it is possible that this may relate to direct prothrombotic endocardial alterations, or subtle differences in LV contraction between scar and dysfunctional but viable myocardium. Irrespective of the mechanism, the concept that presence of thrombus varies according to infarct size suggests that need for prophylactic anticoagulation may vary based on myopathic tissue substrate, a concept that is not reflected in current consensus guidelines (110).

Clinical Applications

In several comparative studies, DE-CMR tissue characterization has been shown to provide improved left ventricular thrombus detection compared to anatomical imaging using either echo or cine-CMR. Tissue-characterization imaging is particularly useful for identification of small intracavitary or mural thrombus, which are typically not detected by anatomical imaging. In addition to direct thrombus detection, DE-CMR also identifies myocardial scar—a risk factor for thrombus that is independent of systolic function and chamber remodeling. Future research is ongoing to assess whether CMR can be used to develop patient-specific predictive models that can guide preventative anticoagulation strategies based on structural substrate for left ventricular thrombus.

■ CONCLUSIONS

Cardiac magnetic resonance imaging provides comprehensive assessment of the post myocardial infarction heart. In addition to assessment of myocardial function, anatomy, and perfusion, CMR provides unique information regarding myocardial tissue characteristics. Tissue characterization imaging via DE-CMR enables high-resolution assessment of infarct myocardium in a non-invasive manner that closely correlates with pathology findings. Established data demonstrates that DE-CMR provides a powerful tool for prediction of post infarct therapeutic response and chamber remodeling. Emerging data suggests that DE-CMR can be used to stratify arrhythmogenic potential and identify thrombotic substrate following myocardial infarction. The ability to provide comprehensive functional, anatomic, and tissue-characterization information within a single test makes CMR a powerful tool for imaging the post myocardial heart.

■ REFERENCES

1. Nicolosi GL, Latini R, Marino P, et al. The prognostic value of predischarge quantitative two-dimensional echocardiographic measurements and the effects of early lisinopril treatment on left ventricular structure and function after acute myocardial infarction in the GISSI-3 Trial. Gruppo Italiano per lo Studio della Sopravvivenza nell'Infarto Miocardico. *Eur Heart J* 1996; 17:1646–56.
2. Burns RJ, Gibbons RJ, Yi Q, et al. The relationships of left ventricular ejection fraction, end-systolic volume index and infarct size to six-month mortality after hospital discharge following myocardial infarction treated by thrombolysis. *J Am Coll Cardiol* 2002; 39:30–6.
3. Carluccio E, Tommasi S, Bentivoglio M, et al. Prognostic value of left ventricular hypertrophy and geometry in patients with a first, uncomplicated myocardial infarction. *Int J Cardiol* 2000; 74:177–83.
4. Foster RE, Johnson DB, Barilla F, et al. Changes in left ventricular mass and volumes in patients receiving angiotensin-converting enzyme inhibitor therapy for left ventricular dysfunction after Q-wave myocardial infarction. *Am Heart J* 1998; 136:269–75.
5. Mewton N, Croisille P, Revel D, et al. Left ventricular post-myocardial infarction remodeling studied by combining MR-tagging with delayed MR contrast enhancement. *Invest Radiol* 2008; 43:219–28.
6. Rademakers F, Van de Werf F, Mortelmans L, Marchal G, Bogaert J. Evolution of regional performance after an acute anterior myocardial infarction in humans using magnetic resonance tagging. *J Physiol* 2003; 546:777–87.
7. Bogaert J, Bosmans H, Maes A, Suetens P, Marchal G, Rademakers FE. Remote myocardial dysfunction after acute anterior myocardial infarction: impact of left ventricular shape on regional function: a magnetic resonance myocardial tagging study. *J Am Coll Cardiol* 2000; 35:1525–34.
8. Dewey M, Muller M, Eddicks S, et al. Evaluation of global and regional left ventricular function with 16-slice computed tomography, biplane cineventriculography, and two-dimensional transthoracic echocardiography: comparison with magnetic resonance imaging. *J Am Coll Cardiol* 2006; 48:2034–44.

9. Annuar BR, Liew CK, Chin SP, et al. Assessment of global and regional left ventricular function using 64-slice multislice computed tomography and 2D echocardiography: a comparison with cardiac magnetic resonance. *Eur J Radiol* 2008; 65:112–9.

10. Grothues F, Smith GC, Moon JC, et al. Comparison of interstudy reproducibility of cardiovascular magnetic resonance with two-dimensional echocardiography in normal subjects and in patients with heart failure or left ventricular hypertrophy. *Am J Cardiol* 2002; 90:29–34.

11. Jacquier A, Higgins CB, Martin AJ, Do L, Saloner D, Saeed M. Injection of adeno-associated viral vector encoding vascular endothelial growth factor gene in infarcted swine myocardium: MR measurements of left ventricular function and strain. *Radiology* 2007; 245:196–205.

12. Carlsson M, Osman NF, Ursell PC, Martin AJ, Saeed M. Quantitative MR measurements of regional and global left ventricular function and strain after intramyocardial transfer of VM202 into infarcted swine myocardium. *Am J Physiol Heart Circ Physiol* 2008; 295:H522–32.

13. de Silva R, Raval AN, Hadi M, et al. Intracoronary infusion of autologous mononuclear cells from bone marrow or granulocyte colony-stimulating factor-mobilized apheresis product may not improve remodelling, contractile function, perfusion, or infarct size in a swine model of large myocardial infarction. *Eur Heart J* 2008; 29:1772–82.

14. Orn S, Manhenke C, Anand IS, et al. Effect of left ventricular scar size, location, and transmurality on left ventricular remodeling with healed myocardial infarction. *Am J Cardiol* 2007; 99:1109–14.

15. Baks T, van Geuns RJ, Biagini E, et al. Recovery of left ventricular function after primary angioplasty for acute myocardial infarction. *Eur Heart J* 2005; 26:1070–7.

16. Myers J, Goebbels U, Dzeikan G, et al. Exercise training and myocardial remodeling in patients with reduced ventricular function: one-year follow-up with magnetic resonance imaging. *Am Heart J* 2000; 139:252–61.

17. Dubach P, Myers J, Bonetti P, et al. Effects of bisoprolol fumarate on left ventricular size, function, and exercise capacity in patients with heart failure: analysis with magnetic resonance myocardial tagging. *Am Heart J* 2002; 143:676–83.

18. Wei JY, Hutchins GM, Bulkley BH. Papillary muscle rupture in fatal acute myocardial infarction: a potentially treatable form of cardiogenic shock. *Ann Intern Med* 1979; 90:149–52.

19. Chatzimavroudis GP, Oshinski JN, Franch RH, Walker PG, Yoganathan AP, Pettigrew RI. Evaluation of the precision of magnetic resonance phase velocity mapping for blood flow measurements. *J Cardiovasc Magn Reson* 2001; 3:11–9.

20. Hundley WG, Li HF, Hillis LD, et al. Quantitation of cardiac output with velocity-encoded, phase-difference magnetic resonance imaging. *Am J Cardiol* 1995; 75:1250–5.

21. Fujita N, Chazouilleres AF, Hartiala JJ, et al. Quantification of mitral regurgitation by velocity-encoded cine nuclear magnetic resonance imaging. *J Am Coll Cardiol* 1994; 23:951–8.

22. Ley S, Eichhorn J, Ley-Zaporozhan J, et al. Evaluation of aortic regurgitation in congenital heart disease: value of MR imaging in comparison to echocardiography. *Pediatr Radiol* 2007; 37:426–36.

23. Thompson LEJ, Crowley AL, Heitner JF, et al. Direct En Face Imaging of Secundum Atrial Septal Defects by Velocity-Encoded Cardiovascular Magnetic Resonance in Patients Evaluated for Possible Transcatheter Closure *Circulation Cardiovascular Imaging* 2008; 1:31–40.

24. Antman EM, Hand M, Armstrong PW, et al. 2007 focused update of the ACC/AHA 2004 guidelines for the management of patients with ST-elevation myocardial infarction: a report of the American College of Cardiology/American Heart Association Task Force on Practice Guidelines. *J Am Coll Cardiol* 2008; 51:210–47.

25. Anderson JL, Adams CD, Antman EM. ACC/AHA 2007 guidelines for the management of patients with unstable angina/non-ST-Elevation myocardial infarction: a report of the American College of Cardiology/American Heart Association Task Force on Practice Guidelines (Writing Committee to Revise the 2002 Guidelines for the Management of Patients With Unstable Angina/Non-ST-Elevation Myocardial Infarction) developed in collaboration with the American College of Emergency Physicians, the Society for Cardiovascular Angiography and Interventions, and the Society of Thoracic Surgeons endorsed by the American Association of Cardiovascular and Pulmonary Rehabilitation and the Society for Academic Emergency Medicine. *J Am Coll Cardiol* 2007; 50:e1–157.

26. Al-Saadi N, Nagel E, Gross M, et al. Noninvasive detection of myocardial ischemia from perfusion reserve based on cardiovascular magnetic resonance. *Circulation* 2000; 101:1379–83.

27. Schwitter J, Nanz D, Kneifel S, et al. Assessment of myocardial perfusion in coronary artery disease by magnetic resonance: a comparison with positron emission tomography and coronary angiography. *Circulation* 2001; 103:2230–5.

28. Chiu CW, So NM, Lam WW, Chan KY, Sanderson JE. Combined first-pass perfusion and viability study at MR imaging in patients with non-ST segment-elevation acute coronary syndromes: feasibility study. *Radiology* 2003; 226:717–22.

29. Nagel E, Klein C, Paetsch I, et al. Magnetic resonance perfusion measurements for the noninvasive detection of coronary artery disease. *Circulation* 2003; 108:432–7.

30. Plein S, Greenwood JP, Ridgway JP, Cranny G, Ball SG, Sivananthan MU. Assessment of non-ST-segment elevation acute coronary syndromes with cardiac magnetic resonance imaging. *J Am Coll Cardiol* 2004; 44:2173–81.

31. Klem I, Heitner JF, Shah DJ, et al. Improved detection of coronary artery disease by stress perfusion cardiovascular magnetic resonance with the use of delayed enhancement infarction imaging. *J Am Coll Cardiol* 2006; 47:1630–8.

32. Costa MA, Shoemaker S, Futamatsu H, et al. Quantitative magnetic resonance perfusion imaging detects anatomic and physiologic coronary artery disease as measured by coronary angiography and fractional flow reserve. *J Am Coll Cardiol* 2007; 50:514–22.

33. Nandalur KR, Dwamena BA, Choudhri AF, Nandalur MR, Carlos RC. Diagnostic performance of stress cardiac magnetic resonance imaging in the detection of coronary artery disease: a meta-analysis. *J Am Coll Cardiol* 2007; 50:1343–53.

34. Schwitter J, Wacker CM, van Rossum AC, et al. MR-IMPACT: comparison of perfusion-cardiac magnetic resonance with single-photon emission computed tomography for the detection of coronary artery disease in a multicentre, multivendor, randomized trial. *Eur Heart J* 2008; 29:480–9.

35. Klem I, Greulich S, Heitner JF, et al. Stress Perfusion Testing for the Detection of Coronary Artery Disease in Women *J Am Coll Cardiol Img* 2008; 1:436–45.

36. Rahimtoola SH. A perspective on the three large multicenter randomized clinical trials of coronary bypass surgery for chronic stable angina. *Circulation* 1985; 72:V123–35.

37. Braunwald E, Rutherford JD. Reversible ischemic left ventricular dysfunction: evidence for the "hibernating myocardium". *J Am Coll Cardiol* 1986; 8:1467-70.

38. Bolli R. Myocardial 'stunning' in man. *Circulation* 1992; 86:1671–91.

39. Vanoverschelde JL, Wijns W, Depre C, et al. Mechanisms of chronic regional postischemic dysfunction in humans. New insights from the study of noninfarcted collateral-dependent myocardium. *Circulation* 1993; 87:1513–23.

40. Buxton DB. Dysfunction in collateral-dependent myocardium. Hibernation or repetitive stunning? *Circulation* 1993; 87:1756–8.

41. Kim RJ, Fieno DS, Parrish TB, et al. Relationship of MRI delayed contrast enhancement to irreversible injury, infarct age, and contractile function. *Circulation* 1999; 100:1992–2002.

42. Simonetti OP, Kim RJ, Fieno DS, et al. An improved MR imaging technique for the visualization of myocardial infarction. *Radiology* 2001; 218:215–23.

43. Sievers B, Elliott MD, Hurwitz LM, et al. Rapid detection of myocardial infarction by subsecond, free-breathing delayed contrast-enhancement cardiovascular magnetic resonance. *Circulation* 2007; 115:236–44.

44. Nguyen TD, Spincemaille P, Cham MD, Weinsaft JW, Prince MR, Wang Y. Free-breathing 3D steady-state free precession coronary magnetic resonance angiography: comparison of diaphragm and cardiac fat navigators. *J Magn Reson Imaging* 2008; 28:509–14.

45. Wagner A, Mahrholdt H, Holly TA, et al. Contrast-enhanced MRI and routine single photon emission computed tomography (SPECT) perfusion imaging for detection of subendocardial myocardial infarcts: an imaging study. *Lancet* 2003; 361:374–9.

46. Mahrholdt H, Wagner A, Holly TA, et al. Reproducibility of chronic infarct size measurement by contrast-enhanced magnetic resonance imaging. *Circulation* 2002; 106:2322–7.

47. Wagner A, Mahrholdt H, Thomson L, et al. Effects of time, dose, and inversion time for acute myocardial infarct size measurements based on magnetic resonance imaging-delayed contrast enhancement. *J Am Coll Cardiol* 2006; 47:2027–33.

48. Wu E, Judd RM, Vargas JD, Klocke FJ, Bonow RO, Kim RJ. Visualisation of presence, location, and transmural extent of healed Q-wave and non-Q-wave myocardial infarction. *Lancet* 2001; 357:21–8.

49. Ricciardi MJ, Wu E, Davidson CJ, et al. Visualization of discrete microinfarction after percutaneous coronary intervention associated with mild creatine kinase-MB elevation. *Circulation* 2001; 103:2780–3.

50. Schaefer S, Malloy CR, Katz J, et al. Gadolinium-DTPA-enhanced nuclear magnetic resonance imaging of reperfused myocardium: identification of the myocardial bed at risk. *J Am Coll Cardiol* 1988; 12:1064–72.

51. Rehwald WG, Fieno DS, Chen EL, Kim RW, Judd RM. Myocardial magnetic resonance imaging contrast agent concentrations after reversible and irreversible ischemic injury. *Circulation* 2002; 105:224–9.

52. Weinmann HJ, Brasch RC, Press WR, Wesbey GE. Characteristics of gadolinium-DTPA complex: a potential NMR contrast agent. *AJR Am J Roentgenol* 1984; 142:619–24.

53. Koenig SH, Spiller M, Brown RD, 3rd, Wolf GL. Relaxation of water protons in the intra- and extracellular regions of blood containing Gd(DTPA). *Magn Reson Med* 1986; 3:791–5.

54. Reimer KA, Jennings RB. Myocardial ischemia, hypoxia and infarction. In: Fozzard HA et al., ed. The Heart and Cardiovascular System. New York: Raven Press; 1992:1875–973.

55. Jennings RB, Schaper J, Hill ML, Steenbergen C, Jr., Reimer KA. Effect of reperfusion late in the phase of reversible ischemic injury. Changes in cell volume, electrolytes, metabolites, and ultrastructure. *Circ Res* 1985; 56:262–78.

56. Whalen DA, Jr., Hamilton DG, Ganote CE, Jennings RB. Effect of a transient period of ischemia on myocardial cells. I. Effects on cell volume regulation. *Am J Pathol* 1974; 74:381–97.

57. McCormick RJ, Musch TI, Bergman BC, Thomas DP. Regional differences in LV collagen accumulation and mature cross-linking after myocardial infarction in rats. *Am J Physiol* 1994; 266:H354–9.

58. Jugdutt BI, Joljart MJ, Khan MI. Rate of collagen deposition during healing and ventricular remodeling after myocardial infarction in rat and dog models. *Circulation* 1996; 94:94–101.

59. Moon JC, Reed E, Sheppard MN, et al. The histologic basis of late gadolinium enhancement cardiovascular magnetic resonance in hypertrophic cardiomyopathy. *J Am Coll Cardiol* 2004; 43:2260–4.

60. Fieno DS, Kim RJ, Chen EL, Lomasney JW, Klocke FJ, Judd RM. Contrast-enhanced magnetic resonance imaging of myocardium at risk: distinction between reversible and irreversible injury throughout infarct healing. *J Am Coll Cardiol* 2000; 36:1985–91.

61. Barkhausen J, Ebert W, Debatin JF, Weinmann HJ. Imaging of myocardial infarction: comparison of magnevist and gadophrin-3 in rabbits. *J Am Coll Cardiol* 2002; 39:1392–8.

62. Amado LC, Gerber BL, Gupta SN, et al. Accurate and objective infarct sizing by contrast-enhanced magnetic resonance imaging in a canine myocardial infarction model. *J Am Coll Cardiol* 2004; 44:2383–9.

63. Gerber BL, Rochitte CE, Melin JA, et al. Microvascular obstruction and left ventricular remodeling early after acute myocardial infarction. *Circulation* 2000; 101:2734–41.

64. Nijveldt R, Beek AM, Hirsch A, et al. Functional recovery after acute myocardial infarction: comparison between angiography, electrocardiography, and cardiovascular magnetic resonance measures of microvascular injury. *J Am Coll Cardiol* 2008; 52:181–9.

65. Wu KC, Kim RJ, Bluemke DA, et al. Quantification and time course of microvascular obstruction by contrast-enhanced echocardiography and magnetic resonance imaging following acute myocardial infarction and reperfusion. *J Am Coll Cardiol* 1998; 32:1756–64.

66. Christian TF, Gibbons RJ, Gersh BJ. Effect of infarct location on myocardial salvage assessed by technetium-99m isonitrile. *J Am Coll Cardiol* 1991; 17:1303–8.

67. Effectiveness of intravenous thrombolytic treatment in acute myocardial infarction. Gruppo Italiano per lo Studio della Streptochinasi nell'Infarto Miocardico (GISSI). *Lancet* 1986; 1:397–402.

68. Randomized trial of intravenous streptokinase, oral aspirin, both, or neither among 17,187 cases of suspected acute myocardial infarction: ISIS-2.ISIS-2 (Second International Study

of Infarct Survival) Collaborative Group. *J Am Coll Cardiol* 1988; 12:3A–13A.

69. Grines CL, Browne KF, Marco J, et al. A comparison of immediate angioplasty with thrombolytic therapy for acute myocardial infarction. The Primary Angioplasty in Myocardial Infarction Study Group. *N Engl J Med* 1993; 328:673–9.

70. Zijlstra F, de Boer MJ, Hoorntje JC, Reiffers S, Reiber JH, Suryapranata H. A comparison of immediate coronary angioplasty with intravenous streptokinase in acute myocardial infarction. *N Engl J Med* 1993; 328:680–4.

71. Choi KM, Kim RJ, Gubernikoff G, Vargas JD, Parker M, Judd RM. Transmural extent of acute myocardial infarction predicts long-term improvement in contractile function. *Circulation* 2001; 104:1101–7.

72. Tarantini G, Razzolini R, Cacciavillani L, et al. Influence of transmurality, infarct size, and severe microvascular obstruction on left ventricular remodeling and function after primary coronary angioplasty. *Am J Cardiol* 2006; 98:1033–40.

73. Beek AM, Kuhl HP, Bondarenko O, et al. Delayed contrast-enhanced magnetic resonance imaging for the prediction of regional functional improvement after acute myocardial infarction. *J Am Coll Cardiol* 2003; 42:895–901.

74. Rubenstein JC, Ortiz JT, Wu E, et al. The use of periinfarct contrast-enhanced cardiac magnetic resonance imaging for the prediction of late postmyocardial infarction ventricular dysfunction. *Am Heart J* 2008; 156:498–505.

75. Gerber BL, Garot J, Bluemke DA, et al. Accuracy of contrast-enhanced magnetic resonance imaging in predicting improvement of regional myocardial function in patients after acute myocardial infarction. *Circulation* 2002; 106:1083–9.

76. Hombach V, Grebe O, Merkle N, et al. Sequelae of acute myocardial infarction regarding cardiac structure and function and their prognostic significance as assessed by magnetic resonance imaging. *Eur Heart J* 2005; 26:549–57.

77. Tarantini G, Razzolini R, Cacciavillani L, et al. Influence of transmurality, infarct size, and severe microvascular obstruction on left ventricular remodeling and function after primary coronary angioplasty. *Am J Cardiol* 2006; 98:1033–40.

78. Shapiro MD, Nieman K, Nasir K, et al. Utility of cardiovascular magnetic resonance to predict left ventricular recovery after primary percutaneous coronary intervention for patients presenting with acute ST-segment elevation myocardial infarction. *Am J Cardiol* 2007; 100:211–6.

79. Wu KC, Zerhouni EA, Judd RM, et al. Prognostic significance of microvascular obstruction by magnetic resonance imaging in patients with acute myocardial infarction. *Circulation* 1998; 97:765–72.

80. Kitagawa K, Sakuma H, Hirano T, Okamoto S, Makino K, Takeda K. Acute myocardial infarction: myocardial viability assessment in patients early thereafter comparison of contrast-enhanced MR imaging with resting (201)Tl SPECT. Single photon emission computed tomography. *Radiology* 2003; 226:138–44.

81. Bello D, Shah DJ, Farah GM, et al. Gadolinium cardiovascular magnetic resonance predicts reversible myocardial dysfunction and remodeling in patients with heart failure undergoing beta-blocker therapy. *Circulation* 2003; 108:1945–53.

82. Eren E, Bozbuga N, Toker ME, et al. Surgical treatment of post-infarction left ventricular pseudoaneurysm: a two-decade experience. *Tex Heart Inst J* 2007; 34:47–51.

83. Konen E, Merchant N, Gutierrez C, et al. True versus false left ventricular aneurysm: differentiation with MR imaging--initial experience. *Radiology* 2005; 236:65–70.

84. Moss AJ, Zareba W, Hall WJ, et al. Prophylactic implantation of a defibrillator in patients with myocardial infarction and reduced ejection fraction. *N Engl J Med* 2002; 346:877–83.

85. Wetstein L, Mark R, Kaplinsky E, et al. Histopathologic factors conducive to experimental ventricular tachycardia. *Surgery* 1985; 98:532–9.

86. Wilber DJ, Lynch JJ, Montgomery D, Lucchesi BR. Postinfarction sudden death: significance of inducible ventricular tachycardia and infarct size in a conscious canine model. *Am Heart J* 1985; 109:8–18.

87. Josephson ME, Zimetbaum P, Huang D, Sauberman R, Monahan KM, Callans DS. Pathophysiologic Substrate for Sustained Ventricular Tachycardia in Coronary Artery Disease. *Jpn Circ J* 1997; 61:459–66.

88. Wetstein L, Mark R, Kaplinsky E, Kaplan A, Sauermelch C, Michelson EL. Histopathologic correlates of inducible ventricular tachycardia in two experimental canine models of myocardial infarction. *Am J Med Sci* 1986; 291:222–31.

89. Gradel C, Jain D, Batsford WP, Wackers FJ, Zaret BL. Relationship of scar and ischemia to the results of programmed electrophysiological stimulation in patients with coronary artery disease. *J Nucl Cardiol* 1997; 4:379–86.

90. Buxton AE, Hafley GE, Lehmann MH, et al. Prediction of sustained ventricular tachycardia inducible by programmed stimulation in patients with coronary artery disease. Utility of clinical variables. *Circulation* 1999; 99:1843–50.

91. De Sutter J, Tavernier R, Van de Wiele C, et al. Infarct size and recurrence of ventricular arrhythmias after defibrillator implantation. *Eur J Nucl Med* 2000; 27:807–15.

92. van der Burg A, Bax JJ, Boersma E, Pauwels E, van der Wall EE, Schalij MJ. Impact of viability, ischemia, scar tissue, and revascularization on outcome after aborted sudden death. *Circulation* 2003; 108:1954–9.

93. Gioia G, Bagheri B, Gottlieb CD, et al. Prediction of outcome of patients with life-threatening ventricular arrhythmias treated with automatic implantable cardioverter-defibrillators using SPECT perfusion imaging. *Circulation* 1997; 95:390–4.

94. Bello D, Fieno DS, Kim RJ, et al. Infarct morphology identifies patients with substrate for sustained ventricular tachycardia. *Journal of the American College of Cardiology* 2005; 45:1104–8.

95. Klem I, Weinsaft J, Heitner JF, et al. The utility of contrast enhanced MRI for screening patients at risk for malignant ventricular tachyarrhythmias. *J Cardiovasc Magn Reson* 2004; 6:84.

96. Nazarian S, Bluemke DA, Lardo AC, et al. Magnetic resonance assessment of the substrate for inducible ventricular tachycardia in non-ischemic cardiomyopathy. *Circulation* 2005; 112:2821–5.

97. Wu E, Ortiz JT, Tejedor P, et al. Infarct size by contrast enhanced cardiac magnetic resonance is a stronger predictor of outcomes than left ventricular ejection fraction or end-systolic volume index: prospective cohort study. *Heart* 2008; 94:730–6.

98. Kwong RY, Chan A, Brown K, et al. Impact of unrecognized myocardial scar detected by cardiac magnetic resonance imaging on event-free survival in patients presenting with signs or symptoms of coronary artery disease. *Circulation* 2006; 113:2733–43.

99. Kim HW, Klem I, Shah DJ, et al. Unrecognized non-Q-wave myocardial infarction: prevalence and prognostic significance in patients with suspected coronary artery disease. *PLoS Med* 2009;6:e1000060.

100. Yan AT, Shayne AJ, Brown KA, et al. Characterization of the per-infarct zone by contrast-enhanced magnetic resonance imaging is a powerful predictor of post-myocardial infarction mortality. *Circulation* 2006; 114:32–9.

101. Witt BJ, Brown RD, Jr., Jacobsen SJ, Weston SA, Yawn BP, Roger VL. A community-based study of stroke incidence after myocardial infarction. *Ann Intern Med* 2005; 143:785–92.

102. Ascione L, Antonini-Canterin F, Macor F, et al. Relation between early mitral regurgitation and left ventricular thrombus formation after acute myocardial infarction: results of the GISSI-3 echo substudy. *Heart* 2002; 88:131–6.

103. Asinger RW, Mikell FL, Elsperger J, Hodges M. Incidence of left-ventricular thrombosis after acute transmural myocardial infarction. Serial evaluation by two-dimensional echocardiography. *N Engl J Med* 1981; 305:297–302.

104. Neskovic AN, Marinkovic J, Bojic M, Popovic AD. Predictors of left ventricular thrombus formation and disappearance after anterior wall myocardial infarction. *Eur Heart J* 1998; 19:908–16.

105. Srichai MB, Junor C, Rodriguez LL, et al. Clinical, imaging, and pathologic characteristics of left ventricular thrombus: A comparison of contrast enhanced magnetic resonance imaging , transthoracic echocardiography and transesophageal echocardiography with surgical or pathological validation. *American Heart Journal* 2006; 152:75–84.

106. Mollet NR, Dymarkowski S, Volders W, et al. Visualization of ventricular thrombi with contrast-enhanced magnetic resonance imaging in patients with ischemic heart disease. *Circulation* 2002; 106:2873–6.

107. Weinsaft J, Kim H, Shah DJ, et al. Detection of Left Ventricular Thrombus by Delayed-Enhancement CMR: Prevalence and Markers in Patients with Systolic Dysfunction. *J Am Coll Cardiol* 2008; 52:148–57.

108. Weinsaft JW, Kim RJ, Ross M, et al. Contrast-enhanced anatomic imaging as compared to contrast-enhanced tissue characterization for detection of left ventricular thrombus. *JACC Cardiovasc Imaging* 2009; 2:969.

109. Pizzetti G, Belotti G, Margonato A, et al. Thrombolytic therapy reduces the incidence of left ventricular thrombus after anterior myocardial infarction. Relationship to vessel patency and infarct size. *Eur Heart J* 1996; 17:421–8.

110. Hunt SA, Abraham WT, Chin MH, et al. ACC/AHA 2005 Guideline Update for the Diagnosis and Management of Chronic Heart Failure in the Adult—Summary Article. A Report of the American College of Cardiology/American Heart Association Task Force on Practice Guidelines (Writing Committee to Update the 2001 Guidelines for the Evaluation and Management of Heart Failure). *Circulation* 2005; 112:1825–52.

Exercise Electrocardiography

3 The Diagnostic and Prognostic Value of Heart Rate

PAUL KLIGFIELD

JOY M. GELBMAN

PETER M. OKIN

OUTLINE

The Chronotropic Response to Exercise   38

Adjustment of ST Segment Depression
for Changing Heart Rate   39

Heart Rate Recovery in the Postexercise
Period   43

Heart Rate Adjustment in the Postexercise
Recovery Period   45

Conclusions   46

References   46

Over the past half century, evaluation of the electrocardiographic response to exercise has been the most widely applied method for the detection of coronary artery disease and the assessment of its functional and prognostic significance. Within 40 years of Einthoven's first publication of the galvanometric recording of the human electrocardiogram in 1902, the fundamental principles of exercise electrocardiography for the identification of myocardial ischemia were established (1). In addition to the technological development of the recording instrument itself, clinical use of the exercise electrocardiogram (ECG) required appreciation of the waveform changes that accompany naturally occurring angina, evolution of methods for provoking ischemia in patients with limited coronary flow reserve, and analysis of electrocardiographic changes induced by exercise in normal

subjects and in patients with coronary artery disease. Much remained to be studied and clarified during the second half of the twentieth century. Emphasis on the quantitative rather than primarily qualitative analysis of the electrocardiogram during exercise-induced ischemia has occupied investigators for decades, as technical improvements in electrocardiographic recording and in treadmill and bicycle methods for the provocation of ischemia made the exercise ECG a fundamental tool of clinical practice.

For patients with interpretable electrocardiograms, ECG exercise testing (the exercise ECG) remains an appropriate method for the initial evaluation of symptomatic patients with suspected coronary artery disease (2–4). The exercise ECG is widely applied for the detection of coronary obstruction, for the assessment of its anatomic and functional severity, for the determination of prognosis, and for guiding therapy. However, the exercise ECG (like all diagnostic tests) has imperfect specificity, sensitivity that varies with the extent of underlying coronary disease and achieved exercise work load, and consequent limited predictive value when standard ECG ST segment depression criteria are used alone for the identification of patients with coronary obstruction (2,3,5,6). Recognition of these limitations has led to the development of novel physiological approaches to exercise ECG interpretation, many of which are based on incorporation of heart rate data that is routinely acquired as part of the ECG signal during exercise and recovery (4,7).

Heart rate is an intrinsic part of the exercise ECG signal that can be easily and accurately measured. Both alone and in combination with ST segment changes, heart rate can provide insight into prognosis, cardiac performance, and the supply–demand balance of the ischemic heart (8–10). Evaluation of heart rate dynamics alone has diagnostic and predictive value, as demonstrated for chronotropic behavior during exercise and heart rate recovery behavior after exercise (11–15). Heart rate has an important relationship to the dynamics of ischemia in patients with coronary artery disease: it is linearly related to the changing myocardial oxygen demand that accompanies progressive exercise (16). As a consequence, adjustment of ST depression for corresponding changes in myocardial oxygen demand that are related to heart rate is physiologically logical (17,18). Resolution of ST segment changes in relation to heart rate during recovery from ischemia also has diagnostic value (14,19–21).

This chapter explores the emerging diagnostic value of heart rate during and after exercise, including chronotropic incompetence, heart rate recovery, and the clinical principles that support heart rate adjustment of ST segment depression during exercise and recovery. Emphasis will be placed on the physiology of exercise-induced myocardial ischemia in relation to changes in the ECG. In selected populations, heart rate based ECG parameters can improve the accuracy of the exercise ECG for the identification of coronary obstruction, for the assessment of the anatomic and functional severity of coronary artery disease, and for the detection of patients at increased risk for future coronary events or death. Many of the recent advances in exercise ECG address the prognostic value of the physiologic response to exercise rather than the diagnostic value of the exercise ECG for the detection of coronary obstruction. In this sense, the exercise ECG has evolved beyond evaluation of the ST segment alone to provide additional assessment and identification of patients at risk (22). These methods are not perfect, but they are sensible and they can improve the usefulness of the exercise ECG.

■ THE CHRONOTROPIC RESPONSE TO EXERCISE

Chronotropic incompetence, defined as a reduced heart rate response to exercise, can be associated with the presence and severity of coronary artery disease independent of ST-segment depression measurements (12). Chronotropic incompetence also has been shown to be predictive of coronary heart disease events and mortality, with an approximately two-fold relative risk (12,13,23,24), even after multivariate adjustment for

left ventricular function and for the extent of ischemic wall motion abnormalities during exercise (25). As a first approximation, chronotropic incompetence may be defined as the inability to exceed 85% of maximal predicted heart rate (12,26,27), Maximal predicted heart rate may be estimated in several ways, the most common being 220 minus the age, in resulting beats per minute (bpm): from this relationship, the maximal predicted heart rate in a 50-year-old person would be 170 bpm (and 85% of maximum would be 144 bpm), while in a 70-year-old person it would be 150 bpm (and 85% would be 127 bpm).

In 1996, Lauer and colleagues examined the prognostic implications of the heart rate response to exercise in a prospective cohort of nearly 1,600 middle-aged male participants in the Framingham Offspring Study who had no evidence of coronary heart disease (12). The study group underwent a submaximal treadmill exercise test using the Bruce protocol. Assessment of the heart rate response included the ability to achieve 85% of maximum predicted heart rate for age, the heart rate increase from resting control to peak exercise, and the ratio of heart rate to metabolic reserve used by stage 2 of exercise. Subjects were followed for 7.7 years for all-cause mortality and the development of coronary heart disease. By proportional hazards analyses, failure to achieve the target heart rate for age was associated with higher total mortality and with increased risk of coronary heart disease (Figure 3.1), even with adjustment

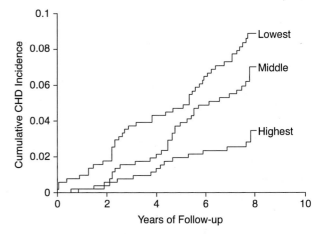

FIGURE 3.1 Kaplan-Meier plot of cumulative coronary heart disease (CHD) incidence according to tertiles of the chronotropic response index, a measure of exercise heart rate response that factors out effects of age, exercise capacity, and resting heart rate. (From Ref. 12, with permission.)

for age, ST segment response, physical activity, and traditional coronary disease risk factors that included diabetes, smoking, hypertension, antihypertensive therapy, and the ratio of total to high-density lipoprotein (HDL) cholesterol. A smaller increase in heart rate with exercise and the ratio of heart rate to stage 2 metabolic reserve were also predictive of total mortality and incident coronary heart disease.

However, chronotropic incompetence also can be estimated by more precise quantitative approaches that incorporate data from both resting heart rate and peak heart rate achieved during exercise, by examining the change in heart rate from rest to peak exercise (the heart rate reserve) (12). Because the proportion of target heart rate achieved depends in part on resting heart rate, the chronotropic response to exercise at any stage of exercise can be assessed as the fraction of heart rate reserve achieved, or the change in heart rate from rest to exercise divided by the difference between the age-predicted target heart rate and the heart rate at rest (28). The chronotropic index is therefore the ratio of heart rate reserve used at peak exercise to the estimated potential metabolic reserve defined by the difference between the maximum predicted heart rate and the resting heart rate (12). As an overall predictor of all-cause mortality, a chronotropic index <80% has been shown to constitute a clinically useful test partition (13,29). The predictive value of the chronotropic index is independent of age, physical fitness, and functional capacity. For example, in a 50-year-old patient not taking a beta blocking drug, the maximum predicted heart rate is 170 bpm (220–age). The maximal predicted heart rate reserve (and ultimately the proportion of heart rate reserve achieved), will depend on the resting heart rate. If the resting heart rate in this patient is 50 bpm, the predicted heart rate reserve will be 170–50, or 120 bpm. If the actual heart rate achieved in this patient is 150 bpm at peak exercise, the peak exercise minus resting rate will be 150–50, or 100 bpm. From this, the chronotropic index will then be 100 bpm/120 bpm, or 83%, a prognostically favorable outcome.

In another study, Lauer and colleagues examined the separate and combined prognostic relationships between chronotropic incompetence and thallium perfusion defects (13). The population included consecutive subjects and patients (1,877 men and 1,076 women) who were referred for symptom-limited treadmill thallium testing and were not taking beta-blockers. Within this group, 316 patients failed to reach 85% of the age

predicted maximum heart rate, and 612 had thallium perfusion defects. After adjustment for age, sex, perfusion defects, and other confounders, failure to reach 85% of maximum predicted heart rate for age was associated with increased mortality (adjusted relative risk 1.84), as was a low chronotropic index (adjusted relative risk 2.19). These findings also were associated with thallium perfusion defects in this population. The combination of both chronotropic incompetence and thallium perfusion defects indicated a particularly high mortality risk.

Although chronotropic incompetence may be a result of ischemia, perhaps involving the SA node, it must be recalled that many drugs taken by cardiac patients, such as beta-blockers and some calcium channel blocking drugs, can also reduce the heart rate response to exercise. This can confound the definition of chronotropic incompetence, as can the termination of exercise at submaximal heart rates in patients with heart disease who become limited by chest pain or shortness of breath. In these situations, apparent chronotropic incompetence may more appropriately be considered a correlate of disease or treatment rather than a finding intrinsic to disease itself. However, the chronotropic index can also be prognostically valuable in patients who are taking beta-blocking drugs when a test partition value of 62% is used (30).

■ ADJUSTMENT OF ST SEGMENT DEPRESSION FOR CHANGING HEART RATE

For half a century, a positive standard ST segment depression response to exercise has been defined as 0.1 mV (1.0 mm at standard gain) or more of additional horizontal or downsloping ST segment depression at peak exercise or in early recovery, beyond any small amount of nonspecific ST segment depression that might be present on the pre-exercise control ECG (2). Upsloping ST segment depression that exceeds 0.1 mV is considered "equivocal," because it occurs with comparable prevalence in normal subjects and in patients with obstructive coronary artery disease. Traditional dependence on an empiric, discrete ST segment threshold reduces the sensitivity of the standard exercise test (2,5,18). If equivocal tests were considered to be positive, exercise ECG sensitivity would be greatly improved, but specificity would be unacceptably reduced.

Anatomic and Physiologic Bases of Exercise-Induced ST Segment Depression

Given an obstructive coronary artery plaque that limits flow reserve during the transient increased myocardial oxygen demand that occurs with exercise, endocardial blood flow becomes compromised more than epicardial blood flow. This results from the higher wall stress that exists at the endocardium, and also from the epicardial to endocardial direction of blood flow that normally exists in the absence of complete obstruction of the extramural coronary arteries. Under normal conditions, phase 2 (the systolic plateau phase) and phase 4 (the end-diastolic resting membrane phase) levels of the endocardial and epicardial action potentials are similar in amplitude (9,31). This results in isoelectric baseline and early repolarization ST segment levels in the nonischemic ECG (32). ST depression during exercise is a consequence of the progressively reduced phase 2 action potential and progressively less negative phase 4 action potential that occurs preferentially in the endocardium (22,33).

It is clear that ST depression during exercise-induced ischemia is dependent not only on the presence of coronary obstruction, but also on the progressive increase in excess myocardial oxygen demand as the exercise workload increases (10,16,34,35). This suggests a physiologically sensible principle: since ST segment depression changes throughout the course of exercise, it must represent more than just the presence or absence of coronary obstruction (18). Because changes in heart rate are closely related to changes in myocardial oxygen demand (8,10,16,35), in the presence of limited coronary blood flow there should be a progressive relationship between the degree of ST depression and increasing heart rate (18,36,37).

These physiologic principles are supported by clinical observation and experience. Consider a patient with no ST depression at a heart rate of 70 bpm at rest who develops 1.0 mm of horizontal ST segment depression at a heart rate of 120 bpm. At this workload, we would agree that ischemia is now present, but we would not argue from our findings that coronary obstruction has developed during the course of the test. If the patient exercised until there was 2.0 mm of ST depression at a heart rate of 140, we would not argue that coronary obstruction is increasing, even though there is more apparent ischemia reflected in the increasing repolarization. And, most important, if only 0.5 mm of ST

segment depression were present earlier in exercise at a heart rate of 100 bpm, we would not conclude from this finding that obstruction were less at slower rates than at the faster rates. From these considerations, it should be evident that a simple measurement of exercise-induced ST segment depression cannot accurately reflect the presence or extent of coronary obstruction without adjustment for the myocardial workload that is present at any point in the test.

These principles also can be examined within an ECG model that explains measured ST segment depression as a function of two distinct aspects of ischemia: ischemic area and ischemic severity (38–40). Ischemic area relates to the extent of myocardium affected by the obstructing coronary lesion during exercise. Severity of ischemia relates to how profoundly ischemic the tissue within the affected myocardium becomes with progressive exercise. For example, there is likely no ischemia at rest or with early exercise, and cell metabolism may be normal. With the early onset of ischemia as myocardial demand exceeds oxygen supply, progressive metabolic abnormalities occur, with mild chemical changes that affect the ECG. At yet greater workloads and increasing heart rate, the metabolic severity of ischemia within the affected myocardium may be profound, with proportionally more change in the ECG (8,10). Accordingly, once ischemia begins, changing ST depression should reflect the increasing metabolic severity of ischemia that is directly related to increasing oxygen demand that is reflected in changing heart rate (34,41). As a result, the ratio of changing ST segment depression to changing heart rate should be directly proportional to the anatomic extent of the ischemic area (18,40).

Heart Rate Adjustment of ST Segment Depression

Plotting ST segment depression against heart rate from exercise test data in patients with coronary disease is physiologically instructive. As peak exercise is approached, the relationship between ST segment depression and heart rate actually does become strongly linear (37) An example of this striking linearity is shown in Figure 3.2, which depicts progressive ST segment depression plotted against heart rate in a patient with three-vessel coronary artery disease. This is consistent with the underlying physiology of ischemia, as increasing heart work becomes proportional to increasing heart rate (16,35). The linearity of ST depression in relation to heart rate at the end of exercise in patients with effort-induced ischemia is seen in the strong correlations that exist between these variables: in one group of consecutive patients with coronary artery disease (37), the mean coefficient of linear correlation at the steepest part of the ST segment–heart rate relationship was 0.96, with nearly all above 0.90. This coefficient of correlation with exercise heart rate is significantly lower in patients with ST segment depression from nonischemic causes, most of which are well below 0.90. These observations support the concept that the ST segment-heart rate relationship can be a useful marker of myocardial ischemia.

Two methods of heart rate adjustment of ST segment depression in exercise phase ECG interpretation have evolved since early application of these principles in England and in Hungary during the 1980s (42–45). The methods include the linear-regression based ST/HR slope and the simpler ST/HR index (Figure 3.2) (17,18,45–47). The ST/HR slope most directly applies

the principles outlined above by searching for a significantly linear relationship between ST depression and heart rate at the end of exercise. Under most conditions, it is more accurate than abbreviated methods of heart rate adjustment of ST depression, but it is also more affected by methodologic problems (18). The ST/HR slope is calculated from the maximal rate of change of ST segment depression relative to heart rate during the period of active ischemia that accompanies higher heart rates at the end of exercise.

In contrast to the regression-based ST/HR slope, the simple ST/HR index represents the average change of ST segment depression relative to heart rate change over the entire course of exercise (17). It does not test the linearity of the ST segment-heart rate relationship at end-exercise, but rather seeks to approximate it with the assumption that ST depression is continuous throughout exercise (48). This approximation introduces error, but that disadvantage is offset in practice by great simplification of the method: rather than a mathematical calculation of regression, all that is required are accurate measurements of ST depression and heart rate at the test endpoint and at a single pre-exercise upright control point. The ST/HR index systematically underestimates the maximal ST/HR slope because there is generally a substantial change in heart rate before ischemia or corresponding ECG changes occur during graded exercise (48), but even so, this simple method is effective for improving the sensitivity of the exercise test for the detection of coronary disease.

Both the ST/HR slope and the ST/HR index are strongly dependent on precise measurement of ST segment depression, even when subthreshold in magnitude. Small changes in ST depression may be important when associated with a correspondingly small change in heart rate (18,49). Other methodologic factors that can affect both of these methods include improved sensitivity with the use of bipolar CM5 and the measurement of ST segment depression at 60 ms after the j point, rather than at the j point (50). The regression-based ST/HR slope requires computer-based calculations and the use of a gently graded treadmill protocol to allow stable data with small heart rate increments to be acquired throughout the course of the exercise test (51). These are not required for the determination of the simple ST/HR index, which can be quite simply calculated without computer assistance and can be recommended for the detection of coronary disease in routine use (18).

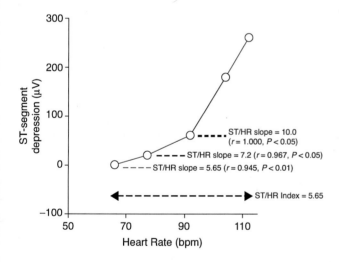

FIGURE 3.2 Heart rate adjustment of ECG ST segment depression. ST depression is shown as positive on the vertical axis. The ST/heart rate (HR) slope is calculated from linear regression that begins at the end of exercise (3 data points) and then progressively incorporates earlier data points in each lead; the highest ST/HR slope with a statistically significant coefficient of correlation for the number of data points involved is selected as the test outcome, in this case 10.0 μV/beat/min because it is the largest of the statistically valid slopes. The ST/HR index is the overall change in ST depression divided by the overall change in heart rate; it approximates and nearly always underestimates the regression-based ST/HR slope because there is usually no ST depression during early exercise in patients with end-exercise ischemia. (From Ref. 18, with permission.)

The Regression-Based ST Segment/Heart Rate Slope

The ST/HR slope is calculated by using linear regression analysis to relate the ST depression measured at 60 msec after the J-point in each lead to the heart rate at the end of each stage of exercise and at peak exercise (18). Because the maximum ST/HR slope is sought in each patient rather than the average slope, regression analysis begins at the end of exercise. Progressively earlier data points are included in subsequent linear regression equations to provide the analysis for each lead (Figure 3.2). The highest of these calculated ST/HR slope values that has a statistically significant coefficient of linear regression becomes the test result for that individual lead. The final test result is taken as the highest ST/HR slope among all the leads (including bipolar CM5 but excluding aVR, aVL, and V1).

An ST/HR slope partition value of 2.4 microvolts/beat per minute (microvolts/bpm) was defined with 95% specificity in clinically normal subjects and a 95% sensitivity in one series of patients with clinically likely or catheterization proven coronary artery disease (17). In this study, upper limits of normal for the heart rate adjusted measures of ST depression were determined by the method of percentile estimation from consecutive clinically normal subjects with normal resting ECGs and no history of angina or other heart disease. This was done to minimize the very important problem of work-up bias when patients with catheterization-proved normal coronary arteries are used for the definition of test specificity. Work-up bias occurs when subjects with abnormal exercise tests are preferentially selected for catheterization, and those with normal coronary arteries (i.e., false positive exercise tests) are then used to evaluate test performance in the catheterized population, leading to inappropriately low specificity (52,53). Interestingly, a recent evaluation by Haggmark and colleagues of pacing-induced vectorcardiographic ST segment measurements in normal subjects without coronary disease found comparable mean values of 20 microvolts per 10 beat change in rate, which was most marked at more rapid rates (54).

Much of the improved sensitivity found for the ST/HR slope arises from correct classification of patients with threshold levels of upsloping ST segment depression who would otherwise be classified as "equivocal," because this upsloping ST depression is also common in normal subjects (17,55). Further, heart rate adjustment

of subthreshold ST depression also results in correct classification of some truly "false negative" tests in which small amounts of depression are linearly associated with correspondingly small changes in exercise heart rate. In addition, the ST/HR slope tends to increase with the anatomic and functional severity of coronary artery disease. In a catheterized population, a partition value of 6.0 microvolts/bpm identified 93% of patients with three-vessel or left main coronary artery disease (17).

An ST/HR slope of more than 6.0 microvolts per beat per minute has therefore served as a useful test partition for the identification of anatomically and functionally extensive coronary disease (18,47,56,57). With high sensitivity but lower specificity, this test partition can serve as a reasonable screen for the exercise ECG identification of three-vessel or left main coronary artery disease (57), and it is more accurate than standard exercise test criteria for identifying extensive coronary obstruction as alternately defined by high Duke jeopardy scores or Gensini scores (56). In addition, higher ST/HR slopes have been found to correlate with larger reductions in left ventricular ejection fraction during exercise radionuclide cineangiography (47).

Thus, the ST/HR slope can significantly improve the sensitivity of the exercise tolerance test for the detection of coronary artery disease with high test specificity. Improvement of exercise test performance for the detection of disease and for the identification of anatomically extensive disease with the ST/HR slope has been found in some, but not all, studies of the method; this may be partially explained by differences in methodology and differences in population selection for evaluation (18,49–51,58,59). Methodological variables that affect the ST/HR slope include location of measurement after the j point, exclusion of ST deviation above the baseline from quantification of ST segment depression, precise measurement of subthreshold ST depression (even when below 1.0 mm), incorporation of bipolar CM5, and use of an exercise protocol that has small heart rate changes between stages (heart rate changes with the standard Bruce protocol are too large to allow enough equilibrated data points for reliable linear regression) (60).

The Simple ST Segment/Heart Rate Index

The ST/HR index represents a simplification of the ST/HR slope method and is calculated by dividing the maximal change in ST segment depression during exercise by the total change in heart rate from rest to peak exercise (Figure 3.2). In the population discussed above (17), an ST/HR index partition value of 1.6 microvolts/bpm was set to result in a specificity of 95% in healthy subjects; with this partition, the simpler method had a sensitivity of 93% for the detection of catheterization proven coronary artery disease (in the same population in whom the higher ST/HR slope partition of 2.4 microvolts/bpm identified 95%). By definition, improved test sensitivity of the ST/HR index occurred in traditional "false negative" responders to the standard test. These include patients with "equivocal" test responses and those with subthreshold ST depression that was correctly adjusted by heart rate. Patients with "false negative" standard tests are predominantly patients with lesser degrees of coronary obstruction, such as single- and double- rather than triple-vessel or left main disease.

For separate identification of three-vessel or left main coronary artery disease by a greater degree of test abnormality, a ST/HR index partition of 3.3 microvolts/bpm was found to identify anatomically severe disease with a sensitivity of 77% (17). Thus, the ST/HR index method appears to approach the performance of the ST/HR slope for identification of coronary disease, but it may not be as useful for assessment of the anatomic severity of disease during treadmill testing. On the other hand, Watanabe et al. found useful predictive value of the ST/HR index during supine bicycle testing for identification of three-vessel disease, and significant correlation with the Gensini score at angiography (61). More recently, a favorable report from Lee and colleagues has supported use of the ST/HR index over ST depression alone for the detection of coronary disease (62). The ST/HR index alone and a summation of index values have also been demonstrated to have enhanced value for prediction of restenosis after percutaneous transluminal coronary angioplasty (63,64). Hamasaki and colleagues developed a new criterion by subtracting the ST/HR index from the ST/HR slope, which has allowed the detection of coronary artery disease in patients on digoxin therapy (65).

The simplicity of the ST/HR index calculation has made it retrospectively applicable to the evaluation of risk in large population studies. Among asymptomatic low risk men and women in Framingham, the simple ST/HR index significantly concentrated the risk of cardiac events (defined as sudden death, myocardial infarction, or new onset angina pectoris) by over threefold during a four-year follow-up (66). In these subjects, standard exercise test criteria based on ST segment depression alone did not significantly concentrate risk. Improved risk stratification by the ST/HR index in this population was even greater in women than in men, and concentration of risk was independent of age and additional standard risk factors.

Similarly, among asymptomatic but higher risk men in the Multiple Risk Factor Intervention Trial (MRFIT) population, the ST/HR index but not standard exercise test criteria significantly concentrated the risk of cardiac death in the usual care group by about fourfold (67). In an evaluation of 5,940 asymptomatic but moderate- to high-risk men from the usual care group of the MRFIT trial who underwent exercise testing, there were 109 coronary artery disease deaths during a seven-year follow-up period. In a Cox proportional hazards model, a positive exercise ECG by standard test criteria was not significantly predictive of coronary mortality (age-adjusted relative risk of 1.5). In contrast, the risk of death from coronary artery disease was significantly increased in those subjects who had an abnormal ST/HR index (age adjusted relative risk 4.1). Even after adjusting for age, diastolic blood pressure, cholesterol, and smoking, the ST/HR index remained a significant independent predictor of coronary death (67). Further, an ST/HR index >1.6 uV/bpm at study entry identified a group of MRFIT men in whom special intervention aimed at reducing coronary risk factors was associated with a greater than 50% reduction of subsequent cardiac death during the seven years of follow-up (Fig. 3.3) (68).

These observations are consistent with improved sensitivity and predictive value of the ST/HR index over standard test interpretation for the detection of ischemia. Perhaps more important, these findings suggest that the ST/HR index is also capable of detecting the presence of prognostically important ischemia.

■ HEART RATE RECOVERY IN THE POSTEXERCISE PERIOD

There is important prognostic information in the behavior of heart rate alone during the recovery phase of exercise testing. Desai et al. have related heart rate recovery to measures of chronotropic incompetence during exercise (69). Since vagally mediated slowing of the heart rate after exercise is known to be enhanced in athletes and reduced in patients with heart failure (70),

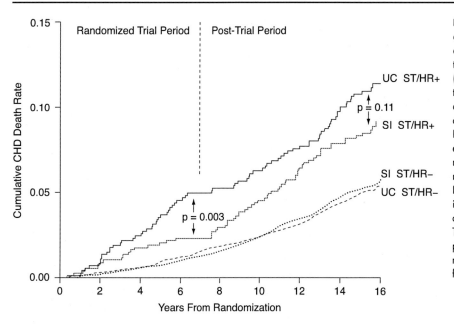

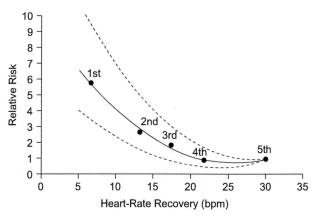

FIGURE 3.3 Cumulative coronary heart disease death rates in the Usual Care (UC) and Special Intervention (SI) patients in the Multiple Risk Factor Intervention Trial (MrFIT), as Kaplan-Meier plots according to intervention group and positive or negative ST/HR index. At the end of 7 years of the randomized trial, an abnormal ST/HR index but not an abnormal standard exercise test significantly concentrated risk of coronary death by fourfold. Of note, among MrFIT men with positive ST/HR indexes, but not with negative ST/HR indexes, special intervention reduced coronary death by nearly half over 7 years. These differences narrowed during the posttrial period, and the differences were not significant at 16 years of extended follow-up. (From Ref. 68.)

it is plausible that prognosis might be related to findings that reflect underlying neurohumoral tone.

Cole and colleagues hypothesized that a reduction in the magnitude of heart rate recovery (HRR) immediately after exercise might be a useful predictor of risk (14). The study population included 2,428 consecutive patients referred for exercise testing without a history of heart failure, coronary revascularization, or pacemakers, and the outcome endpoint was overall mortality. During 6 years of follow-up there were 213 deaths from all causes. A total of 639 patients (26%) had abnormal values for heart rate recovery. By univariate analysis, reduced heart rate recovery was strongly predictive of death (relative risk 4.0). In multivariate analysis, the ability of HRR to predict mortality was maintained after adjustment for age, sex, medications, perfusion defects, standard cardiac risk factors, resting heart rate, change in heart rate during exercise, and work load achieved (adjusted relative risk 2.0). Whether measured as a categorical or continuous variable, a low value for heart rate recovery was highly predictive of death (Figure 3.4).

Abnormal heart rate recovery has been defined as a heart rate that declines 12 or fewer bpm in the first minute after exercise for protocols that use a postexercise cool-down period; for protocols in which exercise is stopped abruptly without a cool-down period, heart rate recovery has been defined as abnormal when the first minute decrease is 18 or fewer bpm (14).

FIGURE 3.4 The relative risk of all-cause mortality during 6 years according to quintile of heart rate recovery during the first minute after exercise. Risk of death is approximately 6 times greater in people with the lowest heart rate recovery. (From Cole CR, Blackstone EH, Pashkow FJ, Snader CE, Lauer MS. Heart-rate recovery immediately after exercise as a predictor of mortality. *N Engl J Med* 1999; 341; 1351–7. © 2001 Massachusetts Medical Society. All rights reserved.)

Even after adjustment for coronary artery disease severity and left ventricular function, abnormal HRR was found to predict 6-year total mortality (71). The mechanism of increased mortality associated with delayed heart rate recovery remains uncertain, but it has been suggested that abnormal heart rate recovery may be related more to autonomic dysfunction than to the presence or extent of coronary artery disease (11). Supporting this suggestion are observations that indicate that heart rate recovery from both maximal and submaximal levels of exercise increase after exercise training, while resting heart rate decreases (72,73).

■ HEART RATE ADJUSTMENT IN THE POSTEXERCISE RECOVERY PERIOD

Early observations by Bruce suggested that ST segment depression caused by myocardial ischemia might have a pattern of postexercise recovery that differs from the pattern that occurs with other causes of exercise-induced repolarization abnormality (74,75). During the past 20 years, it has been demonstrated that heart rate-dependent behavior of ST segment during the recovery phase of the exercise treadmill test also has diagnostic value for the detection of coronary disease (18), based on an asymmetric recovery of ST depression with respect to heart rate in patients with myocardial ischemia. Data can be examined qualitatively as the simple rate-recovery loop (76), or simply quantified as an ST "deficit" between measurement at 3.5 minutes of recovery and the corresponding heart rate during exercise (20,77).

Hollenberg and colleagues incorporated recovery-phase ST behavior with exercise-phase findings by into a treadmill exercise score that is adjusted for heart rate (78,79). Studies during the past decade have confirmed the diagnostic value of combining exercise and recovery phase ST segment data in the heart rate domain. Lehtinen and coworkers introduced a more quantitative analysis of the rate-recovery loop area during a longer period of recovery, known as ST/HR hysteresis (19,80). Combination of exercise and recovery phase ST segment data as an area of the ST segment-heart rate loop appears to be the most accurate and predictive of the current heart rate adjusted methods in routine exercise testing (21,81–83).

The Simple Rate-Recovery Loop

Qualitative rate-recovery loops are constructed by plotting ST segment deviation with reference to changing heart rate throughout treadmill exercise and recovery (Figure 3.5). A simple, qualitative rate recovery loop can be examined using only the data from the first minute of recovery (76). When ST segment depression is plotted in a positive direction against heart rate, normal subjects typically exhibit a clockwise loop of ST segment depression as a function of heart rate during the first minute of recovery, whereas patients with coronary artery disease most commonly exhibit a counterclockwise loop. The rate-recovery loop improves sensitivity of the exercise ECG for the detection of coronary artery disease with no loss in specificity compared with that for standard ST segment depression criteria (18). In contrast to standard ST depression criteria and heart rate-adjusted criteria derived purely from exercise phase data, the sensitivity of the rate-recovery loop appears to be relatively independent of the extent of coronary artery disease. The rate recovery loop has been found to be more useful that ST depression criteria for the identification of restenosis after angioplasty (84). Alone and in combination with the ST/HR index, the rate-recovery loop can improve the prediction of future cardiovascular risk over that with standard ST depression criteria (66).

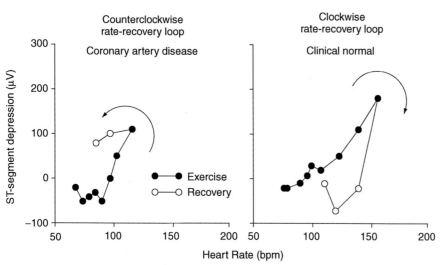

FIGURE 3.5 Rate-recovery loops, with ST depression shown as positive on the vertical axis. With ischemia, recovery phase ST depression at one minute of recovery is greater than ST depression during exercise at the same heart rate, while ST depression in the absence of ischemia demonstrates opposite loop rotation. (From Ref. 18, with permission.)

Quantitative Rate-Recovery Loops

A relatively simple quantification of the rate-recovery loop involves calculation of the ST segment "deficit" between recovery phase ST depression at 3.5 minutes and the ST depression at the corresponding heart rate during exercise (77). ST/HR hysteresis, as developed by Lehtinen and colleagues, integrates the area of ST segment depression with respect to heart rate that is included in the exercise and recovery loop over the heart rate range included in the first three minutes of recovery (19,80,85). This integral is then divided by the heart rate difference (i.e., the maximum heart rate during exercise minus the minimum heart rate during recovery) of the integration interval in order to normalize the result with respect to the postexercise heart rate decline. In one large study, comparison of receiver operating characteristic curves demonstrated that performance of ST/HR hysteresis exceeded that of the ST/HR index, as well as standard test criteria for the detection of coronary artery disease (19). Svensburgh and colleagues have addressed the effect on test performance of the exact range of heart rates included in the rate-recovery area calculation, noting that a large percentage of the loop needs to be considered to optimize diagnosis, especially in women (21). Bigi et al. have examined the entire rate-recovery loop by defining a stress-recovery index as the difference in areas under the full exercise and recovery phase ST heart rate plots (81). The stress-recovery index has been found to be more accurate than other standard ST segment and heart rate adjusted test methods for the identification of anatomically extensive coronary disease after myocardial infarction (81), for the prediction of mortality after myocardial infarction (82), and for the prediction of all cause mortality in hypertensive patients with chest pain (83).

The simple rate-recovery loop and the quantitative rate-recovery area are both dependent on the asymmetry of the exercise phase and recovery phase ST segment change with respect to heart rate in patients with ischemia (34). The mechanism underlying asymmetry of ST change during exercise and recovery is unclear. In addition to slower clearing of ischemic metabolites during recovery than their production during exercise, a delay in ST segment resolution in relation to decreasing heart rate during recovery may be explained in part by neurohormonal influences on vascular tone. Neuropeptide Y is a long-lasting and potent vasoconstrictor that is costored and released with norepinephrine during sympathetic activity. However, neuropeptide Y is eliminated from its site of action and from the blood more slowly than is norepinephrine. An interesting study by Gullestad and colleagues has shown that an exercise-induced increase in neuropeptide Y during ischemia can be closely correlated with prolongation of ST segment depression during the recovery phase of exercise (20). This association suggests that neuropeptide Y may contribute to the relative delay of ST depression with respect to heart rate during the recovery phase of ischemia in patients with coronary artery disease.

■ CONCLUSIONS

Despite ongoing major advances in other forms of noninvasive imaging, the simple exercise treadmill test remains the most accessible and affordable method for the initial evaluation of suspected ischemia in most people. Incorporation of heart rate information into exercise testing can improve the performance of the exercise ECG for the detection of coronary disease, for the assessment of its severity, and for prediction of risk. The best way to use heart rate information in exercise testing requires continued evaluation and evolution. The complexity of measurement and calculation required by some of these methods, such as the ST/HR slope and the ST/HR rate-recovery loop areas, are daunting, but these disadvantages can be overcome by computer-assisted electrocardiography (85,86). Other methods, such as the simple ST/HR index, can be easily examined from precisely measured ST segment findings; this precision can be enhanced by accurate computer-based methods. Estimation of chronotropic competence and heart rate recovery require only simple calculations based on heart rate alone. Whether the ST/HR rate-recovery loop area, or other combinations of available or as yet undiscovered methods, will provide optimal combination of information contained in both exercise and recovery data remains to be seen. No matter how it will be best incorporated into routine testing, it is clear that heart rate is a critical element in the evaluation of the exercise electrocardiogram.

■ REFERENCES

1. Kligfield P. Historical notes: The early evolution of the exercise electrocardiogram. In: Schalij M, Janse MJ, van Oosterom A,

Wellens HJJ, van der Wall EE, eds. *Einthoven 2002*. Leiden: The Einthoven Foundation; 2002.

2. Goldschlager N, Selzer A, Cohn K. Treadmill stress tests as indicators of presence and severity of coronary artery disease. *Ann Intern Med*. 1976; 85:277–86.

3. Chaitman BR. The changing role of the exercise electrocardiogram as a diagnostic and prognostic test for chronic ischemic heart disease. *J Am Coll Cardiol* 1986; 8:1195–210.

4. Kligfield P, Okin PM. Evolution of the exercise electrocardiogram. *Am J Cardiol* 1994; 73:1209–10.

5. Borer JS, Brensike JF, Redwood DR, et al. Limitations of the electrocardiographic response to exercise in predicting coronary-artery disease. *N Engl J Med* 1975; 293:367–71.

6. Epstein SE. Value and limitations of the electrocardiographic response to exercise in the assessment of patients with coronary artery disease. Controversies in cardiology II. *Am J Cardiol* 1978; 42:667–74.

7. Kligfield P. Rehabilitation of the exercise electrocardiogram. *Ann Intern Med* 1998; 128:1035–7.

8. Mirvis DM, Ramanathan KB. Alterations in transmural blood flow and body surface ST segment abnormalities produced by ischemia in the circumflex and left anterior descending coronary arterial beds of the dog. *Circulation* 1987; 76:697–704.

9. Holland RP, Brooks H. Precordial and epicardial surface potentials during Myocardial ischemia in the pig. A theoretical and experimental analysis of the TQ and ST segments. *Circ Res* 1975; 37:471–80.

10. Mirvis DM, Ramanathan KB, Wilson JL. Regional blood flow correlates of ST segment depression in tachycardia-induced myocardial ischemia. *Circulation* 1986; 73:365–73.

11. Chaitman BR. Abnormal heart rate responses to exercise predict increased long-term mortality regardless of coronary disease extent: the question is why? *J Am Coll Cardiol* 2003; 42:839–41.

12. Lauer MS, Okin PM, Larson MG, Evans JC, Levy D. Impaired heart rate response to graded exercise. Prognostic implications of chronotropic incompetence in the Framingham Heart Study. *Circulation* 1996; 93:1520–6.

13. Lauer MS, Francis GS, Okin PM, Pashkow FJ, Snader CE, Marwick TH. Impaired chronotropic response to exercise stress testing as a predictor of mortality. *JAMA* 1999; 281:524–9.

14. Cole CR, Blackstone EH, Pashkow FJ, Snader CE, Lauer MS. Heart-rate recovery immediately after exercise as a predictor of mortality. *N Engl J Med* 1999; 341:1351–7.

15. Cole CR, Foody JM, Blackstone EH, Lauer MS. Heart rate recovery after submaximal exercise testing as a predictor of mortality in a cardiovascularly healthy cohort. *Ann Intern Med* 2000; 132:552–5.

16. Kitamura K, Jorgensen CR, Gobel FL, Taylor HL, Wang Y. Hemodynamic correlates of myocardial oxygen consumption during upright exercise. *J Appl Physiol* 1972; 32:516–22.

17. Kligfield P, Ameisen O, Okin PM. Heart rate adjustment of ST segment depression for improved detection of coronary artery disease. *Circulation* 1989; 79:245–55.

18. Okin PM, Kligfield P. Heart rate adjustment of ST segment depression and performance of the exercise electrocardiogram: a critical evaluation. *J Am Coll Cardiol* 1995; 25:1726–35.

19. Lehtinen R, Sievanen H, Viik J, Turjanmaa V, Niemela K, Malmivuo J. Accurate detection of coronary artery disease by integrated analysis of the ST-segment depression/heart rate patterns during the exercise and recovery phases of the exercise electrocardiography test. *Am J Cardiol* 1996; 78:1002–6.

20. Gullestad L, Jorgensen B, Bjuro T, et al. Postexercise ischemia is associated with increased neuropeptide Y in patients with coronary artery disease. *Circulation* 2000; 102:987–93.

21. Svensbergh A, Johansson M, Pahlm O, Brudin LH. ST-recovery loop of exercise-induced ST deviation in the identification of coronary artery disease: which parameters should we measure? *J Electrocardiol* 2004; 37:275–83.

22. Kligfield P, Lauer MS. Exercise electrocardiogram testing: beyond the ST segment. *Circulation* 2006; 114:2070–82.

23. Lauer MS, Mehta R, Pashkow FJ, Okin PM, Lee K, Marwick TH. Association of chronotropic incompetence with echocardiographic ischemia and prognosis. *J Am Coll Cardiol* 1998; 32:1280–6.

24. Sandvik L, Erikssen J, Ellestad M, et al. Heart rate increase and maximal heart rate during exercise as predictors of cardiovascular mortality: a 16-year follow-up study of 1960 healthy men. *Coron Artery Dis* 1995; 6:667–79.

25. Elhendy A, Mahoney DW, Khandheria BK, Burger K, Pellikka PA. Prognostic significance of impairment of heart rate response to exercise: impact of left ventricular function and myocardial ischemia. *J Am Coll Cardiol* 2003; 42:823–30.

26. Dresing TJ, Blackstone EH, Pashkow FJ, Snader CE, Marwick TH, Lauer MS. Usefulness of impaired chronotropic response to exercise as a predictor of mortality, independent of the severity of coronary artery disease. *Am J Cardiol* 2000; 86:602–9.

27. Elhendy A, van Domburg RT, Bax JJ, et al. The functional significance of chronotropic incompetence during dobutamine stress test. *Heart* 1999; 81:398–403.

28. Okin PM, Lauer MS, Kligfield P. Chronotropic response to exercise. Improved performance of ST-segment depression criteria after adjustment for heart rate reserve. *Circulation* 1996; 94:3226–31.

29. Azarbal B, Hayes SW, Lewin HC, Hachamovitch R, Cohen I, Berman DS. The incremental prognostic value of percentage of heart rate reserve achieved over myocardial perfusion single-photon emission computed tomography in the prediction of cardiac death and all-cause mortality: superiority over 85% of maximal age-predicted heart rate. *J Am Coll Cardiol* 2004; 44:423–30.

30. Khan MN, Pothier CE, Lauer MS. Chronotropic incompetence as a predictor of death among patients with normal electrograms taking beta blockers (metoprolol or atenolol). *Am J Cardiol* 2005; 96:1328–33.

31. Richeson JF, Akiyama T, Schenk E. A solid angle analysis of the epicardial ischemic TQ-ST deflection in the pig. A theoretical and experimental study. *Circ Res* 1978; 43:879–88.

32. Yan GX, Lankipalli RS, Burke JF, Musco S, Kowey PR. Ventricular repolarization components on the electrocardiogram: cellular basis and clinical significance. *J Am Coll Cardiol* 2003; 42:401–9.

33. Kligfield P. ST segment analysis in exercise stress testing. In: Zareba W, Maison-Blanche P, Locati EH, eds. *Noninvasive Electrocardiology in Clinical Practice*. Armonk, NY: Futura; 2001:227–256.

34. Detry JM, Piette F, Brasseur LA. Hemodynamic determinants of exercise ST-segment depression in coronary patients. *Circulation* 1970; 42:593–9.

35. Holmberg S, Serzysko W, Varnauskas E. Coronary circulation during heavy exercise in control subjects and patients with coronary heart disease. *Acta Med Scand* 1971; 190:465–80.

36. Linden RJ, Mary DA. Limitations and reliability of exercise electrocardiography tests in coronary heart disease. *Cardiovasc Res* 1982; 16:675–710.

37. Kligfield P, Okin PM. Linearity of the ST segment relationship to heart rate during exercise in coronary artery disease and in normal subjects. *Japanese Heart Journal* 1994; 35 Suppl:109–110.

38. Holland RP, Arnsdorf MF. Solid angle theory and the electrocardiogram: physiologic and quantitative interpretations. *Prog Cardiovasc Dis* 1977; 19:431–57.

39. Holland RP, Brooks H. TQ-ST segment mapping: critical review and analysis of current concepts. *Am J Cardiol* 1977; 40:110–29.

40. Okin PM, Kligfield P. Solid-angle theory and heart rate adjustment of ST-segment depression for the identification and quantification of coronary artery disease. *Am Heart J* 1994; 127:658–67.

41. Watanabe T, Akutsu Y, Yamanaka H, et al. Exercise-induced ST-segment depression: imbalance between myocardial oxygen demand and myocardial blood flow. *Acta Cardiol* 2000; 55:25–31.

42. Elamin MS, Mary DA, Smith DR, Linden RJ. Prediction of severity of coronary artery disease using slope of submaximal ST segment/heart rate relationship. *Cardiovasc Res* 1980; 14:681–91.

43. Berenyi I, Hajduczki IS, Boszormenyi E. Quantitative evaluation of exercise-induced ST-segment depression for estimation of degree of coronary artery disease. *Eur Heart J* 1984; 5:289–94.

44. Hajduczki I, Berenyi I, Enghoff E, Malmberg P, Erikson U. Qualitative and quantitative evaluation of the exercise electrocardiogram in assessing the degree of coronary heart disease. *J Electrocardiol* 1985; 18:55–62.

45. Kardash M, Elamin MS, Mary DA, et al. The slope of ST segment/heart rate relationship during exercise in the prediction of severity of coronary artery disease. *Eur Heart J* 1982; 3:449–58.

46. Detrano R, Salcedo E, Passalacqua M, Friis R. Exercise electrocardiographic variables: a critical appraisal. *J Am Coll Cardiol* 1986; 8:836–47.

47. Kligfield P, Okin PM, Ameisen O, Borer JS. Evaluation of coronary artery disease by an improved method of exercise electrocardiography: the ST segment/heart rate slope. *Am Heart J* 1986; 112:589–98.

48. Kligfield P, Ameisen O, Okin PM. Relation of the exercise ST/HR slope to simple heart rate adjustment of ST segment depression. *J Electrocardiol* 1987; 20 Suppl:135–40.

49. Okin PM, Kligfield P. Effect of precision of ST-segment measurement on identification and quantification of coronary artery disease by the ST/HR index. *J Electrocardiol* 1992; 24 Suppl:62–7.

50. Okin PM, Bergman G, Kligfield P. Effect of ST segment measurement point on performance of standard and heart rate-adjusted ST segment criteria for the identification of coronary artery disease. *Circulation* 1991; 84:57–66.

51. Okin PM, Ameisen O, Kligfield P. A modified treadmill exercise protocol for computer-assisted analysis of the ST segment/heart rate slope: methods and reproducibility. *J Electrocardiol* 1986; 19:311–8.

52. Okin PM, Kligfield P. Population selection and performance of the exercise ECG for the identification of coronary artery disease. *Am Heart J* 1994; 127:296–304.

53. Froelicher VF, Lehmann KG, Thomas R, et al. The electrocardiographic exercise test in a population with reduced workup bias: diagnostic performance, computerized interpretation, and multivariable prediction. Veterans Affairs Cooperative Study in Health Services #016 (QUEXTA) Study Group. Quantitative Exercise Testing and Angiography. *Ann Intern Med* 1998; 128:965–74.

54. Haggmark S, Haney MF, Jensen SM, Johansson G, Naslund U. ST-segment deviations during pacing-induced increased heart rate in patients without coronary artery disease. *Clin Physiol Funct Imaging* 2005; 25:246–52.

55. Sansoy V, Watson DD, Beller GA. Significance of slow upsloping ST-segment depression on exercise stress testing. *Am J Cardiol* 1997; 79:709–12.

56. Okin PM, Kligfield P, Ameisen O, Goldberg HL, Borer JS. Identification of anatomically extensive coronary artery disease by the exercise ECG ST segment/heart rate slope. *Am Heart J* 1988; 115:1002–13.

57. Kligfield P, Okin PM, Goldberg HL. Value and limitations of heart rate-adjusted ST segment depression criteria for the identification of anatomically severe coronary obstruction: test performance in relation to method of rate correction, definition of extent of disease, and beta-blockade. *Am Heart J* 1993; 125:1262–8.

58. Okin PM, Kligfield P. Effect of exercise protocol and lead selection on the accuracy of heart rate-adjusted indices of ST-segment depression for detection of three-vessel coronary artery disease. *J Electrocardiol* 1989; 22:187–94.

59. Haggmark S, Haney MF, Johansson G, Reiz S, Naslund U. Contributions of myocardial ischemia and heart rate to ST segment changes in patients with or without coronary artery disease. *Acta Anaesthesiol Scand* 2008; 52:219–28.

60. Okin PM, Kligfield P. On the matter of method in exercise testing. *Am Heart J* 1994; 127:1673–6.

61. Watanabe M, Yokota M, Miyahara T, et al. Clinical significance of simple heart rate-adjusted ST segment depression in supine leg exercise in the diagnosis of coronary artery disease. *Am Heart J* 1990; 120:1102–10.

62. Lee JH, Cheng SL, Selvester R, Ellestad MH. Kligfield-Okin index: revisiting the correction of ST depression for delta heart rate. *Am J Cardiol* 2000; 85:1022–4.

63. Hamasaki S, Arima S, Tahara M, et al. Increase in the delta ST/delta heart rate (HR) index: a new predictor of restenosis after successful percutaneous transluminal coronary angioplasty. *Am J Cardiol* 1996; 78:990–5.

64. Hamasaki S, Abematsu H, Arima S, et al. A new predictor of restenosis after successful percutaneous transluminal coronary angioplasty in patients with multivessel coronary artery disease. *Am J Cardiol* 1997; 80:411–5.

65. Hamasaki S, Nakano F, Arima S, et al. A new criterion combining ST/HR slope and deltaST/deltaHR index for detection of coronary artery disease in patients on digoxin therapy. *Am J Cardiol* 1998; 81:1100–4.

66. Okin PM, Anderson KM, Levy D, Kligfield P. Heart rate adjustment of exercise-induced ST segment depression. Improved risk stratification in the Framingham Offspring Study. *Circulation* 1991; 83:866–74.

67. Okin PM, Grandits G, Rautaharju PM, et al. Prognostic value of heart rate adjustment of exercise-induced ST segment

depression in the multiple risk factor intervention trial. *J Am Coll Cardiol* 1996; 27:1437–43.

68. Okin PM, Prineas RJ, Grandits G, et al. Heart rate adjustment of exercise-induced ST-segment depression identifies men who benefit from a risk factor reduction program. *Circulation* 1997; 96:2899–904.

69. Desai MY, De la Pena-Almaguer E, Mannting F. Abnormal heart rate recovery after exercise as a reflection of an abnormal chronotropic response. *Am J Cardiol* 2001; 87:1164–9.

70. Imai K, Sato H, Hori M, et al. Vagally mediated heart rate recovery after exercise is accelerated in athletes but blunted in patients with chronic heart failure. *J Am Coll Cardiol* 1994; 24:1529–35.

71. Vivekananthan DP, Blackstone EH, Pothier CE, Lauer MS. Heart rate recovery after exercise is a predictor of mortality, independent of the angiographic severity of coronary disease. *J Am Coll Cardiol* 2003; 42:831–8.

72. Kligfield P, McCormick A, Chai A, Jacobson A, Feuerstadt P, Hao SC. Effect of age and gender on heart rate recovery after submaximal exercise during cardiac rehabilitation in patients with angina pectoris, recent acute myocardial infarction, or coronary bypass surgery. *Am J Cardiol* 2003; 92:600–3.

73. Hao SC, Chai A, Kligfield P. Heart rate recovery response to symptom-limited treadmill exercise after cardiac rehabilitation in patients with coronary artery disease with and without recent events. *Am J Cardiol* 2002; 90:763–5.

74. Bruce R, McDonough J. Stress testing in screening for cardiovascular disease. *Bull N Y Acad Med* 1969; 45:1288–1305.

75. Bruce R. Exercise testing of patients with coronary heart disease: principles and normal standards for evaluation. *Ann Clin Res* 1971; 3:323–332.

76. Okin PM, Ameisen O, Kligfield P. Recovery-phase patterns of ST segment depression in the heart rate domain. Identification of coronary artery disease by the rate-recovery loop. *Circulation* 1989; 80:533–41.

77. Bjuro T, Gullestad L, Endresen K, et al. Evaluation of ST-segment changes during and after maximal exercise tests in one-, two- and three-vessel coronary artery disease. *Scand Cardiovasc J* 2004; 38:270–7.

78. Hollenberg M, Budge WR, Wisneski JA, Gertz EW. Treadmill score quantifies electrocardiographic response to exercise and improves test accuracy and reproducibility. *Circulation* 1980; 61:276–85.

79. Hollenberg M, Zoltick JM, Go M, et al. Comparison of a quantitative treadmill exercise score with standard electrocardiographic criteria in screening asymptomatic young men for coronary artery disease. *N Engl J Med* 1985; 313:600–6.

80. Lehtinen R. ST/HR hysteresis: exercise and recovery phase ST depression/heart rate analysis of the exercise ECG. *J Electrocardiol* 1999; 32 Suppl:198–204.

81. Bigi R, Maffi M, Occhi G, Bolognese L, Pozzoni L. Improvement in identification of multivessel disease after acute myocardial infarction following stress-recovery analysis of ST depression in the heart rate domain during exercise. *Eur Heart J* 1994; 15:1240–6.

82. Bigi R, Cortigiani L, Gregori D, De Chiara B, Fiorentini C. Exercise versus recovery electrocardiography in predicting mortality in patients with uncomplicated myocardial infarction. *Eur Heart J* 2004; 25:558–64.

83. Bigi R, Cortigiani L, Gregori D, De Chiara B, Parodi O, Fiorentini C. Exercise versus recovery electrocardiography for predicting outcome in hypertensive patients with chest pain. *J Hypertens* 2004; 22:2193–9.

84. Parrens E, Douard H, Couffinal T, Bordier P, Tourtoulou V, Broustet JP. The exercise-recovery loop and exercise slope of ST segment changes/heart rate in the diagnosis of coronary disease and restenosis after angioplasty. *Arch Mal Coeur Vaiss* 1994; 87:1283–8.

85. Lehtinen R, Vanttinen H, Sievanen H, Malmivuo J. A computer program for comprehensive ST-segment depression/heart rate analysis of the exercise ECG test. *Comput Methods Programs Biomed* 1996; 50:63–71.

86. Okin PM, Kligfield P. Computer-based implementation of the ST-segment/heart rate slope. *Am J Cardiol* 1989; 64:926–30.

4

ECG Left Ventricular Hypertrophy
Detection and Prognosis

SETH R. BENDER
PETER M. OKIN

ECG Detection of LVH   51
Regression of ECG LVH   60
Conclusion   65
References   65

Left ventricular hypertrophy (LVH), a common complication of hypertensive, coronary and valvular heart disease, is strongly associated with increased cardiovascular morbidity and mortality. Thus, the accurate identification, risk stratification. and treatment of patients with LVH are imperative. This chapter will review the role of the electrocardiogram in the diagnosis and prognosis of patients with LVH.

■ ECG DETECTION OF LVH

Characteristic ECG Manifestations of LVH

LVH results in characteristic alterations to myocardial depolarization and repolarization. As a result, the ECG has long been a useful tool for the identification of LVH. The first literature on ECG detection of LVH dates to the early 20th century. Over the years, many ECG criteria have been put forth for detection of LVH (Table 4.1). These criteria make use of common characteristic ECG abnormalities seen in patients with LVH: patterns that mainly reflect increased QRS amplitudes, delayed ventricular activation, and abnormal repolarization, but also left-axis deviation and left-atrial abnormality.

QRS Complex Voltage Amplitude

Increased QRS complex amplitude is perhaps the most intuitive ECG finding associated with LVH. Increased LV mass, whether via increased wall thickness and/or increased LV chamber size, produces an increased size of the electrical activation boundary of the heart resulting in increased QRS voltages. However, many conditions, both intrinsic (myocardial or pericardial pathologies) and extrinsic (COPD, obesity) to the heart can attenuate this relationship. In addition, QRS amplitudes vary with age, gender, and ethnicity. In general, increased QRS voltages are highly specific but poorly sensitive for LVH (1).

Abnormal Repolarization

In the setting of LVH, the typical "LV strain pattern" of asymmetric T-wave inversions and ST depressions in the lateral leads are thought to reflect increased myocardial cell hypertrophy, and to possibly be due to subendocardial ischemia and/or disorganized repolarization of hypertrophied myocardial cells. This ECG strain pattern of abnormal repolarization has been shown to be an independent marker of more severe LVH and worse prognosis (2,3).

QRS Prolongation and Delayed Ventricular Activation

Although the mechanisms for QRS prolongation and delayed intrinsicoid deflection in LVH have not been determined, these findings may be related to the longer time required to activate myocardium that is increasingly

■ **Table 4.1** Common electrocardiogram criteria for identifying left ventricular hypertrophy

Name	Criteria	Threshold
Sokolow-Lyon voltage	$SV_1 + RV_{5/6}$	>35 mm
Gubner and Ungerleider	RI + SIII	>22 mm
12-Lead voltage	Sum of Max (R, S) amplitude in each lead	>179 mm
Framingham criteria	RI + SIII >2.5 mV $SV_{1/2} + RV_{5/6}$ >3.5 mV $SV_{1/2/3}$ >2.5 mV + $RV_{4/5/6}$ >2.5 mV	Probable – any voltage Definite – any voltage *plus* LV strain
Cornell voltage	R-wave aVL + SV_3	>28 mm (men) >20 mm (women)
Adjusted Cornell voltage	Men: RaVL + SV_3 + 0.0174 × (age × 49) + 0.191 × (BMI × 26.5) Women: RaVL + SV_3 + 0.0387 × (age × 50) + 0.212 × (BMI × 24.9)	>28 mm >20 mm
Cornell product	Cornell Voltage (*plus 8 in women*) × QRS duration	>2,440 mm × msec
Romhilt-Estes score	Any limb-lead R or S >2.0 mV or $SV_{1/2}$ >3.0 mV or $RV_{5/6}$ >3.0 mV (3 points) LV strain pattern (3 points) with digitalis (1 point) LAE (3 points) LAD >30° (2 points) QRS duration >90 msec (1 point) Intrinsicoid >50 msec in $V_{5/6}$ (1 point)	Probable ≥4 points Definite ≥5 points
Perugia index (each 1 point)	Modified Cornell Voltage Men >24 mm Women >20 mm Romhilt-Estes score ≥5 Typical strain pattern	≥1 point
Cornell/Strain index	Modified Cornell Voltage Typical strain pattern	≥1 point
Novacode LV mass index (LVMI)	**White and black men:** LVMI = 0.01(RV_5) + 0.02(Q or SV_1) + 0.028(max SIII or QIII) + 0.182(Tneg V_6) – 0.148(Tpos aVR) + 1.049(QRS duration) – 36.43 **White women:** LVMI = 0.018(RV_5) + 0.053(max SV_5 or QV_5) – 0.112(max SI or QI) + 0.108(Tpos V1) + 1.7(Tneg aVF) – 0.094(Tpos V_6) + 88.44 **Black women:** LVMI = 0.022(RaVL) + 0.018 (RV_6 + SV_2) – 0.014(RV_2) – 0.069 (max SV_5 or QV_5) + 0.199 (Tneg aVL) + 0.746 (QRS duration) – 22.31	>131 g/m² (men) >110 g/m² (women)
Minnesota Code	Voltage 3–1 and 3–3 Abnormal repolarization 4.1 to 4.3 or 5.1 to 5.3	

distant from specialized conduction tissue, decreased conduction velocity in hypertrophied myocardium, or changes in the activation sequence and the relative conductivity of fibrotic intracellular and extracellular spaces. Alone, QRS duration has poor sensitivity for LVH. However, when combined with QRS voltage, its relationship to LVH is more robust (4).

Left Atrial Abnormality

Left atrial abnormality, denoted by more pronounced and prolonged terminal negative deflection of the P-wave in V1, has also been associated with LVH. This is thought to be a consequence of increased left atrial pressure caused by decreased LV diastolic relaxation and increased LV end diastolic pressure.

Left Axis Deviation

Left axis deviation has also been correlated with LV mass. As the left ventricle enlarges the heart takes a more horizontal position thus shifting the axis of the heart leftward.

ECG Criteria for the Identification of LVH

Many early ECG LVH criteria make use of QRS voltages alone. Among the earliest ECG criteria for the identification of LVH were Gubner-Ungerleider voltage criteria, Sokolow-Lyon voltage criteria, and the Romhilt-Estes point score. Gubner-Ungerleider and Sokolow-Lyon criteria were derived from correlation analysis of the amplitudes of standard limb leads or precordial leads, and the diagnosis of LVH is made if the sum of the QRS amplitudes of interest is greater than a cut off threshold established from a control population (4,5).

The Romhilt-Estes point score system considers QRS amplitudes, left axis deviation, left atrial abnormality, intrinsicoid delay, QRS duration, and the presence of the ECG strain pattern; it assigns weighted points for the presence of each abnormality. Generally, LVH is considered possibly present when the score is 4 points and definitely present if the score is 5 or more points. However, test performance characteristics can be altered by changing the threshold point value (6,7).

Although the above criteria have the advantage of being easy to calculate and interpret, their performance has been poor when applied to general populations, with sensitivities ranging from 20% to less than 50% (8–11). The poor performance of these criteria are at least in part due to biases in the original derivation cohorts, the lack of separate threshold values for men and women and varying severity of anatomic hypertrophy in the study populations, but may also reflect the inherent inaccuracy of these ECG characteristics for LVH. Indeed, Devereux et al. (8) compared the accuracy of Sokolow-Lyon criteria and the Romhilt-Estes point score with that of a commercial computer algorithm, and that of physician judgment for identifying echocardiographic LVH. They found that physician judgment out-performed both ECG criteria and the computer algorithm. This suggests that additional information about LVH, not detected by commonly applied criteria but recognized by experienced electrocardiographers, may be present on the ECG.

Cornell Voltage Criteria

The need for improved criteria for ECG detection of LVH prompted development of Cornell voltage criteria (12,13), which were derived from and validated in cohorts of patients with echocardiographic and anatomic LV mass measurements. Analysis revealed that R-wave amplitude in aVL and S-wave amplitude in V_3 independently correlated with LV mass index. This relationship was true in both men and women, however, voltages were significantly lower in woman than men. As a result, sex-specific diagnostic cutoff values of the sum of voltages of RaVL and SV_3 were implemented: >2.8 mV (28 mm) for men and 2.0 mV (20 mm) for woman. Compared to Sokolow-Lyon voltage criteria and the Romhilt-Estes score (≥4 points), in normal subjects, Cornell voltage criteria maintain high levels of specificity (100%, 94%, and 96%, respectively) while significantly improving test sensitivity (22%, 33%, and 42%, respectively) (12,13).

Voltage-Duration Product and Area Improve Accuracy

Performance of voltage criteria can be improved by incorporating a measure of QRS duration. Findings from two less accessible modalities, vectorcardiography and 126-lead dipole electrocardiography, suggested that the measure of the area under the QRS complex, the time-voltage integral, could improve ECG assessment of LV mass. In the absence of a readily available method for measurement of QRS area, the simple product of QRS duration with various ECG voltage criteria was evaluated as an approximation of the true area. Simple voltage-duration products, used in surrogate of the more complex integral calculation, significantly improved sensitivity of Sokolow-Lyon, 12-lead sum, and Cornell voltage criteria. At a matched specificity of 96%, sensitivity for the Cornell product was 51% compared with only 36% for Cornell voltage. Similar improvements in sensitivity were found for Sokolow-Lyon product and 12-lead product criteria (14,15). Additional improvements in sensitivity can be achieved by considering the true area under the QRS complex, but further testing of this approach using measurements from clinically available ECG carts will be required (16).

Signal Averaged Electrocardiography Improves Detection

The signal-averaged electrocardiogram (SAECG) is a computerized technique for detecting subtle abnormalities from the surface ECG, computed by performing the arithmetic mean of multiple ECG complexes. Thus SAECG increases the signal-to-noise ratio of cardiac potentials and enables the detection of much smaller signals than would otherwise be discernible from the surface ECG. The time voltage integral of the horizontal plane SAECG QRS vector significantly improved detection of LVH compared with conventional voltage criteria (17). However, utility of this modality is hampered by its complexity and limited general availability.

Perugia Score and Cornell/Strain Index: Tests in Parallel to Improve Sensitivity

A further effort to improve ECG identification of LVH led to the development of the Perugia score. Perugia criteria for LVH are met if a patient meets at least one of the following well-characterized ECG LVH criteria: Cornell voltage (modified to cutoffs of 2.4 mV for men and 2.0 mV for women), the presence of a typical strain pattern. or Romhilt-Estes score ≥5. By combining these three ECG criteria for LVH, the Perugia score increases test sensitivity (34% versus 21% for Sokolow-Lyon voltage) and accuracy (73% versus 66% for Sokolow-Lyon voltage) without a significant change in specificity (93% versus 89% for Sokolow-Lyon voltage) (18,19). The Cornell/Strain Index, proposed by the same investigators, consists of the presence of either modified Cornell Voltage criteria or typical stain pattern and also improves sensitivity with little loss of specificity when compared to traditional criteria (20).

Multivariate Analyses to Improve Accuracy

Equations derived from multivariate regression analysis offer another technique for simultaneously accounting for multiple predictors of ECG LVH. For example, using linear multivariate regression analysis to adjust for body mass index and age enhanced the sensitivity of a number of commonly used ECG voltage criteria and all specificities in a subset for Framingham participants (21,22). Similarly, examination of the Cornell criteria validation cohort revealed that in addition to the significant QRS voltages, gender, QRS duration, T-wave amplitude in V1, and terminal negative P-wave forces in V1 were independent predictors of LV mass, with the resulting multivariate formula improving test sensitivity and accuracy (12).

Unfortunately, these regression equations have proven too cumbersome for routine manual calculation and clinical application. However, computerized multivariable analyses such as the Novacode ECG LV mass index have been demonstrated to improve both identification of LVH and risk stratification (23).

Additional Factors that Can Affect ECG Identification of LVH

Age

Data from the Framingham Heart Study reveal that the sensitivity of the Framingham criteria increases with age while there is a concomitant decrease in specificity (24).

Sex

Men have significantly longer QRS durations and greater ECG voltages than women (25). As a result, many common ECG criteria that use identical, fixed, voltage partitions for both sexes, such as Sokolow-Lyon voltage and Romhilt-Estes score, have decreased sensitivity in women. Interestingly, criteria using separate threshold values for men and women, such as the Cornell criteria (12,13) and Perugia score (18), only partially mitigate this effect. In fact, when evaluated continuously, as opposed to using a threshold, the sensitivities of many ECG LVH indices, including SAECG (15), were significantly lower in women at all levels of specificity, even after adjustment for gender differences in body size and LV mass. These differences in test performance may partially reflect gender differences in lean body mass (26).

Body Habitus

Body habitus can affect ECG detection of LVH in several ways. Obesity and increases in body mass index are associated with increased risk of anatomic LVH, however the excess soft tissue between the myocardium and the ECG electrodes act to attenuate QRS voltage amplitudes in some leads (24). As a consequence, sensitivity of Sokolow-Lyon voltage criteria is reduced in obese patients and enhanced in lean individuals, whereas test specificity is high in the obese and quite low in lean patients. In contrast, accuracy of Cornell voltage and Cornell product criteria is essentially independent of BMI (27–29). In addition, both cachexia and mastectomy are associated with increases in QRS amplitudes (30), possibly reflecting a relative decrease in distance from electrode to myocardium.

Ethnicity

Multiple studies have demonstrated that the accuracy of ECG LVH criteria is not consistent across ethnicities. ECG LVH is two to four times more prevalent among African American than white adults even after adjustment for differences in blood pressure. In contrast, studies using echocardiography show less striking differences. The reason for this discrepancy can be explained by higher normal precordial QRS voltages in blacks, the wide-spread dependence on Sokolow-Lyon voltage criteria, and the failure to adjust voltage thresholds for ethnicity (31). When Lee and colleagues compared the sensitivity and specificity of ECG LVH criteria in African American and white patients, five commonly used ECG LVH criteria had significantly lower specificities in blacks, resulting in an increase in false positive diagnoses (32). However, this effect is very much dependent on the use of ECG criteria with fixed thresholds. When ECG voltage criteria were analyzed as continuous variables as opposed to dichotomous thresholds, to account for difference in "normal" voltages, these apparent ethnic differences in test performance mostly disappear (33). Although less extensively studied, ECG LVH criteria appear to have different performance characteristics in Hispanic populations as well (31,34). Use of multivariate regression equations correcting for differences between ethnicities represents one strategy to improve the detection of LVH across ethnic groups (31,35).

In summary, the ECG offers an indirect assessment of LVH manifested by several characteristic ECG changes. Multiple important factors may alter the relationship between ECG criteria and the presence of anatomic LVH. As a result, ECG criteria tend to best detect more severe LVH and are highly specific but modestly sensitive despite the use of multiple strategies to improve detection. Despite this apparent limitation, ECG LVH remains a powerful tool for identifying patients at high risk of cardiovascular complications.

ECG LVH: Prognostic Implications

LVH is a well characterized marker of preclinical cardiovascular disease (36), and when detected on ECG, LVH is a particularly ominous sign and a harbinger of significant risk. In fact, ECG LVH criteria identify patients with more severe increases in LV mass than those with LVH by echocardiography in the absence of ECG LVH (2). As a result, ECG LVH identifies a population of patients at an especially high risk of cardiovascular morbidity and mortality (37).

The Framingham Heart Study provided some of the first substantial evidence that subjects with ECG LVH are at significantly increased risk of adverse CV outcome. During the first 14 years of follow-up, 44% of deaths occurred in patients with "probable" or "definite" ECG LVH. "Definite" ECG LVH was associated with a three-to-fourfold increased risk of death, a greater risk of dying than in patients with previous myocardial infarction. In addition to increased mortality, patients with ECG LVH were considerably more likely to suffer from a myriad of CV complications including angina, coronary artery disease, myocardial infarction, congestive heart failure, stroke, peripheral arterial disease, and sudden death (37–39).

Over the four decades since the initial Framingham data, a large body of evidence has been compiled supporting the utility of ECG LVH as predictor of cardiovascular outcome. A review by Vakili et al. (40) demonstrated a strong and consistent relationship between the presence of ECG LVH at baseline and subsequent cardiovascular morbidity (hazard ratio [HR] 1.6–4.0) and all-cause mortality (HR 1.5–6.8). Importantly, these findings persisted across various ECG LVH criteria and clinical populations, as well as differences in gender and ethnicity.

Additional analyses have further enhanced our knowledge of the prognostic value of ECG LVH by examining various ECG LVH indices and outcomes. The Heart Outcomes Prevention Evaluation trial (HOPE)

(41) evaluated the predictive value of Sokolow-Lyon voltage criteria in 9,541 men and woman greater than 55 years of age with known CV disease and additional risk factors (Figure 4.1). ECG LVH was present in 793 (8.3%) of subjects and was associated with a statistically significant increase in death (15.6% versus 10.8%), major cardiovascular events (19.0% versus 15.6%), and incident heart failure (6.1% versus 2.9%), and remained an independent predictor of all-cause mortality, cardiovascular death, and incident heart failure in multivariate analyses. These findings provide support for the use of a commonly used simple criterion to accurately identify patients at increased risk.

The Copenhagen City Heart Study, however, found mixed results when evaluating the prognostic utility of ECG LVH voltage in isolation. This observational prospective cohort study examined the relative predictive value of ECG LVH by voltage and repolarization abnormalities in isolation and combination in 10,982 Danish men and women. Analysis revealed that men older than 55 years who met voltage criteria for ECG LVH were at increased risk for fatal and nonfatal myocardial infarction (RR 1.94) and ischemic heart disease (RR 1.58). However, voltage-only LVH was not predictive of outcome in men younger than 55 years. In contrast, when both voltage and abnormal repolarization were considered in combination, patients with both features were at a significantly greater 7- and 21-year risk of fatal or nonfatal MI (RR 2.8, 95% CI 1.7–4.8; 1.9, 1.3–2.7) ischemic heart disease (RR 3.6, 95% CI 2.5–5.3; 2.2, 1.7–2.8), and death (RR 3.0, 95% CI 1.9–4.7; 1.9, 1.5–2.5). The relative risks associated with ECG LVH and abnormal repolarization in combination were greater than those for either ECG LVH by voltage or abnormal repolarization alone (42).

Additional studies have compared the prognostic capabilities of various ECG criteria, including those that consider only QRS voltage as well as more complex, multifactorial criteria. Analysis from the Progetto Ipertensione Umbria Monotoraggio Ambulatoriale (PIUMA) registry (19) examined prognostic value of several common ECG LVH criteria (Sokolow-Lyon, Romhilt-Estes, Perugia, Framingham, and LV Strain) in 1,717 previously untreated hypertensive patients (Figure 4.2). The adjusted HRs (95% CI) for cardiovascular morbidity ranged from 2.6 (1.7–4.1) for a Romhilt-Estes score of ≥5 to 1.2 (0.8–1.8) for Sokolow-Lyon voltage. The results for cardiovascular mortality were similar with adjusted HRs ranging from 4.9 (2.2–11.1) for Romhilt-Estes score ≥4 to 1.8 (0.7–4.6)

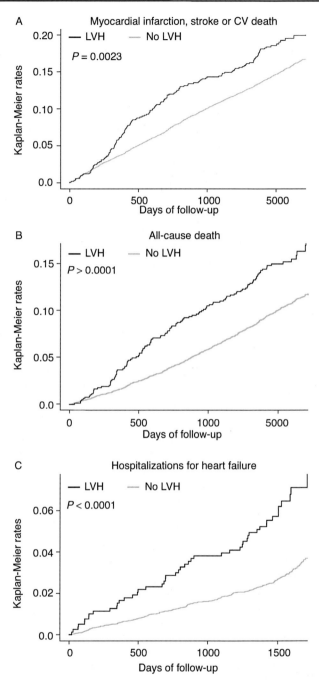

FIGURE 4.1 Kaplan-Meier estimates of the composite of myocardial infarction, stroke, or death from cardiovascular causes (A), of all-cause death (B), and of hospitalizations for heart failure (C) in patients with and without ECG-LVH by Sokolow-Lyon Voltage in the HOPE trial. (From Ref. 41, with permission.)

for Sokolow-Lyon voltage. Of note, both of the voltage criteria studied (Sokolow-Lyon and Cornell) had nonsignificant HRs for cardiovascular morbidity and mortality, while criteria that incorporated measures of

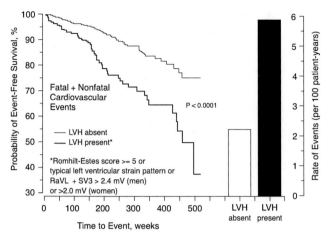

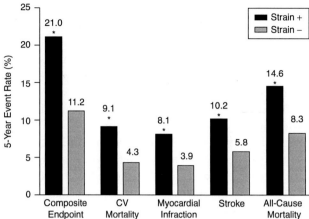

FIGURE 4.2 Event-free survival curves for total cardiovascular events in the PUIMA cohort grouped by the presence or absence of LVH according to Perugia score (*left*). The rate of major cardiovascular morbid events was significantly higher in the subset with LVH (*right*). For the subset with LVH, Romhilt-Estes score ≥5, or typical left ventricular strain pattern, or RaVL + SV3 >2.4 mV (men) or >2.0 mV (women). (From Ref. 18, with permission.)

FIGURE 4.3 Five-year event rates according to the presence or absence of strain on the baseline ECG in the LIFE study. (**P* <0.001 versus patients without strain.) (From Ref. 45, with permission.)

repolarization had HRs that were all significant with the exception of a nonsignificant prediction of mortality by Framingham criteria.

A second comparative analysis (43) yielded similar results. Seventeen commonly used ECG LVH criteria, including simple voltage indices, voltage duration products, point-scoring systems, and more complex regression models were evaluated in 46,950 consecutive veterans. After adjusting for age, heart rate, and BMI, the presence of ECG LVH was associated with a 1.4 to 3.7 increased risk of mortality depending on the criteria used. In general, ECG LVH criteria that included assessment of both voltage and morphology were more predictive of CV mortality than simple voltage criteria. In further analysis, the presence of characteristic "LV strain" and abnormal P-wave morphology were associated with the highest hazards of CV mortality.

These findings suggest a significant impact of abnormal repolarization on the prognosis of patients with LVH. In fact, in Framingham Heart Study patients with "probable," voltage-only LVH, much of the increased risk was mitigated by controlling for additional CV risk factors. In contrast, the presence of repolarization abnormalities in combination with voltage criteria, termed "definite" LVH, remained an independent risk factor for morbidity and mortality after controlling for covariates (44).

The prognostic value of ECG strain was further evaluated among 8,854 hypertensive patients with ECG LVH who underwent aggressive antihypertensive therapy as part of the Losartan Intervention For Reduction in Endpoints (LIFE) trial (Figure 4.3) (45). All of the patients enrolled had LVH determined by either Sokolow-Lyon or Cornell voltage-duration product criteria. LV strain was present in 971 (11.0%) of patients. After controlling for standard CV risk factors, baseline blood pressure, and severity of ECG LVH, ECG strain remained a significant predictor of CV mortality (HR 1.6, 95% CI 1.2–2.0), fatal and nonfatal myocardial infarction (HR 1.6, 95% CI 1.2–2.1), and a composite endpoint of CV death, nonfatal MI or stroke (HR 1.3, 95% CI 1.1–1.6). Thus ECG strain is a marker of increased CV risk in the setting of aggressive blood pressure control independent of the severity of baseline ECG LVH.

The predictive value of abnormal repolarization in combination with echocardiographic LVH (Echo-LVH) was examined in the Strong Heart Study (46). In this prospectively followed cohort of American Indians, ST-segment depression (STD) ≥50 μV was present in 133 participants (6.1%) and was associated with a > six-fold increased risk of CV death and with a nearly four-fold increased risk of all-cause mortality. After adjustment for known CV risk factors, both STD ≥50 μV and Echo-LVH remained independent significant predictors of CVD and all-cause mortality. Combined Echo-LVH and ECG STD improved risk stratification compared with either Echo-LVH or STD alone for CVD and all-cause mortality. After adjustment for covariates, the presence of both ECG-STD and Echo-LVH remained a significant predictor of CVD and all-cause mortality, associated with a 6.3-fold increased risk of CVD death and a 4.6-fold increased risk of all-cause mortality (47).

These findings highlight the prognostic and pathophysiologic significance of abnormal repolarization in the setting of LVH. The presence of ECG strain identifies patients with more severe cardiovascular disease and increased risk of CV morbidity and mortality. The Framingham investigators have posited that the increase in QRS voltage may be primarily related to the chronicity and severity of hypertension, while repolarization abnormalities reflect actual pathologic changes in the myocardium (44). This is further supported by data from the LIFE trial demonstrating that patients with ECG strain have a higher prevalence and greater severity of anatomic LVH than those with voltage ECG LVH alone (2,48).

ECG LVH and CV Morbidity

The presence of ECG LVH is clearly associated with an increased risk of CV risk. The impact of ECG LVH on several particular CV outcomes merits separate discussion.

Stroke

First shown in the Framingham cohort, LVH has been shown to be an important risk factor for stroke. More recent analyses revealed that ECG LVH by the Perugia score was associated with a nearly 80% increase in cerebrovascular events after adjustment for CV risk factors (49). The increased risk of stroke independent of blood pressure and other CV risk factors suggests that ECG LVH may reflect longitudinal exposure to the combined effects of multiple CV risk factors, not solely hypertension (50).

Additional data suggests that ECG LVH predicts stroke independent of the presence of echocardiographic LVH. In a case-control study, patients with first ischemic stroke were more likely to have ECG-LVH by Sokolow-Lyon criteria, Cornell voltage, and Cornell product. The presence of both echocardiographic LVH and Cornell voltage LVH was associated with a 3.5-fold increase in risk of stroke. Of note, after adjustment for echocardiographic LVH, Cornell voltage criteria

remained a significant predictor of stroke (OR 1.73, 95% CI 1.14–2.88). (51) These observations add to the notion that ECG LVH detects a particularly high-risk population.

Heart Failure

As previously noted, the HOPE trail demonstrated a clear relationship between the presence of Sokolow-Lyon voltage and new onset heart failure (41). Furthermore, given the relation of ECG strain to disease severity, it is not surprising that ECG strain predicts the development of heart failure. Among the 8,686 LIFE study patients without heart failure at study enrollment, ECG strain was present in 923 (10.6%), while new onset heart failure occurred in 265 (3.0%), 26 of whom had CHF-related death. In univariate Cox analyses, ECG strain was a significant predictor of new-onset CHF (HR 3.3, 95% CI 2.5–4.3) and of CHF mortality (HR 4.7, 95% CI 2.1–10.6). In Cox multivariable analyses controlling for baseline difference between patients with and without new-onset CHF, in-treatment differences in blood pressure, severity of ECG LVH, and the impact of treatment with losartan versus atenolol on outcomes, ECG strain remained a significant predictor of incident CHF (HR 1.8, 95% CI 1.3–2.5) and CHF-related death (HR 2.8, 95% CI 1.0–7.6) (52). Of note, additional analysis from LIFE trial revealed that patients with albuminuria in addition to ECG strain were at a further increased risk of developing new-onset heart failure (HR 2.8, 95% CI 1.8–4.4) (53).

Analysis of the absolute magnitude of ST segment deviation above or below the isometric baseline in leads V5 and V6 in 2,059 Strong Heart Study participants with no history of CHF provides further evidence of the value of repolarization for stratifying risk of CHF. The 77 subjects (3.7%) who developed heart failure had greater baseline severity of ECG LVH by Sokolow-Lyon voltage and Cornell product, as well as greater baseline ST segment depression. In univariate analyses, ST segment depression was a significant predictor of new-onset heart failure, with each 10 μV increase in ST depression associated with a 31% greater risk of developing heart failure (HR 1.3, 95% CI 1.2–1.4). ST segment depression remained a significant predictor of incident heart failure after controlling for age, gender, diabetes, coronary heart disease, albuminuria, and other baseline risk factors (HR 1.2, 95% CI 1.1–1.3 per 10 μV increase). Of note, the association between ST depression and new-onset heart failure was similar in participants with and without Cornell product LVH (54).

Despite the known association of LV strain with LVH and LV systolic dysfunction independent of coronary heart disease (2), no association with diastolic heart failure was found in a subgroup of LIFE patients (55).

Sudden Death

Observations from large cohort studies suggest that patients with ECG LVH are at increased risk of sudden cardiac death (SCD) (56,57). Increased ventricular ectopy (58) and nonsustained ventricular tachycardia (59) have been offered as indirect evidence of increase arrhythmic death in patients with ECG LVH. A prospective analysis of 59 untreated hypertensive patients found that SCD was associated with both ECG-LVH and Lown's arrhythmia score, but not QT dispersion (60).

Atrial Fibrillation

LVH has been linked to the development of atrial fibrillation. ECG LVH was a univariate predictor of new onset atrial fibrillation in the Framingham cohort and the Manatoba Follow-up study. However, this relationship was not significant in multivariate analysis accounting for other known CV risk factors, nor was ECG LVH predictive in analysis in the PIUMA registry (61–64).

ECG LVH in Selected Populations

Patients with Heart Failure

The relation of ECG LVH to morbidity and mortality in patients with *established* heart failure was examined in 7,599 patients with symptomatic heart failure enrolled in the Candesartan in Heart Failure: Assessment of Reduction in Mortality and Morbidity (CHARM) study. ECG LVH was determined by the individual site investigators without the use of uniform standard criteria and was present in 15.7% of patients. ECG LVH was an independent predictor of the composite primary outcome of CV related death or unplanned hospitalization for symptomatic heart failure (RR 1.3, 95% CI 1.0–1.6). In addition, ECG LVH was associated with increased risk of cardiovascular death (RR 1.5, 95% CI 1.1–2.0), hospitalization due to heart failure (RR 1.2, 95% CI 0.9–1.5), and composite major cardiovascular events (1.4, 95% CI 1.1–1.6) (65).

Patients with Acute MI/Unstable Angina

Patients with acute coronary syndrome and concomitant ECG LVH are a group at particularly high risk. In a subgroup analysis of Diltiazem Reinfarction Study Group patients with confirmed non-Q-wave acute myocardial infarction in whom ECG LVH was determined by voltage criteria alone, patients with LVH had smaller elevations in biomarkers and similar short-term prognosis. However, at one year of follow-up, patients with ECG LVH were more likely to have reinfarction (24% versus 12%, P <0.005) or death (19% versus 9% P <0.044). Multivariate regression analysis adjusting for significant univariate predictors revealed the relative risk of reinfarction and death for patients with ECG LVH were 1.7 and 2.1 respectively (66). Similarly, Yotsukura et al. found that the presence of Sokolow-Lyon voltage criteria for LVH on a preinfarction ECG was predictive of both in-hospital mortality (21.8% versus 9.6% P <0.05) and mortality 1 year after hospital discharge (8.8% versus 1.8% P <0.05) (67). In multivariate analysis, ECG LVH was an independent predictor of one-year mortality in patients over 70 years of age. Interestingly, this relationship was not observed when considering LVH on early postinfarction or discharge ECG, and these findings may reflect the impact of MI on performance of ECG LVH criteria.

Further insight is provided by the Global Utilization of Strategies to Open Occluded Arteries (GUSTO) IV ACS trial. Of the 7,443 patients with acute coronary syndrome and admission ECGs, 586 patients (7.6%) met Cornell voltage criteria and had evidence of LV strain, of which 74% were women. Patients with ECG LVH by these criteria were at significantly increased risk of 30-day and one-year mortality (5% versus 3%, P = 0.046, and 14% versus 7%, P <0.001, respectively). After adjustment for baseline characteristics, LVH remained associated with an increased risk of one-year mortality in women (HR 1.4 95% CI 1.0–1.9), but not men. Of note, patients with LVH were significantly less likely to undergo invasive procedures (68).

Older Patients

Because the prevalence of LVH increases with age (37), older patients represent a particularly important group to evaluate. The Bronx Longitudinal Aging Study examined the prognostic significance of ECG LVH in patients older than 75. EGG LVH was determined by the Minnesota Code, a diagnostic coding system that accounts for abnormalities in both voltage and repolarization (Table 4.1). ECG LVH was present in 9.2% of participants at baseline and was associated with increased rates of all-cause mortality, CV mortality and myocardial infarction. Furthermore, significantly increased risks of all cause mortality, CV mortality and myocardial infarction were observed in an additional 8.5% of participants who developed new ECG LVH during the trial (69). In a population of elderly Swedish men, ECG-LVH defined by Cornell product predicted total mortality independently of echocardiographic measurements of LV mass (HR 2.89, 95% CI 1.41–5.96) (70).

In summary, ECG LVH is potent, independent marker of increased risk cardiovascular morbidity and mortality. Increased risk is seen when using a multitude of ECG criteria. However, criteria that include assessment of repolarization seem to be particularly predictive of increased risk. ECG LVH identifies high risk across all patient groups and is particularly ominous in certain clinical situations and patient groups. Having established that ECG LVH is an important tool in the identification of patients at risk, the following section will review the prognostic implications of ECG LVH regression.

■ REGRESSION OF ECG LVH

Antihypertensive Therapy

Therapy targeted to reduce blood pressure can also result in LVH regression. In the Hypertension Detection and Follow-Up Program, a study of 10,940 hypertensive adults, the incidence of new ECG LVH by Minnesota code criteria was lower in subjects randomly assigned to more intensive stepped-care (SC) antihypertensive therapy than to the community based referred-care (RC) (5.6% versus 6.6%, P <0.05). Moreover, when patients with tall R waves and ECG LVH were combined, regression of these findings was more common in SC than in RC patients (54.3% versus 42.9%, P >0.01) (71). Similar results were seen in the Multiple Risk Factor Intervention Trial (MRFIT) (72) and the Treatment of Mild Hypertension Study (TOMHS) (73). However, these studies are limited due to a failure to control for blood pressure differences between arms or show a clinically significant difference when changes in blood pressure were taken into account (71–73).

Stemming from evidence that the renin-angiotensin system (RAS) is an important pathophysiological mediator of LVH (74–76) and that RAS inhibition may lead to increased LVH regression compared to other antihypertensive therapies, investigators evaluated a blood pressure independent relationship of RAS inhibition and the regression of LVH (77–79). The Heart Outcomes Prevention Evaluation (HOPE) study (80) demonstrated that compared with placebo, treatment with the angiotensin converting enzyme inhibitor, ramipril, was associated with a lower likelihood of development or persistence of ECG LVH by Sokolow-Lyon voltage and with a greater likelihood of prevention or regression of ECG LVH, even after adjusting for a greater decrease in BP with ramipril therapy. However, the HOPE study did not compare ramipril with another active treatment, had a very low prevalence of ECG LVH at baseline, did not adjust for the severity of baseline ECG LVH, and only analyzed Sokolow-Lyon LVH as a dichotomous variable as opposed to the magnitude of change in voltage.

The Losartan Intervention for Reductions in Endpoints (LIFE) study was the first study adequately powered to compare regression of ECG LVH between two active treatment arms. Losartan based antihypertensive therapy achieved greater reductions in ECG LVH by both Cornell voltage-duration product and Sokolow-Lyon voltage compared to treatment with atenolol. This difference was noted at 6 months of treatment (–200 versus –69 mm × msec, and –2.5 versus –0.7 mm, respectively, P <0.001 for both) and persisted during up to 5 years of follow-up. Increased LVH regression with losartan-based therapy was independent of baseline severity of ECG LVH and hypertension and of any therapy-related differences in changes in BP. In fact, at all time points through 5 years of study treatment, losartan therapy was associated with significantly lower prevalences of ECG LVH, as well as with greater decreases in the prevalence of ECG LVH from study baseline by both Cornell product and Sokolow-Lyon voltage. Importantly, greater regression of ECG LVH with losartan as compared with atenolol was observed in women and men, younger and older patients, those with and without diabetes, and in whites and nonwhites (81).

The greater reduction in ECG LVH with losartan in the setting of similar reductions in BP with both therapies supports a potential antihypertrophic effect of losartan, possibly mediated by direct blockade of myocardial effects of angiotensin II.

Improves Outcome

A number of studies have demonstrated that regression of and/or prevention of progression to ECG LVH was associated with a reduced risk of CV morbidity (80,82,83). An observational study of 524 participants in the Framingham Heart Study with ECG LVH by various criteria at a qualifying examination found that a significant decline in Cornell voltage or LV strain pattern was associated with lower risk of CV disease, whereas a significant increase in Cornell voltage or LV strain pattern identified individuals at increased risk of CV disease (83).

The Heart Outcomes Prevention Evaluation (HOPE) trial further supported the hypothesis that regression of electrocardiographic LVH improves prognosis (80). The combined end point of either regression of ECG LVH or prevention of progression to ECG LVH in response to ramipril-based therapy was associated with reduced risk of death (5.4% versus 8.9%, P <0.0001), MI (8.7% versus 10.9%, P = 0.042), stroke (3.5% versus 4.7%, P = 0.079), and congestive heart failure (9.3% versus 15.4%, P <0.0001). However, the usefulness of these findings is limited by the low prevalence of ECG LVH in the HOPE trial (8.2%), the absence of adjustment for other clinical variables in outcome analyses, and the absence of specific data addressing the value of changes in Sokolow-Lyon voltage for predicting outcome.

The LIFE trial, consisting of a population selected for the presence of ECG-LVH, adds significant information about the prognostic importance of serial measurement of electrocardiographic LVH during antihypertensive treatment (Fig. 4.4). Lower in-treatment values of both Cornell-voltage duration product and Sokolow-Lyon voltage during antihypertensive therapy were strongly associated with decreased risk of CV morbidity and mortality. After controlling for treatment with losartan or atenolol, baseline Framingham risk score, baseline ECG-LVH, and baseline and in-treatment BP in multivariate analysis, one standard deviation lower (1,050 mm·msec) Cornell product was associated with a 14.5% decreased risk of composite end-point, 22.0% lower risk of CV death and 10% decrease in the rates of both MI and stroke over a mean follow-up of 4.8 years. Similarly, a one-standard deviation lower (10.5 mm) Sokolow-Lyon voltage resulted in similar reduction of endpoints (16.6%, 20.4%, 10%, and 18.8%, respectively). Interestingly, serial measures of both Cornell product and Sokolow-Lyon voltage remained in the adjusted Cox models for all end points, such that the combination of lower in-treatment values of both electrocardiographic LVH criteria was associated with a greater than 29% reduction in the composite end point of CV morbidity and mortality. These data demonstrate that lower values of electrocardiographic LVH by Cornell product and/or Sokolow-Lyon voltage criteria during antihypertensive therapy are associated with a lower likelihood of CV morbidity and mortality, independent of treatment modality and of decreases in BP. In addition, serial measurements of electrocardiographic LVH criteria appear valuable for assessing CV risk over time in patients with hypertension suggesting that antihypertensive therapy targeted at regression or prevention of electrocardiographic LVH by these criteria may improve prognosis (84).

In separate analyses from LIFE, regression of ECG LVH was associated with decreased risks of new onset atrial fibrillation (AF) (85), sudden cardiac death (SCD) (86), and new onset heart failure (54).

The relationship of LVH to the risk of developing atrial fibrillation has been demonstrated in population-based studies (61–63,87) and among hypertensive patients (64,88) using both electrocardiographic measures of LVH (61–64,88) and echocardiographic left ventricular mass (64,87). Analysis from the LIFE trial examined the effect of ECG LVH regression on the incidence of atrial fibrillation. New-onset AF occurred in fewer patients with in-treatment regression or continued absence of ECG LVH than patients with persistence or development of ECG LVH by Cornell product criteria (14.9 versus 19.0 per 1,000 patient-years). In multivariable Cox analyses, lower in-treatment Cornell product LVH treated as a time-varying covariate was associated with a 12.4% lower rate of new-onset AF (HR 0.88; 95% CI 0.80–0.97) for every one standard deviation (1,050 mm·msec) lower Cornell product. This relationship was also significant when Cornell product LVH (>2,440 mm·msec) was analyzed a dichotomous variable (HR 0.83; 95% CI 0.71–0.98). Of note, losartan-based therapy had an independent protective effect on the development of AF (HR, 0.83; 95% CI 0.71–0.97). These findings demonstrate that regression of electrocardiographic LVH during antihypertensive therapy is associated with a lower likelihood of new-onset AF, independent of blood pressure lowering and of the beneficial effect of losartan-based therapy on the development of AF (85).

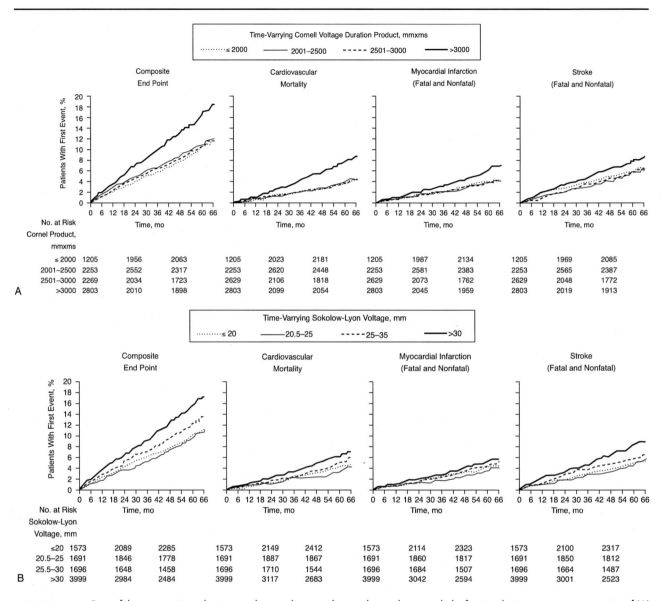

FIGURE 4.4 Rate of the composite end point, cardiovascular mortality, stroke, and myocardial infarction by time-varying categories of (A) Cornell product and (B) Sokolow-Lyon Voltage in the LIFE study. (From Ref. 85, with permission.)

Studies have consistently shown that ECG LVH is strongly associated with higher prevalences of premature ventricular contractions and complex ventricular arrhythmias (59,89,90), as well as increased risk for sudden cardiac death (SCD) (91–94). The LIFE study evaluated the association of ECG LVH regression with SCD. SCD occurred in 190 (2.1%) of LIFE patients over mean follow-up of 4.8 years. Patients who experienced SCD were older, had more comorbid disease, and greater baseline ECG LVH. In univariate Cox regression analysis, a one-standard deviation lower in-treatment ECG LVH was associated with a 28% and 26% lower risk of SCD for both Cornell product and Sokolow-Lyon voltage, respectively. Together, a one-standard deviation lower Cornell product and Sokolow-Lyon voltage was associated with a 43% lower risk of SCD. After adjustment for differences in baseline characteristics and known risk factors for SCD, one-standard deviation lower in-treatment Cornell product and Sokolow-Lyon voltage remained predictive of SCD (19% and 18%, respectively, and 30% for both). In tiered analysis, patients with in-treatment CP <2,000 mm·msec was associated with an estimated 66% decrease in SCD compared to patients with CP >3,000 mm/msec at 4 years (86).

LVH on electrocardiography predicts incident heart failure in both hypertensive and normotensive individuals (80,95,96), and prevention of electrocardiographic LVH appears to attenuate the risk for new-onset heart failure in high-risk patients (80). In the LIFE trial, after controlling for other risk factors for heart failure, in-treatment blood pressures, and treatment effects, greater-than-median reduction of ECG LVH by Cornell product (≥236 mm·msec) on serial assessment of ECGs was associated with a 36% lower incidence of heart failure (HR 0.64, 95% CI 0.47–0.89). When examined as a continuous variable, in multivariate analysis, every one-standard deviation greater reduction in Cornell product (817 mm·msec) was associated with a 19% decrease in incident heart failure (HR 0.81, 95% CI 0.74–0.89). This data demonstrates that in-treatment reduction of electrocardiographic LVH significantly reduces the risk of new-onset heart failure, independent of the effects of blood pressure, baseline severity of ECG LVH, and other risk factors for heart failure (54).

Finally, regression of ECG LVH in hypertensive patients has been shown to be associated with a decrease in new onset diabetes mellitus. Over the course of the LIFE trial 562 patients (7%) developed new onset diabetes. Patients who developed new diabetes were more likely to have had prior antihypertensive treatment, were less likely to have been randomized to losartan-based therapy, were more obese, had higher Framingham risk scores, serum glucose, creatinine and uric acid levels, and lower total and HDL cholesterol levels but were similar with respect to age, gender, race, history of ischemic heart disease, congestive heart failure, myocardial infarction, stroke and peripheral vascular disease, and albuminuria. In addition, patients who developed new diabetes had slightly higher baseline systolic and diastolic blood pressures, and higher baseline prevalence of LVH by Cornell product criteria (72% versus 66%, P <0.001). New-onset diabetes mellitus developed in 330 patients with persistent LVH during treatment (17.1 per 1,000 patient-years) and in 232 with resolution or continued absence of Cornell product LVH (14.3 per 1,000 patient-years). In Cox analyses which adjusted for the known effect of losartan versus atenolol treatment on diabetes incidence in LIFE (97), in-treatment resolution or continued absence of LVH by Cornell product was associated with a 38% (HR 0.62, 95% CI 0.50–0.78)

lower incidence of diabetes, compared with in-treatment persistence or development of ECG LVH. After further adjustment for differences in baseline characteristics, in-treatment resolution or continued absence of LVH by Cornell product criteria remained associated with a 26% (HR 0.74, 95% CI 0.58–0.93) lower incidence of new diabetes (98).

The above studies focus on regression of ECG voltage and product as modifiers of outcome. However, it is important to also consider the prognostic effect of serial change in repolarization patterns. Verdecchia et al. (99) evaluated the hypothesis that serial changes in ECG LVH voltage and repolarization abnormalities independently determine outcome (Fig. 4.5) in 496 patients with hypertension and ECG LVH by Perugia score followed prospectively for a composite of CV endpoints. In multivariate regression analysis, in-treatment LVH regression, as a dichotomous variable, was associated with decreased risk (HR 0.42, 95% CI 0.23–0.77). However, when the major determinants of the Perugia score, modified Cornell voltage criteria and strain were entered into multivariate analysis, only the in-treatment absence of abnormal repolarization was associated with improved outcome (HR 0.42, 95% CI 0.28–0.78).

Recent analysis of data from LIFE study (100,101) offers further information regarding the prognostic significance of serial changes in repolarization and its relation to regression of ECG LVH voltage. LIFE patients were categorized into one of four groups: ECG strain absent on both baseline and year 1 ECGs (85.3% of patients), regression from baseline to year 1 (3.3%), persistent on both ECGs (7.4%) and absent at baseline but present by year 1 (3.9%). The persistence or development of new ECG strain was associated with greater echocardiographic LV mass index and a higher prevalence of LVH. During 3.8 ± 0.8 years of follow-up after the year-1 ECG, CV death occurred in 236 patients (3.2%), myocardial infarction (MI) in 198 (2.7%), stroke in 313 (4.2%), the LIFE composite endpoint of the first occurrence of these three events in 600 patients (8.1%), sudden cardiac death in 92 patients (1.2%), and death from any cause in 486 patients (6.6%). In univariate Cox analyses, development of new ECG strain pattern was associated with the highest risk of all endpoints, with nearly three to fivefold increased risks compared with the absence of strain on both ECGs. In contrast, regression of strain between baseline and year 1 was associated with nonsignificant or marginally significant increased risk of events. Persistence of ECG strain

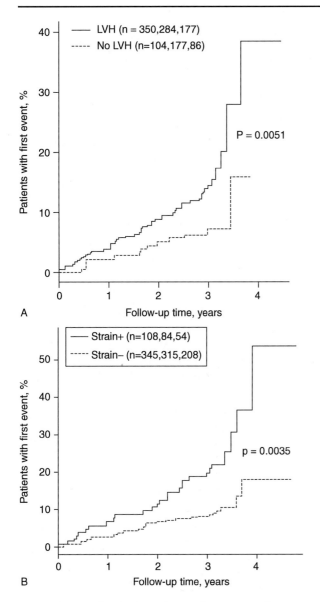

FIGURE 4.5 Composite cardiovascular event rate by time varying categories of presence or absence of LVH by Perugia score (A) and repolarization abnormalities (B). Numbers in parentheses are of at-risk patients for each category of time-varying LVH or repolarization abnormalities at 1, 2, and 3 years of follow-up. (From Ref. 99, with permission.)

significant. Importantly, in-treatment ECG LVH by Cornell product or Sokolow-Lyon voltage remained significant predictors of all endpoints in these multivariable models, supporting the notion that regression of both ECG LVH voltage and strain modify outcome independently.

Special Considerations

Gender

Gender differences in LVH regression were detected in the LIFE trial. During follow-up, women had significantly less reduction in Cornell product (–149 ± 823 versus –251 ± 890 mm·msec) and Sokolow-Lyon Voltage (–3.0 ± 6.8 versus –4.8 ± 7.7 mm) than men (P <0.001 for both). This finding persisted after adjustment for baseline ECG-LVH, baseline and change in BP, treatment group and age. Women were less likely to have had a greater than median level of regression of Cornell product and Sokolow-Lyon voltage (32% and 15% less likely, respectively). Thus, women have less regression of ECG LVH than men in response to antihypertensive therapy, independent of baseline gender differences in severity of ECG LVH and after accounting for antihypertensive treatment and blood pressure changes (102). These results are consistent with observed gender differences seen in LV remodeling to hemodynamic loads (103,104).

Diabetic Patients

Diabetes is a well-recognized stimulus for hypertrophy (105,106) that may be, in part, the result of independent effects of insulin resistance on left ventricle (LV) growth (107). In addition, there appear to be synergistic effects of diabetes and hypertension on LV structure and function (105,108), with the combination of the two conditions associated with greater prevalences of LVH and subnormal LV function than either alone (105). Data from the LIFE study, in which the prevalence of diabetes mellitus was 13%, support the hypothesis that patients with diabetes have greater LVH, less regression in response to antihypertensive therapy, and subsequently have worse outcomes. In LIFE, diabetic patients had greater baseline LVH by Cornell product (72% versus 66%, P <0.001) and less regression of Cornell product LVH (–138 ± 866 versus –204 ± 854 mm·msec, P <0.001) during mean follow-up of 4.8 years. At study completion 56% of patients with diabetes had ECG LVH compared to 48.1% of nondiabetics (P <0.001).

on both baseline and year 1 ECGs was associated with approximately two-fold–higher risks of these endpoints. After adjusting for baseline differences, development of new ECG strain remained associated with an approximately 2- to 2.4-fold increased risk of all endpoints, while the risk associated with regression or persistence of ECG strain was attenuated and no longer statistically

The deleterious effects of diabetes in patients with LVH extend to outcome. In the same analysis, patients with diabetes had significantly higher rates of the LIFE composite end point (20.3% versus 10.7%), CV death (8.3% versus 4.2%), stroke (9.7% versus 5.3%), myocardial infarction (7.6% versus 3.7%), and total mortality (14.0% versus 8.1%), P- <0.001 for all. These differences remained significant after adjustment for possible covariates. Further, in-treatment regression of ECG LVH was not associated with improvement in prognosis in diabetic patients, while a 17%–35% reduction in risks of CV mortality, myocardial infarction, and stroke, the LIFE composite end point, and all-cause mortality was observed in nondiabetics (109).

■ CONCLUSION

The ECG is a vital tool in the detection and risk stratification of patients with LVH. When present, ECG LVH has ominous prognosis implications. This grim picture can be in part modified by the regression of ECG LVH. We recommend that an ECG for the detection of LVH should be obtained in all patients at risk of cardiovascular disease in the setting of both primary and secondary prevention, particularly those with hypertension, diabetes, heart failure, and/or myocardial infarction. Furthermore, patients found to have evidence of ECG LVH should receive aggressive antihypertensive therapy to achieve regression of LVH and consequentially improvement in outcome.

As reviewed in this chapter, several factors may alter the performance of ECG LVH criteria. In addition, commonly used ECG LVH criteria are not validated and may be less reliable in patients with a paced ventricular rhythm and right or left buddle branch blocks—although patients with left bundle branch blocks often have anatomic LVH. In these scenarios, other diagnostic modalities such as echocardiography should be considered.

■ REFERENCES

1. Bacharova L and Kyselovic J, Electrocardiographic diagnosis of left ventricular hypertrophy: is the method obsolete or should the hypothesis be reconsidered? *Med Hypotheses* 2001; 57: 487–490.

2. Okin PM, Devereux RB, Nieminen MS, et al., Relationship of the electrocardiographic strain pattern to left ventricular structure and function in hypertensive patients: the LIFE study. Losartan Intervention For End point. *J Am Coll Cardiol* 2001; 38: 514–520.

3. Salles G, Cardoso C, Nogueira AR, et al., Importance of the electrocardiographic strain pattern in patients with resistant hypertension. *Hypertension* 2006; 48: 437–442.

4. Sokolow M and Lyon TP, The ventricular complex in left ventricular hypertrophy as obtained by unipolar precordial and limb leads. *Am Heart J* 1949; 37: 161–186.

5. Gubner RS and Ungerleider HE, Electrocardiographic criteria of left ventricular hypertrophy. *Arch Intern Med* 1943; 72: 196–206.

6. Romhilt DW, Bove KE, Norris RJ, et al., A critical appraisal of the electrocardiographic criteria for the diagnosis of left ventricular hypertrophy. *Circulation* 1969; 40: 185–195.

7. Romhilt DW and Estes EH, Jr., A point-score system for the ECG diagnosis of left ventricular hypertrophy. *Am Heart J* 1968; 75: 752–758.

8. Devereux RB, Casale PN, Eisenberg RR, et al., Electrocardiographic detection of left ventricular hypertrophy using echocardiographic determination of left ventricular mass as the reference standard. Comparison of standard criteria, computer diagnosis and physician interpretation. *J Am Coll Cardiol* 1984; 3: 82–87.

9. Devereux RB, Phillips MC, Casale PN, et al., Geometric determinants of electrocardiographic left ventricular hypertrophy. *Circulation* 1983; 67: 907–911.

10. Pewsner D, Juni P, Egger M, et al., Accuracy of electrocardiography in diagnosis of left ventricular hypertrophy in arterial hypertension: systematic review. *BMJ* 2007; 335: 711.

11. Reichek N and Devereux RB, Left ventricular hypertrophy: relationship of anatomic, echocardiographic and electrocardiographic findings. *Circulation* 1981; 63: 1391–1398.

12. Casale PN, Devereux RB, Alonso DR, et al., Improved sex-specific criteria of left ventricular hypertrophy for clinical and computer interpretation of electrocardiograms: validation with autopsy findings. *Circulation* 1987; 75: 565–572.

13. Casale PN, Devereux RB, Kligfield P, et al., Electrocardiographic detection of left ventricular hypertrophy: development and prospective validation of improved criteria. *J Am Coll Cardiol* 1985; 6: 572–580.

14. Molloy TJ, Okin PM, Devereux RB, et al., Electrocardiographic detection of left ventricular hypertrophy by the simple QRS voltage-duration product. *J Am Coll Cardiol* 1992; 20: 1180–1186.

15. Okin PM, Roman MJ, Devereux RB, et al., Electrocardiographic identification of increased left ventricular mass by simple voltage-duration products. *J Am Coll Cardiol* 1995; 25: 417–423.

16. Okin PM, Roman MJ, Devereux RB, et al., Time-voltage QRS area of the 12-lead electrocardiogram: detection of left ventricular hypertrophy. *Hypertension* 1998; 31: 937–942.

17. Okin PM, Roman MJ, Devereux RB, et al., Electrocardiographic diagnosis of left ventricular hypertrophy by the time-voltage integral of the QRS complex. *J Am Coll Cardiol* 1994; 23: 133–140.

18. Schillaci G, Verdecchia P, Borgioni C, et al., Improved electrocardiographic diagnosis of left ventricular hypertrophy. *Am J Cardiol* 1994; 74: 714–719.

19. Verdecchia P, Schillaci G, Borgioni C, et al., Prognostic value of a new electrocardiographic method for diagnosis of left ventricular hypertrophy in essential hypertension. *J Am Coll Cardiol* 1998; 31: 383–390.

20. Verdecchia P, Angeli F, Reboldi G, et al., Improved cardiovascular risk stratification by a simple ECG index in hypertension. *Am J Hypertens* 2003; 16: 646–652.

21. Norman JE, Jr. and Levy D, Improved electrocardiographic detection of echocardiographic left ventricular hypertrophy: results of a correlated data base approach. *J Am Coll Cardiol* 1995; 26: 1022–1029.

22. Norman JE, Jr., Levy D, Campbell G, et al., Improved detection of echocardiographic left ventricular hypertrophy using a new electrocardiographic algorithm. *J Am Coll Cardiol* 1993; 21: 1680–1686.

23. Rautaharju PM, Park LP, Chaitman BR, et al., The Novacode criteria for classification of ECG abnormalities and their clinically significant progression and regression. *Journal of Electrocardiology* 1998; 31: 157–187.

24. Levy D, Labib SB, Anderson KM, et al., Determinants of sensitivity and specificity of electrocardiographic criteria for left ventricular hypertrophy. *Circulation* 1990; 81: 815–820.

25. Simonson E, Sex Differences in the the Electrocardiogram. *Circulation* 1960; 22: 598–601.

26. Okin PM, Roman MJ, Devereux RB, et al., Gender differences and the electrocardiogram in left ventricular hypertrophy. *Hypertension* 1995; 25: 242–249.

27. Okin PM, Jern S, Devereux RB, et al., Effect of obesity on electrocardiographic left ventricular hypertrophy in hypertensive patients: the losartan intervention for endpoint (LIFE) reduction in hypertension study. *Hypertension* 2000; 35: 13–18.

28. Okin PM, Roman MJ, Devereux RB, et al., ECG identification of left ventricular hypertrophy. Relationship of test performance to body habitus. *J Electrocardiol* 1996; 29 Suppl: 256–261.

29. Okin PM, Roman MJ, Devereux RB, et al., Electrocardiographic identification of left ventricular hypertrophy: test performance in relation to definition of hypertrophy and presence of obesity. *J Am Coll Cardiol* 1996; 27: 124–131.

30. LaMonte CS and Freiman AH, The electrocardiogram after mastectomy. *Circulation* 1965; 32: 746–754.

31. Rautaharju PM, Zhou SH and Calhoun HP, Ethnic differences in ECG amplitudes in North American white, black, and Hispanic men and women. Effect of obesity and age. *J Electrocardiol* 1994; 27 Suppl: 20–31.

32. Lee DK, Marantz PR, Devereux RB, et al., Left ventricular hypertrophy in black and white hypertensives. Standard electrocardiographic criteria overestimate racial differences in prevalence. *JAMA* 1992; 267: 3294–3299.

33. Okin PM, Wright JT, Nieminen MS, et al., Ethnic differences in electrocardiographic criteria for left ventricular hypertrophy: the LIFE study. Losartan Intervention For Endpoint. *Am J Hypertens* 2002; 15: 663–671.

34. Perez MV, Yaw TS, Myers J, et al., Prognostic value of the computerized ECG in Hispanics. *Clin Cardiol* 2007; 30: 189–194.

35. Havranek EP, Froshaug DB, Emserman CD, et al., Left ventricular hypertrophy and cardiovascular mortality by race and ethnicity. *Am J Med* 2008; 121: 870–875.

36. Devereux RB, Koren MJ, de Simone G, et al., Left ventricular mass as a measure of preclinical hypertensive disease. *Am J Hypertens* 1992; 5: 175S-181S.

37. Kannel WB, Left ventricular hypertrophy as a risk factor: the Framingham experience. *J Hypertens Suppl* 1991; 9: S3–8; discussion S8–9.

38. Kannel WB, Gordon T, Castelli WP, et al., Electrocardiographic left ventricular hypertrophy and risk of coronary heart disease. The Framingham study. *Ann Intern Med* 1970; 72: 813–822.

39. Kannel WB, Gordon T and Offutt D, Left ventricular hypertrophy by electrocardiogram. Prevalence, incidence, and mortality in the Framingham study. *Ann Intern Med* 1969; 71: 89–105.

40. Vakili BA, Okin PM and Devereux RB, Prognostic implications of left ventricular hypertrophy. *Am Heart J* 2001; 141: 334–341.

41. Lonn E, Mathew J, Pogue J, et al., Relationship of electrocardiographic left ventricular hypertrophy to mortality and cardiovascular morbidity in high-risk patients. *Eur J Cardiovasc Prev Rehabil* 2003; 10: 420–428.

42. Larsen CT, Dahlin J, Blackburn H, et al., Prevalence and prognosis of electrocardiographic left ventricular hypertrophy, ST segment depression and negative T-wave; the Copenhagen City Heart Study. *Eur Heart J* 2002; 23: 315–324.

43. Hsieh BP, Pham MX and Froelicher VF, Prognostic value of electrocardiographic criteria for left ventricular hypertrophy. *Am Heart J* 2005; 150: 161–167.

44. Kannel WB, Prevalence and natural history of electrocardiographic left ventricular hypertrophy. *Am J Med* 1983; 75: 4–11.

45. Okin PM, Devereux RB, Nieminen MS, et al., Electrocardiographic strain pattern and prediction of cardiovascular morbidity and mortality in hypertensive patients. *Hypertension* 2004; 44: 48–54.

46. Lee ET, Welty TK, Fabsitz R, et al., The Strong Heart Study. A study of cardiovascular disease in American Indians: design and methods. *Am J Epidemiol* 1990; 132: 1141–1155.

47. Okin PM, Roman MJ, Lee ET, et al., Combined echocardiographic left ventricular hypertrophy and electrocardiographic ST depression improve prediction of mortality in American Indians: the Strong Heart Study. *Hypertension* 2004; 43: 769–774.

48. Okin PM, Devereux RB, Fabsitz RR, et al., Quantitative assessment of electrocardiographic strain predicts increased left ventricular mass: the Strong Heart Study. *J Am Coll Cardiol* 2002; 40: 1395–1400.

49. Verdecchia P, Porcellati C, Reboldi G, et al., Left ventricular hypertrophy as an independent predictor of acute cerebrovascular events in essential hypertension. *Circulation* 2001; 104: 2039–2044.

50. Benjamin EJ and Levy D, Why is left ventricular hypertrophy so predictive of morbidity and mortality? *Am J Med Sci* 1999; 317: 168–175.

51. Kohsaka S, Sciacca RR, Sugioka K, et al., Additional impact of electrocardiographic over echocardiographic diagnosis of left ventricular hypertrophy for predicting the risk of ischemic stroke. *Am Heart J* 2005; 149: 181–186.

52. Okin PM, Devereux RB, Nieminen MS, et al., Electrocardiographic strain pattern and prediction of new-onset congestive heart failure in hypertensive patients: the Losartan Intervention for Endpoint Reduction in Hypertension (LIFE) study. *Circulation* 2006; 113: 67–73.

53. Okin PM, Wachtell K, Devereux RB, et al., Combination of the electrocardiographic strain pattern and albuminuria for the

prediction of new-onset heart failure in hypertensive patients: the LIFE study. *Am J Hypertens* 2008; 21: 273–279.

54. Okin PM, Devereux RB, Harris KE, et al., Regression of electrocardiographic left ventricular hypertrophy is associated with less hospitalization for heart failure in hypertensive patients. *Ann Intern Med* 2007; 147: 311–319.

55. Palmieri V, Okin PM, Bella JN, et al., Electrocardiographic strain pattern and left ventricular diastolic function in hypertensive patients with left ventricular hypertrophy: the LIFE study. *J Hypertens* 2006; 24: 2079–2084.

56. Kannel WB, Doyle JT, McNamara PM, et al., Precursors of sudden coronary death. Factors related to the incidence of sudden death. *Circulation* 1975; 51: 606–613.

57. Haider AW, Larson MG, Benjamin EJ, et al., Increased left ventricular mass and hypertrophy are associated with increased risk for sudden death. *J Am Coll Cardiol* 1998; 32: 1454–1459.

58. Messerli FH, Ventura HO, Elizardi DJ, et al., Hypertension and sudden death. Increased ventricular ectopic activity in left ventricular hypertrophy. *Am J Med* 1984; 77: 18–22.

59. McLenachan JM, Henderson E, Morris KI, et al., Ventricular arrhythmias in patients with hypertensive left ventricular hypertrophy. *N Engl J Med* 1987; 317: 787–792.

60. Saadeh AM and Jones JV, Predictors of sudden cardiac death in never previously treated patients with essential hypertension: long-term follow-up. *J Hum Hypertens* 2001; 15: 677–680.

61. Benjamin EJ, Levy D, Vaziri SM, et al., Independent risk factors for atrial fibrillation in a population-based cohort. The Framingham Heart Study. *JAMA* 1994; 271: 840–844.

62. Benjamin EJ, Wolf PA, D'Agostino RB, et al., Impact of atrial fibrillation on the risk of death: the Framingham Heart Study. *Circulation* 1998; 98: 946–952.

63. Krahn AD, Manfreda J, Tate RB, et al., The natural history of atrial fibrillation: incidence, risk factors, and prognosis in the Manitoba Follow-Up Study. *Am J Med* 1995; 98: 476–484.

64. Verdecchia P, Reboldi G, Gattobigio R, et al., Atrial fibrillation in hypertension: predictors and outcome. *Hypertension* 2003; 41: 218–223.

65. Hawkins NM, Wang D, McMurray JJ, et al., Prevalence and prognostic implications of electrocardiographic left ventricular hypertrophy in heart failure: evidence from the CHARM programme. *Heart* 2007; 93: 59–64.

66. Boden WE, Kleiger RE, Schechtman KB, et al., Clinical significance and prognostic importance of left ventricular hypertrophy in non-Q-wave acute myocardial infarction. *Am J Cardiol* 1988; 62: 1000–1004.

67. Yotsukura M, Suzuki J, Yamaguchi T, et al., Prognosis following acute myocardial infarction in patients with ECG evidence of left ventricular hypertrophy prior to infarction. *J Electrocardiol* 1998; 31: 91–99.

68. Westerhout CM, Lauer MS, James S, et al., Electrocardiographic left ventricular hypertrophy in GUSTO IV ACS: an important risk marker of mortality in women. *Eur Heart J* 2007; 28: 2064–2069.

69. Kahn S, Frishman WH, Weissman S, et al., Left ventricular hypertrophy on electrocardiogram: prognostic implications from a 10-year cohort study of older subjects: a report from the Bronx Longitudinal Aging Study. *J Am Geriatr Soc* 1996; 44: 524–529.

70. Sundstrom J, Lind L, Arnlov J, et al., Echocardiographic and electrocardiographic diagnoses of left ventricular hypertrophy predict mortality independently of each other in a population of elderly men. *Circulation* 2001; 103: 2346–2351.

71. Five-year findings of the Hypertension Detection and Follow-up Program. Prevention and reversal of left ventricular hypertrophy with antihypertensive drug therapy. Hypertension Detection and Follow-up Program Cooperative Group. *Hypertension* 1985; 7: 105–112.

72. MacMahon S, Collins G, Rautaharju P, et al., Electrocardiographic left ventricular hypertrophy and effects of antihypertensive drug therapy in hypertensive participants in the Multiple Risk Factor Intervention Trial. *Am J Cardiol* 1989; 63: 202–210.

73. Neaton JD, Grimm RH, Jr., Prineas RJ, et al., Treatment of Mild Hypertension Study. Final results. Treatment of Mild Hypertension Study Research Group. *JAMA* 1993; 270: 713–724.

74. Everett AD, Tufro-McReddie A, Fisher A, et al., Angiotensin receptor regulates cardiac hypertrophy and transforming growth factor-beta 1 expression. *Hypertension* 1994; 23: 587–592.

75. Schlaich MP, Schobel HP, Langenfeld MR, et al., Inadequate suppression of angiotensin II modulates left ventricular structure in humans. *Clin Nephrol* 1998; 49: 153–159.

76. Pachori AS, Numan MT, Ferrario CM, et al., Blood pressure-independent attenuation of cardiac hypertrophy by AT(1)R-AS gene therapy. *Hypertension* 2002; 39: 969–975.

77. Dahlof B, Left ventricular hypertrophy and angiotensin II antagonists. *Am J Hypertens* 2001; 14: 174–182.

78. Schlaich MP and Schmieder RE, Left ventricular hypertrophy and its regression: pathophysiology and therapeutic approach: focus on treatment by antihypertensive agents. *Am J Hypertens* 1998; 11: 1394–1404.

79. Dahlof B, Pennert K and Hansson L, Reversal of left ventricular hypertrophy in hypertensive patients. A metaanalysis of 109 treatment studies. *Am J Hypertens* 1992; 5: 95–110.

80. Mathew J, Sleight P, Lonn E, et al., Reduction of cardiovascular risk by regression of electrocardiographic markers of left ventricular hypertrophy by the angiotensin-converting enzyme inhibitor ramipril. *Circulation* 2001; 104: 1615–1621.

81. Okin PM, Devereux RB, Jern S, et al., Regression of electrocardiographic left ventricular hypertrophy by losartan versus atenolol: The Losartan Intervention for Endpoint reduction in Hypertension (LIFE) Study. *Circulation* 2003; 108: 684–690.

82. Prineas RJ, Rautaharju PM, Grandits G, et al., Independent risk for cardiovascular disease predicted by modified continuous score electrocardiographic criteria for 6-year incidence and regression of left ventricular hypertrophy among clinically disease free men: 16-year follow-up for the multiple risk factor intervention trial. *J Electrocardiol* 2001; 34: 91–101.

83. Levy D, Salomon M, D'Agostino RB, et al., Prognostic implications of baseline electrocardiographic features and their serial changes in subjects with left ventricular hypertrophy. *Circulation* 1994; 90: 1786–1793.

84. Okin PM, Devereux RB, Jern S, et al., Regression of electrocardiographic left ventricular hypertrophy during antihypertensive treatment and the prediction of major cardiovascular events. *JAMA* 2004; 292: 2343–2349.

85. Okin PM, Wachtell K, Devereux RB, et al., Regression of electrocardiographic left ventricular hypertrophy and decreased incidence of new-onset atrial fibrillation in patients with hypertension. *JAMA* 2006; 296: 1242–1248.

86. Wachtell K, Okin PM, Olsen MH, et al., Regression of electrocardiographic left ventricular hypertrophy during antihypertensive therapy and reduction in sudden cardiac death: the LIFE Study. *Circulation* 2007; 116: 700–705.

87. Vaziri SM, Larson MG, Benjamin EJ, et al., Echocardiographic predictors of nonrheumatic atrial fibrillation. The Framingham Heart Study. *Circulation* 1994; 89: 724–730.

88. Wachtell K, Lehto M, Gerdts E, et al., Angiotensin II receptor blockade reduces new-onset atrial fibrillation and subsequent stroke compared to atenolol: the Losartan Intervention For End Point Reduction in Hypertension (LIFE) study. *J Am Coll Cardiol* 2005; 45: 712–719.

89. Levy D, Anderson KM, Savage DD, et al., Risk of ventricular arrhythmias in left ventricular hypertrophy: the Framingham Heart Study. *Am J Cardiol* 1987; 60: 560–565.

90. Schillaci G, Verdecchia P, Borgioni C, et al., Association between persistent pressure overload and ventricular arrhythmias in essential hypertension. *Hypertension* 1996; 28: 284–289.

91. Chiang BN, Perlman LV, Fulton M, et al., Predisposing factors in sudden cardiac death in Tecumseh, Michigan. A prospective study. *Circulation* 1970; 41: 31–37.

92. Cupples LA, Gagnon DR and Kannel WB, Long- and short-term risk of sudden coronary death. *Circulation* 1992; 85: I11–18.

93. Kannel WB and Abbott RD, A prognostic comparison of asymptomatic left ventricular hypertrophy and unrecognized myocardial infarction: the Framingham Study. *Am Heart J* 1986; 111: 391–397.

94. Kannel WB and Schatzkin A, Sudden death: lessons from subsets in population studies. *J Am Coll Cardiol* 1985; 5: 141B–149B.

95. Aronow WS and Ahn C, Association of electrocardiographic left ventricular hypertrophy with the incidence of new congestive heart failure. *J Am Geriatr Soc* 1998; 46: 1280–1281.

96. Levy D, Larson MG, Vasan RS, et al., The progression from hypertension to congestive heart failure. *JAMA* 1996; 275: 1557–1562.

97. Lindholm LH, Ibsen H, Borch-Johnsen K, et al., Risk of new-onset diabetes in the Losartan Intervention For Endpoint reduction in hypertension study. *J Hypertens* 2002; 20: 1879–1886.

98. Okin PM, Devereux RB, Harris KE, et al., In-treatment resolution or absence of electrocardiographic left ventricular hypertrophy is associated with decreased incidence of new-onset diabetes mellitus in hypertensive patients: the Losartan Intervention for Endpoint Reduction in Hypertension (LIFE) Study. *Hypertension* 2007; 50: 984–990.

99. Verdecchia P, Reboldi G, Angeli F, et al., Prognostic value of serial electrocardiographic voltage and repolarization changes in essential hypertension: the HEART Survey study. *Am J Hypertens* 2007; 20: 997–1004.

100. Okin PM OL, Viitasalo M, Toivonen L, Kjeldsen SE, Nieminen MS, Edelman JM, Dahlöf B, Devereux RB, Development of new electrocardiographic strain pattern is associated with an increased risk of cardiovascular morbidity and mortality during antihypertensive treatment: The LIFE Study. *Circulation* 2006; 114: 576.

101. Okin PM OL, Viitasalo M, Toivonen L, Kjeldsen SE, Nieminen MS, Edelman JM, Dahlöf B, Devereux RB, Development of new electrocardiographic strain pattern during antihypertensive therapy is associated with increased risk of sudden cardiac death: the LIFE Study. *J Am Coll Cardiol* 2007; 49: 331A.

102. Okin PM, Gerdts E, Kjeldsen SE, et al., Gender differences in regression of electrocardiographic left ventricular hypertrophy during antihypertensive therapy. *Hypertension* 2008; 52: 100–106.

103. Weinberg EO, Thienelt CD, Katz SE, et al., Gender differences in molecular remodeling in pressure overload hypertrophy. *J Am Coll Cardiol* 1999; 34: 264–273.

104. Luchner A, Brockel U, Muscholl M, et al., Gender-specific differences of cardiac remodeling in subjects with left ventricular dysfunction: a population-based study. *Cardiovasc Res* 2002; 53: 720–727.

105. Bella JN, Devereux RB, Roman MJ, et al., Separate and joint effects of systemic hypertension and diabetes mellitus on left ventricular structure and function in American Indians (the Strong Heart Study). *Am J Cardiol* 2001; 87: 1260–1265.

106. Palmieri V, Bella JN, Arnett DK, et al., Effect of type 2 diabetes mellitus on left ventricular geometry and systolic function in hypertensive subjects: Hypertension Genetic Epidemiology Network (HyperGEN) study. *Circulation* 2001; 103: 102–107.

107. Phillips RA, Krakoff LR, Dunaif A, et al., Relation among left ventricular mass, insulin resistance, and blood pressure in nonobese subjects. *J Clin Endocrinol Metab* 1998; 83: 4284–4288.

108. Taegtmeyer H, McNulty P and Young ME, Adaptation and maladaptation of the heart in diabetes: Part I: general concepts. *Circulation* 2002; 105: 1727–1733.

109. Okin PM, Devereux RB, Gerdts E, et al., Impact of diabetes mellitus on regression of electrocardiographic left ventricular hypertrophy and the prediction of outcome during antihypertensive therapy: the Losartan Intervention For Endpoint (LIFE) Reduction in Hypertension Study. *Circulation* 2006; 113: 1588–1596.

Diabetes

5

RICHARD B. DEVEREUX
GIOVANNI DE SIMONE

OUTLINE

Coronary Artery Disease   69

Pathophysiology/Risk Factors   72

Cerebrovascular Disease   79

Cardiomyopathy   80

Conclusion   83

References   83

Over the past several decades, progress in reducing smoking and in controlling hypertension and dyslipidemia has resulted in steady reduction in age-adjusted rates of cardiovascular disease (CVD) mortality (Figures 5.1–5.4) (1–6). However, at the same time, the rising tide of obesity in the United States and other industrialized countries (Figure 5.5) (7–8) has led to an increase in the prevalence of diabetes mellitus (DM) of epidemic proportions (9) (Figure 5.6). The prevalence of diabetes now exceeds 10% in U.S. adults 40 to 59 years old and approaches 25% in those 60 and older (Figure 5.7) (10). Epidemiological studies have shown that diabetes is a potent independent risk factor for both small-vessel and large-vessel CVD (11–12), with a lag phase of 10 years or more between the onset of diabetes and rise in CVD events. After this lag phase, diabetic adults suffer two- to threefold more CVD events than their nondiabetic counterparts. CVD accounts for up to 80% of deaths in diabetic patients, most of which are due to ischemic heart disease (13). Therefore, the American Heart Association has concluded that "diabetes is a cardiovascular disease" (14).

Although the CVD burden associated with diabetes is obvious, the causal pathways are incompletely understood, and there is considerable uncertainty as to how to stratify CVD risk in individual patients and about the optimal therapeutic approach to minimize cardiovascular (CV) events. Major CV effects of diabetes are accelerated coronary artery disease, high risk of stroke, and specific diabetic cardiomyopathy. In this chapter, we review the manifestations of diabetic heart disease, their relation to CV events, and the impact of treatment on diabetes-associated CVD.

■ CORONARY ARTERY DISEASE

Accelerated coronary artery disease (CAD), accounts for up to 75% of deaths in diabetic patients, with substantial associated disability and expense (15). Extensive epidemiological data document diabetes to be an independent risk factor for CAD in men and even more so in women (11–12,16). In a seminal study (17), diabetic patients with no history of CAD were found, on average, to have long-term rates of myocardial infarction and CV death comparable to those of nondiabetic patients with prior myocardial infarction. To make matters worse, once diabetics develop clinical CAD, they suffer higher mortality than do nondiabetic CAD patients (18). Although CV mortality is declining in the general U.S. population due to reduction in CV risk factors and improved therapies, the decline has been smaller in diabetic versus. nondiabetic men (−13% vs. −36%), and, worse yet, CV mortality actually increased in diabetic women (+27% vs. −23%) (19). While overall heart disease mortality decreased by 52% from 1970 to 2002, deaths associated with diabetes rose by 45% (20).

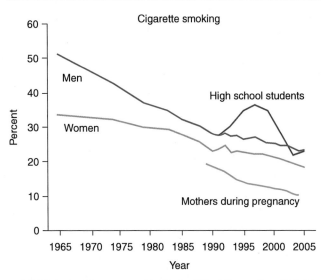

FIGURE 5.1   Cigarette smoking in the United States. (From Ref. 1.)

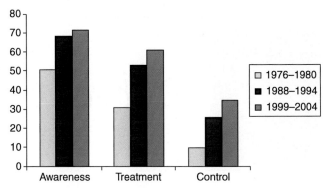

FIGURE 5.2   Hypertension awareness, treatment, and control in the United States (National Health and Nutrition Examination Surveys). (Adapted from Refs. 2 and 3, with permission.)

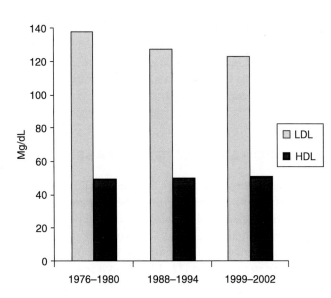

FIGURE 5.3   LDL and HDL cholesterol levels in U.S. adults. (From Ref. 4.)

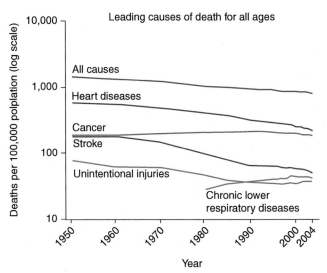

FIGURE 5.4   Leading causes of death for all ages in the United States, 1950–2004. (From Ref. 5.)

Myocardial Infarction

Patients with diabetes have a higher risk of myocardial infarction (MI) compared with the general population. In fact, in several populations the incidence of MI among patients with diabetes who did not have CAD has been similar to nondiabetic patients with preexisting CAD (17). Diabetes is associated with a higher case-fatality rate during the first year after acute MI after adjusting for confounding variables (21), in both men (24% vs. 14%) and women (33% vs. 11%) (22).

The one-year mortality after acute coronary syndrome (UA/NSTEMI or STEMI) is significantly higher in diabetic than in nondiabetic patients (11.2 vs. 6.8, adjusted HR = 1.33 [1.20–1.48]) (Figure 5.8) (18). In addition, diabetic patients with symptoms of MI are more likely to die before reaching the hospital (sudden deaths) than their nondiabetic counterparts (23). Mechanisms of this high sudden death rate have not been established, but might be in part related to diabetes-associated microvascular disease and to diabetic heart muscle disease manifested by left ventricular hypertrophy (LVH) and impaired LV contractility and relaxation, independent of large-artery CAD, and to potential repeated myocardial insults due to silent ischemic episodes (24).

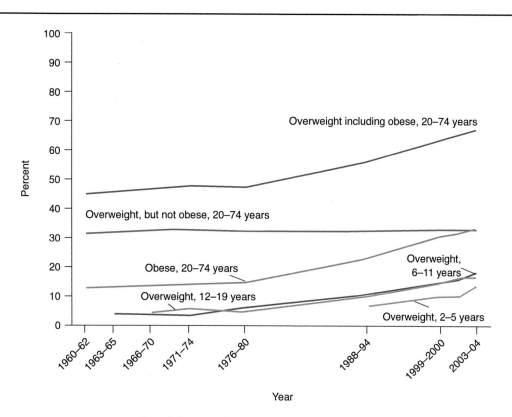

FIGURE 5.5 Overweight and obesity in the United States, 1960–2004. (From Ref. 7.)

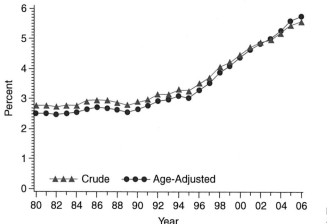

FIGURE 5.6 Rising prevalence of diabetes in the United States, 1980–2006. (From Ref. 10.)

FIGURE 5.7 Diabetes prevalence in the United States by age, 2007. (From Ref. 10.)

Silent Ischemia

Myocardial ischemia due to coronary atherosclerosis is more commonly "silent" (without anginal symptoms) in diabetic than in nondiabetic patients. As a result, diabetic patients are likely to have more advanced multivessel atherosclerosis before ischemic symptoms occur and treatment is instituted. Diabetic patients have higher prevalences of asymptomatic ischemia on both exercise stress tests and ambulatory ECG monitoring in most (25–26), but not all (27) studies. In a necropsy study (28), nearly 80% of diabetic subjects without clinically apparent coronary heart disease (CHD) exhibited high-grade coronary atherosclerosis and more than 50% had

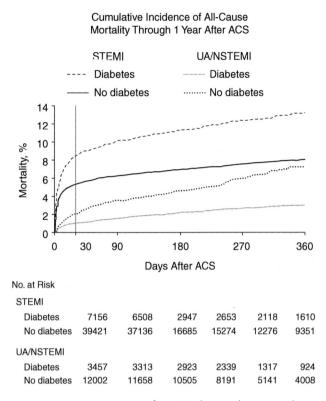

Cumulative Incidence of All-Cause Mortality Through 1 Year After ACS

No. at Risk						
STEMI						
Diabetes	7156	6508	2947	2653	2118	1610
No diabetes	39421	37136	16685	15274	12276	9351
UA/NSTEMI						
Diabetes	3457	3313	2923	2339	1317	924
No diabetes	12002	11658	10505	8191	5141	4008

FIGURE 5.8 By one year after ACS, the cumulative mortality in patients with diabetes versus those without diabetes was higher in UA/NSTEMI (7.2% vs. 3.1%, P <0.001) and STEMI (13.2% vs. 8.1%, P <0.001), and accrues at a higher rate in patients with diabetes than in patients without diabetes. The relative increase in mortality for the patients with diabetes following UA/STEMI exceeds that of STEMI (P = 0.004) for interaction between diabetes status and ACS stratum. Vertical dotted line represents 30 days following either UA/NSTEMI (2.1% vs. 1.1%, P <0.001) or STEMI (8.5% vs. 5.4%, P <0.001). (ACS, acute coronary syndromes; STEMI, ST-segment elevation myocardial infarction; UA/NSTEMI, unstable angina/non-STEMI.) (From Ref. 18, with permission.)

multivessel disease. In the absence of diabetes, women had less atherosclerosis than men, but this advantage was lost when diabetes was present. Interestingly, the degree of coronary atherosclerotic lesions in diabetic subjects without clinical CAD was similar to that found in nondiabetic subjects with clinical history of CHD.

The increased rate of silent ischemia may be due to diabetes-associated autonomic neuropathy, impairing both sympathetic and parasympathetic innervation of the heart (29). Painless ischemia is significantly more frequent in patients with neuropathy than in those without it (38% vs. 5%) (30). The resultant impaired pain perception makes angina an insensitive symptom of ischemic heart disease in many diabetic patients. Up to one-quarter

of asymptomatic patients with type 2 diabetes may have evidence of significant CAD by myocardial perfusion imaging, coronary calcium scoring, or multislice computed tomographic coronary arteriography (31). Because totally asymptomatic patients with diabetes have at least an intermediate probability of CAD, this prevalence might justify screening by noninvasive testing, such as stress myocardial perfusion imaging (32), especially considering the evidence of potential reduction of perfusion defects with treatment. In the Detection of Ischemia in Asymptomatic Diabetics (DIAD-2) study, diabetic patients underwent adenosine-stress myocardial perfusion imaging at baseline and after 3 years of follow-up. The number with abnormal perfusion scans decreased from 71 to 43, associated with increased use of statins, aspirin, and ACE inhibitors. This suggests that asymptomatic ischemia in diabetic patients can be reversed by aggressive medical management (33). However, a more aggressive diagnostic approach including coronary angiography does not seem to be generally needed (34).

■ PATHOPHYSIOLOGY/RISK FACTORS

The increased CV event rate in diabetes is at least partially due to independent contributions of other major CV risk factors (11–12,35). Most patients with type 2 DM have insulin resistance, commonly with the metabolic syndrome cluster of hypertension, central obesity, hyperinsulinemia, glucose intolerance, and dyslipidemia (36–40).

Diabetes is also associated with coagulopathy and endothelial dysfunction, predisposing to thrombosis and vasospasm in the presence of atherosclerotic damage to arterial intima (41–42). However, the relationship between diabetes, other established risk factors, and the risk of CV events are complex. In early analyses in populations in which 5% or fewer had diabetes, diabetes was considered as a monolithic condition that had a direct multiplicative effect on the risks imparted by other CV risk factors. However, more recent studies in large populations of diabetic individuals have demonstrated a strong gradient of rates of subsequent CVD events, from low levels in diabetic adults with only one or no other risk factor to levels approaching or exceeding those in nondiabetic adults with overt CHD in the presence of three or more concomitant risk factors (43–46) (Figure 5.9). Thus, all individuals with diabetes cannot be assumed to have the same risk of CV events; instead, careful attention

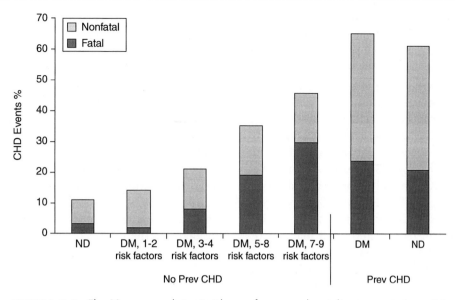

FIGURE 5.9 The 10-year cumulative incidence of coronary heart disease events in participants without or with previous (Prev) CHD. (From Ref. 43, with permission.)

needs to be paid to identifying the impact on CV event rate associated with individual risk factors and their combinations, as a basis for choosing interventions to mitigate those risks. Among participants without CHD at baseline (Figure 5.9), the incidence of CHD was minimally higher in participants with DM and more than two risk factors, including male gender, LDL cholesterol >100 mg/dl, albuminuria (>300 mg/g creatinine), hypertension, HDL <40 mg/dl, triglycerides >150 mg/dl, current smoking, fourth quartile of fibrinogen (>352 mg/dl), and diabetes duration >20 years, than in nondiabetic participants, and rose progressively in the presence of more CHD risk factors.

Dyslipidemia

Early data from the Multiple Risk Factor Intervention Trial (MRFIT) showed a curvilinear relationship between total cholesterol and CHD death in diabetic men that was parallel but with about fourfold higher mortality than that in men without diabetes (47). Type 2 diabetic patients often have an atherogenic dyslipidemia characterized by elevated levels of very low-density lipoprotein (VLDL) triglycerides; small, dense low-density lipoprotein (LDL) cholesterol particles; and low levels of high-density lipoprotein (HDL) cholesterol, each of which may aggravate the atherogenic effect of the commonly elevated serum LDL cholesterol level. Because of frequent changes of glycemic control of

diabetic patients and their effects on lipoprotein levels, the American Diabetes Association has recommended that fasting levels of LDL, HDL, total cholesterol, and triglycerides be measured annually in adult patients.

Intervention Trials

No clinical trial data are available specifically testing whether lipid-lowering treatment reduces CHD events in diabetic patients, although analyses of subsets of diabetic individuals in clinical trials of lipid-lowering treatment suggest benefit from treating hyperlipidemia. The Helsinki Heart Study found a nonsignificant trend toward lower CHD incidence in diabetic subjects (3.4% vs. 10.5%, P = NS) treated with gemfibrozil versus placebo (48), especially in the subset with high triglycerides and low HDL cholesterol. In the Fenofibrate Intervention and Event Lowering in Diabetes (FIELD) study (49), fenofibrate did not reduce risk of primary outcome of coronary events, but this finding could be influenced by the higher rate of statin therapy in patients taking placebo. In subgroup analyses of the Scandinavian Simvastatin Survival Study (4S) (50) and the Cholesterol and Recurrent Events (CARE) trial (51), aggressive LDL-lowering therapy reduced recurrent CVD events by about 25% in patients with type 2 diabetes. Among 1,501 participants with diabetes and CHD in the Treating to New Targets (TNT) study (52), more aggressive statin therapy with attained mean LDL cholesterol levels of 77 versus 99 mg/dL resulted in a 25% reduction of CHD events (hazard ratio [HR] 0.75, 95% CI 0.58–0.97, P = 0.026) and more than 30% decrease in cerebrovascular events HR = 0.69, 95% CI 0.48–0.98, P = 0.037) with a 15% reduction of all CV events HR0.85, 95% CI 0.73–1.00, P = 0.044). A recent meta-analysis examined the effect of statin treatment on CV outcomes in 18,686 diabetic participants and 71,370 without diabetes in 14 randomized trials of statin therapy (53). During a mean follow-up of 4.3 years, there were 3,247 major vascular events in people with diabetes. There was a 9% proportional reduction in all-cause mortality per mmol/L reduction in LDL cholesterol in participants with diabetes (P = 0.02), similar to a 13% reduction in those without diabetes (P <0.0001). This finding reflected a 13% reduction in vascular mortality (P = 0.008) in participants with diabetes. There were significant 21% proportional reductions in major vascular events per mmol/L reduction in LDL cholesterol in people with or without diabetes (both P <0.0001). In diabetic participants there were reductions in myocardial infarction or coronary death by 22%, coronary revascularization by 25%, and stroke by 21% (all P <0.0003). After 5 years, 42 (95% CI 30-55) fewer people with diabetes had major vascular events per 1,000 undergoing statin therapy.

Based on the most recent National Cholesterol Education Program (Adult Treatment Panel III) guidelines, diabetes is regarded as equivalent to overt CHD due to the high risk of new CHD within 10 years, with a treatment goal of reducing LDL cholesterol to <100 mg/dL (37). This goal should be achieved by addition of drug therapy after maximal dietary therapy. Statins are first-line drug therapy for LDL cholesterol reduction. Triglyceride levels >200 mg/dL should be treated with niacin or fibrate therapy. Combining a statin and a fibrate in the treatment of combined hyperlipidemia needs to be carefully considered given the documented, although infrequent, occurrence of rhabdomyolysis with this combination. Nicotinic acid can effectively reduce triglyceride and raise HDL levels, and the mildly increased glucose levels associated with its use did not blunt the reduction of MI by nicotinic acid in the Coronary Drug Project (54).

Hypertension

Hypertension is a well-established major risk factor for CVD. The prevalence of hypertension in diabetic patients is at least twofold higher than in nondiabetic adults. In the Strong Heart Study, the risk of developing hypertension after 8 years of follow-up was 2.6-fold higher in participants with initial normal glucose tolerance and optimal blood pressure who were found to be diabetic after four years, compared to those maintaining normal glucose levels (55). However, the association between diabetes and hypertension is not clear in terms of cause versus effect. While there is evidence of the effect of diabetes on arterial stiffness (56) and microvascular dysfunction (54), there is also emerging evidence of a possible reverse causation, as subjects with hypertension exhibit an about twofold higher risk of developing diabetes than subjects with normal blood pressure (57), which appears to be independent of therapy.

The combination of diabetes with hypertension is particularly harmful. In addition to increasing risk for coronary events, hypertension also increases the risk of stroke, nephropathy, and retinopathy in diabetes. In MRFIT, the rate of CVD mortality was nearly three times higher at each level of systolic blood pressure in diabetic as compared to nondiabetic hypertensive men (47).

Thus, not only is hypertension more prevalent in diabetic individuals, it also has a greater impact on the risks of CAD. Clinical trials in hypertensive patients with type 2 diabetes have shown that blood pressure control using several classes of medication is an extremely effective and important preventive therapy (58–60).

Of interest, several large recent randomized hypertension treatment trials have shown greater rates of new-onset diabetes in patients treated by regimens based on beta blockers or diuretics than in patients receiving regimens based on renin-angiotensin-aldosterone system inhibitors or calcium channel blockers (61–63). There is evidence that maintenance of serum potassium levels may blunt the effect of diuretics to impair glucose metabolism (64). In one large series of treated hypertensive patients, moderate self-reported physical activity (>30 minutes twice a week) was associated with a 34% lower rate of new-onset diabetes, independent of the type of treatment and other risk factors for diabetes (65).

Intervention Trials

Clinical trial data all support the need to aggressively treat hypertension in patients with type 2 diabetes. The Hypertension Optimal Treatment (HOT) (66) trial evaluated the effect of aggressive versus less aggressive lowering of diastolic blood pressure using felodipine, a calcium channel–blocking agent. A 51% reduction in CV events was seen in diabetic patients when diastolic pressure was treated to a mean of 82.6 mm Hg as compared to those treated to a diastolic pressure of 90 mm Hg. In the Systolic Hypertension in the Elderly Trial (67), antihypertensive treatment with chlorthalidone produced a 34% reduction in CVD events in diabetic participants. A study of tight blood pressure control within the UK Prospective Diabetes Study (UKPDS) (60), predominately using atenolol or captopril, showed that a difference of 10/5 mm Hg was associated with a 24% reduction in combined microvascular and macrovascular endpoints.

Accumulating evidence suggests that inhibitors of the renin-angiotensin-aldosterone system may be particularly effective in preventing CV events in hypertensive diabetic patients. The Appropriate Blood Pressure Control in Diabetes (ABCD) trial (68) and the Fosinopril versus Amlodipine Cardiovascular Events Randomized Trial (FACET) (69) found that the incidence of CVD events was lower by 8% ($P = 0.01$) and 7% ($P = 0.03$), respectively, in those randomized to an angiotensin-converting enzyme (ACE) inhibitor than in those treated with dihydropyridine calcium channel blockers. In fact, the ABCD trial was terminated one year earlier than scheduled because the independent Data and Safety Monitoring Committee became concerned with the disparity between the two treatment arms in the number of major coronary events. The Heart Outcomes Prevention Evaluation (HOPE) and the MICRO-HOPE substudy (61) demonstrated that ACE inhibitors lowered the risk of CV death by 37% and total mortality by 24% in patients with diabetes. After adjusting for the change in clinic blood pressure, the risks of CV and total mortality were still reduced by 25% ($P = 0.0004$). Similarly, in the LIFE study, treatment based on the angiotensin-receptor blocker losartan was associated with a 25% reduction in overall CV morbidity and mortality and a 40% reduction in CV death compared to treatment based on the beta blocker atenolol (70). Smaller, albeit still beneficial, reductions of 9% to 14% in a spectrum of micro- and macrovascular events was seen with a fixed ACE inhibitor–diuretic combination in the Action in Diabetes and Vascular Disease Study (ADVANCE) (71).

The HOPE study also demonstrated that ACE inhibitors reduced the risk of overt nephropathy (by 24%) as well as microalbuminuria ($P = 0.02$). Albuminuria is not only a manifestation of nephropathy, but may be considered a renal marker of CVD (72). Another finding, confirmed in subsequent studies evaluating treatment regimens using ACE inhibitors or angiotensin receptor blockers (61–63), is that there was a reduction by one-third in new-onset diabetes in those not diabetic at baseline over the 4.5 years of the HOPE study. Although ACE inhibitors may worsen renal function in patients with bilateral renal artery stenosis or stenosis of the artery to a single functioning kidney and may cause hyperkalemia, they can be used safely with careful titration and measurement of electrolytes and creatinine. Given the powerful protective effect on a range of important CV outcomes and renal function, ACE inhibitors are emerging as first line antihypertensive treatment in diabetic patients. Furthermore, angiotensin II receptor antagonists also have strong reno-protective effects in patients with type 2 diabetes (73–74).

Independent of the agent used, aggressive blood pressure control should be a high priority. Current guidelines in the United States and Europe recommend a target blood pressure of less than 130/85 mm Hg in subjects with diabetes. However, the continued high rates of CV events in individuals with diabetes despite current approaches to treatment has stimulated investigation of whether treatment to lower goals for both blood pressure and LDL cholesterol would be of clinical benefit. While the large Action to Control Cardiovascular Risk in Diabetes (ACCORD) study has not yet reported its findings on the effect of more aggressive blood pressure lowering on CV outcomes, the Stop Atherosclerosis in Native Diabetics Study (SANDS) trial has already documented that treatment over three years to more aggressive goals of LDL cholesterol ≤70 mg/dL and systolic blood pressure ≤115 mm Hg resulted in regression versus progression of carotid intimal-medial thickness and greater regression of LV hypertrophy than treatment to goals espoused in current guidelines (75) (Table 5.1).

Hyperglycemia

Chronic hyperglycemia can directly impair vascular endothelial function, which is thought to be an underlying mechanism of increased vascular events in diabetes. Accumulation of advanced glycation end products (AGEs) in the vessel wall, formed by the glycation of proteins and lipoproteins, leads to increased vessel stiffness, lipoprotein binding, macrophage recruitment, reduced nitric oxide production, and proliferation of

■ **Table 5.1** Baseline and follow-up carotid and cardiac measures in the SANDS study				
	Mean (95% CI)			
	Aggressive	**Standard**	**Difference**	*P* Value
Carotid (*n* = 499) Intimal medial thickness, mm				
Baseline	0.808 (0.78–0.83)	0.797 (0.78–0.82)		
36 months	0.796 (0.77–0.82)	0.837 (0.81–0.86)		
Mean change, 36 months	−0.012 (−0.03–0.003)[a]	0.038 (0.02–0.06)[a,b]	0.05	<0.001[c]
Arterial cross-sectional area, mm²				
Baseline	17.36 (16.7–18.0)	17.33 (16.8–17.9)		
36 months	17.53 (17.0–18.1)	18.39 (17.8–19.0)		
Mean change, 36 months	−0.02 (−0.33–0.30)[a]	1.05 (0.73–1.38)[a,b]	1.07	<0.001[d]
Plaque score (0–8)				
Baseline	1.85 (1.64–2.05)	1.84 (1.64–2.03)		
36 months	2.38 (2.17–2.59)	2.34 (2.13–2.55)		
Mean change, 36 months	0.54 (0.39–0.68)[b]	0.50 (0.36–0.65)[b]	0.03	0.75
Cardiac (*n* = 453) Left ventricular mass, g				
Baseline	156.7 (152–162)	156.1 (151–161)		
36 months	149.3 (145–154)	152.5 (147–157)		
Mean change, 36 months	−8.0 (−10.9–5.1)[b]	−3.3 (−6.2–0.35)	4.8	0.02
Ejection fraction, %				
Baseline	60.5 (60–61)	59.8 (59–61)		
36 months	59.7 (59–60.3)	59.1 (58–60)		
Mean change, 36 months	20.7 (21.4–0)	20.74 (21.5–0)	0.03	0.95

[a]The changes at 36 months in intimal medial thickness and in arterial cross-sectional area remained significantly different between the two groups under the Bonferroni-adjusted significance level 0.007 (= 0.05/7).
[b]Significant within-group change (*P* value <0.01)
[c]*P* values from the worst-rank analyses for intimal medial thickness were 0.691 at 18 months and <0.0001 at 36 months.
[d]*P* values from the worst-rank analyses for arterial cross-sectional area were 0.194 at 18 months and <0.0001 at 36 months.
[e]Significant within-group change (*P* value <0.05)
Source: Adapted from Ref. 75, with permission.

vascular smooth muscle cells (76). All of these contribute to abnormal vasomotion and increased atherogenesis and risk of arterial thrombosis. Data from clinical trials show that the degree of hyperglycemia in diabetic patients correlates with the risk and severity of microvascular complications, and improving hyperglycemia reduces this risk incrementally. Whether this is a direct effect of hyperglycemia or consequence of a chronic exposure eliciting more complex metabolic consequences is not clear (77). However, the relationship between glycemic control and macrovascular complications is even more remote.

Early observational studies of the relationship between hyperglycemia and the risk of CVD in the diabetic population yielded conflicting results (78–82). Data from the Diabetes Control and Complications Trial (DCCT) (83) identified a trend toward reduction in CV events in the intensive versus conventional treatment group (0.5 event per 100 patient years vs. 0.8 event, 95% CI, –10 to 68%). However, the study was conducted among relatively young patients with type 1 diabetes and was not powered to test the prevention of CV events. The study did find significant risk reductions for microvascular complications in the intensively treated group (by 76% for development of retinopathy, 39% for micro-albuminuria and 60% for clinical neuropathy). The UKPDS, initiated in the 1970s, reported the effects of intensive treatment of hyperglycemia using sulfonylurea agents, insulin, or metformin in newly diagnosed type 2 diabetic patients over a 10-year period (84). Despite the fact that the hemoglobin A1c was lower in the intensively treated group (7.0% vs. 7.9%, approaching the American Diabetes Association goal of <7%), the differences in myocardial infarction (14.7 events per 1,000 patient-years vs. 17.4 events; $P = 0.052$) and stroke (5.6 events per 1,000 patient-years vs. 5.0 events per 1,000 patient years; $P = 0.52$) were not significantly lower compared with the conventional treatment group. The development of microvascular disease was, however, significantly reduced (by 25%, $P <0.01$). This study was powered to demonstrate whether improved glycemic control would reduce CV events, but demonstrated only a modest reduction in myocardial infarction and none for stroke.

More recent randomized studies with greater power have yielded divergent results with regard to the effect of intensive long-term glycemic control on CV events (85–88). In the ACCORD study (86), 10,251 patients with type 2 diabetes (mean age 62.2 years) with a median glycated hemoglobin level of 8.1% were randomly assigned to receive intensive therapy (targeting a glycated hemoglobin level <6.0%) or standard therapy (targeting a level from 7.0 to 7.9%). The primary outcome was a composite of nonfatal myocardial infarction, nonfatal stroke, or death from CV causes. At one year, median glycated hemoglobin levels of 6.4% and 7.5% were achieved in the intensive-therapy group and the standard-therapy group, respectively. During follow-up, the primary outcome occurred in 352 patients in the intensive-therapy group, as compared with 371 in the standard-therapy group (HR, 0.90; 95% CI, 0.78–1.04; $P = 0.16$). At the same time, 257 patients in the intensive-therapy group died, as compared with 203 patients in the standard-therapy group (HR, 1.22; 95% CI, 1.01–1.46; $P = 0.04$). Hypoglycemia requiring assistance and weight gain of more than 10 kg was more frequent with intensive therapy ($P <0.001$). Thus, in this population, the use of intensive therapy to target normal glycated hemoglobin levels for 3.5 years increased mortality and did not significantly reduce major CV events. In a study of 1,791 military veterans with type 2 diabetes, despite a median HgA1C of 6.9% versus 8.4% with intensive versus standard treatment, there were no differences between groups in a composite endpoint of macrovascular events ($P = 0.14$) or in all-cause mortality ($P = 0.62$) (85). Contrasting results were obtained in the ADVANCE study (87) of 11,140 patients with type 2 diabetes randomized to either standard glucose control or intensive glucose control (to achieve a glycated hemoglobin value ≤6.5%). After a median of five years of follow-up, the mean glycated hemoglobin level was lower in the intensive-control group (6.5%) than in the standard-control group (7.3%). Intensive control reduced the incidence of combined major macrovascular and microvascular events (18.1%, vs. 20.0%; HR, 0.90; 95% CI, 0.82 to 0.98; $P = 0.01$), as well as that of major microvascular events (9.4% vs. 10.9%; HR, 0.86; 95% CI, 0.77–0.97; $P = 0.01$), primarily because of a reduction in the incidence of nephropathy (4.1% vs. 5.2%; HR, 0.79; 95% CI, 0.66–0.93; $P = 0.006$), with no significant effect on retinopathy ($P = 0.50$) or on major macrovascular events, death from CV causes, or death from any cause (HRs with intensive control, 0.88 to 0.93, $P = 0.12$–0.32). In the Prospective Pioglitazone Clinical Trial in Macro Vascular Events (PROACTIVE) study (88), patients randomized to receive pioglitazone on top of their existing glucose-lowering and CV medications had an 18% lower incidence of a composite endpoint of all-cause mortality, nonfatal myocardial infarction, non-fatal stroke or acute coronary syndromes in the more aggressively treated patient group. A recent meta-analysis (89) of 29 randomized studies of tight glucose control versus usual care in 8,432 adult intensive care unit patients found no impact of tighter glucose control on mortality or need for dialysis, but did identify a 24% reduction in the risk of septicemia and a fivefold increase in the risk of hypoglycemia requiring treatment. Thus, aggressive treatment of hyperglycemia in diabetes has been shown to be extremely beneficial in prevention of microvascular disease. However, whether reducing HgA1c to <7% will reduce the excess risk of CV disease in diabetic patients over and above the benefit of aggressively treating other established risk factors remains uncertain.

Procoagulant State

Multiple abnormalities in platelet function, coagulation, fibrinolysis, and blood viscosity have been described in diabetic patients. Abnormal platelet adhesion and aggregation, increased fibrinogen, factor VII and increased plasminogen activator inhibitor-1 levels are well recognized (90). These alterations in the coagulation system are particularly seen in those with the metabolic syndrome or Syndrome X. For these reasons, the American Diabetes Association has recommended that aspirin treatment be considered in diabetic patients with two or more risk factors in addition to those with established CVD.

Cigarette Smoking, Obesity, and Physical Activity

Cigarette smoking is a leading risk factor for CVD. In MRFIT (47), cigarette smoking was a powerful determinant of CVD mortality in men with diabetes and had an additive effect when superimposed on other risk factors. Among the more than 11,000 participants in the Swedish National Diabetes Register, current smoking and higher body mass index both strongly predicted the occurrence of nearly 1,500 incident CV events (both P <0.002), independent of effects of other risk factors (91). Weight reduction and regular physical activity have beneficial effects on glycemic control, hypertension, dyslipidemia, and insulin resistance.

Management of Coronary Artery Disease in Diabetic Patients

The available data indicate that smoking cessation and optimal control of both arterial pressure and lipid levels are of substantial benefit, in addition to effective glycemic control, for prevention of CAD events in diabetic patients. Use of aspirin and nephroprotection by ACE inhibitors or angiotensin receptor blockers also appear to reduce the rate of CV events in patients with diabetes (73). After myocardial infarction, optimal glucose control with insulin therapy in diabetic patients was shown to produce a significant 30% reduction in mortality at 12 months as compared to usual glycemic control (92). Beta blockers are also effective in mortality reduction after myocardial infarction in diabetic patients. Pooled trial results show a 37% reduction in CVD mortality in diabetic patients compared with 13% found in all treated groups (93). Thus, management of diabetic patients with acute myocardial infarction should include optimal glycemic control with insulin, immediate coronary reperfusion, aspirin, and early beta blockade.

Coronary Revascularization

Either coronary artery bypass graft surgery (CABG) or percutaneous coronary angioplasty (PTCA) may be used for revascularization in patients with diabetes. Diabetes is not associated with increased perioperative mortality during bypass graft surgery, although the frequency of wound infection and the length of hospital stay are increased. Although the initial rate of success of PTCA is similar in diabetics and nondiabetics, there is an increased rate of restenosis during the next six months when diabetes is present. The mechanism of restenosis is thought to be due to exaggerated neointimal hyperplasia rather than increased vessel remodeling (94). Whether the use of more technologically advanced stenting procedures will lead to improved outcomes in diabetes remains to be answered by future clinical trials.

Several trials have examined the outcome of PTCA compared to CABG in diabetic patients with multivessel CAD. The Bypass Angioplasty Revascularization Investigation (BARI) (95) demonstrated that 5-year survival was only 65.5% in diabetic patients randomly assigned to PTCA compared to 80.6% survival in the CABG group, as compared to virtually identical five-year mortality rates in patients without diabetes. After 10 years of follow-up in the BARI study (96), in the subgroup of patients with untreated diabetes, survival rates were nearly identical by randomization to PTCA (77.0%) versus CABG (77.3%, P = 0.59). In the subgroup with treated diabetes, the group assigned to CABG continued to have higher survival than the group assigned to PTCA (57.8% vs. 45.5%, P = 0.025). One limitation of this study, however, was the lack of the use of stents in the angioplasty group, since stenting may improve outcomes in patients with diabetes. The question of whether use of stents has improved the relative benefit of angioplasty versus bypass surgery for diabetic patients is being addressed in the ongoing randomized BARI-2 study (97). One explanation for the higher mortality associated with PTCA is that diabetes is usually associated with more diffuse coronary disease and the vessels are of smaller caliber. It is also likely that angioplasty leaves a higher proportion of ischemic myocardium than does bypass grafting. In keeping with this hypothesis, in a meta-analysis of four trials that compared 263 diabetic patients to 965 nondiabetic patients who underwent single-vessel stenting, repeat revascularization of the stented lesion was performed more frequently during the first year in patients with diabetes (16.0% vs. 10.9%, P = 0.01) but not thereafter (1.8% vs. 1.3% per year) in patients with and without diabetes, whereas repeat revascularization of other coronary segments was more frequent in patients with diabetes during the entire five years of follow-up (32.2% vs. 24.1%, P = 0.005). Cardiac death or MI was also more frequent among diabetic patients (5-year rates, 25.4% vs. 17.9%, P = 0.008) and remained significant after adjustment for all differences in baseline characteristics (HR 1.5, 95% CE, 1.1–2.0, P = 0.01) (98). The issue of whether the findings of the BARI trial are consistent with other revascularization trials has been raised. The Emory Angioplasty Versus Surgery Trial (EAST) (99) found no difference in mortality in diabetic patients treated with PTCA compared with coronary bypass surgery. However, diabetic patients fared no worse than nondiabetic patients in general, which suggests that the diabetic patients in this study represented an unusually low-risk group. Also, EAST involved fewer diabetic patients than did BARI and had limited statistical power to detect a treatment difference. In the recently-published BARI-2 Diabetes trial, there was no significant difference in the rates of death and major cardiovascular events between patients undergoing prompt revascularization and those undergoing medical therapy or between strategies of insulin sensitization and insulin provision (137).

A recent meta-analysis of 13 randomized clinical trials and 16 registries including over 12,500 diabetic patients comparing treatment with the two major types of drug-eluting stents (100) found similar, moderate rates of subsequent target vessel revascularization (5.8–8.6%) or major adverse cardiac events (10.1–15.4%) with both types of drug-eluting stents. However, this analysis was limited by lack of comparative data for outcomes with coronary bypass surgery. Until more definitive data are available, available studies suggest that the form of revascularization to treat multivessel coronary disease in diabetes can be individually tailored to patients, taking into account the clinical and angiographic suitability for each procedure. Those patients with more severe disease should undergo surgery and those with milder forms of disease can be treated with angioplasty plus stenting.

■ CEREBROVASCULAR DISEASE

Parallel to its strong effect on the development of CAD, diabetes is also a strong risk factor for stroke. In a case-control study in the Cincinnati region (101), diabetes increased ischemic stroke incidence at all ages, especially under age 55 in African Americans and under age 65 in whites. This study estimated that 37% to 42% of all ischemic strokes in both African Americans and whites are attributable to effects of diabetes alone or in combination with hypertension. In the biracial, middle-aged population of the ARIC study, 26% of stroke cases over 13 years were attributed to diabetes (102). In the population-based sample of American Indian participants in the Strong Heart Study (103), 306 (6.8%) of 4,507 participants without prior stroke suffered a first stroke within 10 years of follow-up. Diabetes at baseline was associated with a twofold higher rate of subsequent stroke, independent of older age, higher diastolic blood pressure, smoking, and albuminuria; in alternative models fasting glucose and HbA1$_C$ were independent predictors of stroke as were hypertension and prehypertension as categorical variables. In several studies of patients with hypertension and other markers of high risk, treatment with regimens based on newer antihypertensive agents has been associated with 20% to 25% lower rates of incident stroke in patients with concomitant diabetes (60,70,104). In the LIFE study, losartan-based therapy was associated with an approximately

25% lower rate of subsequent stroke among patients with diabetes at baseline, although this result did not attain statistical significance (70). In ASCOT (60), in the large subpopulation (*n* = 5,137) with DM in the trial's blood pressure-lowering arm, amlodipine-based treatment reduced the incidence of fatal and nonfatal strokes 25% (*P* = 0.017). In ACCOMPLISH, among 6,946 hypertensive patients with diabetes, those randomized to treatment with amlodipine plus benazepril had a 21% lower rate (95% CI 8–32%, *P* = 0.003) of a composite endpoint of CV events and CV death than those randomized to hydrochlorothiazide plus benazapril (104).

■ **CARDIOMYOPATHY**

The poor prognosis in patients with diabetes after myocardial infarction or other CHD events is related to both a high case-fatality rate due to CHD and an increased susceptibility to develop heart failure. In the Framingham study population, diabetic men had more than twice the frequency of heart failure than their nondiabetic counterparts, while diabetic women had a fivefold increased risk of developing heart failure (105). This excessive risk of heart failure persisted despite correcting for age, hypertension, obesity, hypercholesterolemia, other conventional risk factors and recognized CAD at baseline. However, it remained unclear whether the excess incidence of heart failure in diabetic individuals was due to their high rate of incident myocardial infarction. In the Cardiovascular Health Study, DM was an independent risk factor for heart failure in participants either with or without CHD (106). Recently, de Simone et al. (107) documented in a large population-based sample that diabetes was associated with a 1.5-fold higher incidence of heart failure after accounting for incident myocardial infarction as a competing risk, in addition to control for a wide array of established risk factors (Figure 5.10). It has been proposed that a specific diabetic cardiomyopathy exists, independent of CAD or other coexisting confounding factors, characterized by alteration of left ventricular (LV) geometry and function. There are now considerable experimental, pathological, and epidemiological

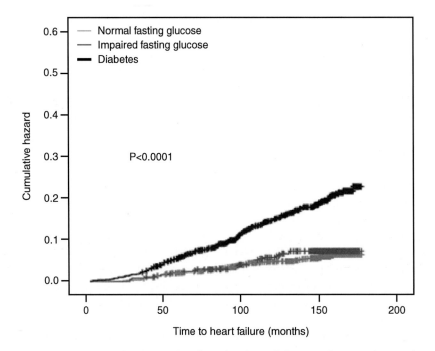

FIGURE 5.10 Kaplan-Meier plot of incident heart failure in subjects with normal (light gray line and symbols) or impaired (dark gray line and symbols) fasting glucose or diabetes (black line and symbols). (From Ref. 107, with permission.)

data to support the existence of "diabetic cardiomyopathy." The existence of a subclinical or early form of diabetic cardiomyopathy is suggested by documentation of abnormal LV structure and function detected by echocardiography in newly diagnosed type 2 diabetes (108). The process of alteration of the myocardium may occur before the degree of abnormality of glucose metabolism reaches the level required for the diagnosis of diabetes.

Left Ventricular Hypertrophy

The association of LV hypertrophy and risk of CV morbidity and mortality is well established (109). In one landmark study, LV hypertrophy was associated with a greater relative risk for all-cause mortality than the number of stenotic coronary arteries or the LV ejection fraction (110). In animal models (111), rats with streptozotocin-induced diabetes demonstrate increased LV mass. The combination of hypertension and DM is synergistic in rats, leading to higher mortality, as it does in humans. This finding is confirmed in pathologic studies, which showed that human diabetic hearts have higher LV mass unrelated to the extent of coronary artery disease and hypertension (112). Other abnormalities noted in human diabetic hearts include increased microvascular tone, interstitial fibrosis, and edema.

In epidemiological studies, diabetes has been shown to be independently associated with higher prevalence of LV hypertrophy in both the Framingham population and the Strong Heart Study (113–114). In the latter study, the combination of hypertension and diabetes, which frequently coexist, was associated with a higher prevalence of LV hypertrophy (38%) than found in individuals with either diabetes or hypertension (19–24%) or with neither (11%) (115). In 1,950 hypertensive patients in the population-based HyperGEN study (116), the 386 (20%) with diabetes had a higher prevalence of LV hypertrophy (38 vs. 26%, $P = 0.03$) and lower myocardial function, as evidenced by reduced LV midwall shortening ($P < 0.001$). Recently, evaluation of a population-based sample of adolescents and young adults has shown that diabetes is associated with an increased prevalence of LV hypertrophy even at young ages (117). In a population of 1,810 diabetic adults, CV mortality was significantly higher (HR = 2.36, 95% CI, 1.18–4.69) in diabetic participants with echocardiographic LV hypertrophy as opposed to those without, after adjusting for age, gender, body mass index, hypertension, smoking, and plasma creatinine

(118). Furthermore, electrocardiographic repolarization abnormalities that are influenced by LV hypertrophy as well as underlying CAD have been shown to predict CV and all-cause mortality (119). In addition to increasing LV mass, diabetes also impacts cardiac remodeling, with an associated increase in relative wall thickness, a measure of concentricity of LV geometry (114).

The association between diabetes and LV hypertrophy may be bidirectional. Recent analyses in a large population of patients with moderately severe hypertension have shown that individuals with diabetes at baseline had less reduction of LV hypertrophy—whether measured by electrocardiography (120) or echocardiography (121)—than their nondiabetic counterparts despite even greater reduction of blood pressure in the former group. Similarly, in 6,793 nondiabetic hypertensive patients in this same population, those with two or more metabolic abnormalities (including obesity, high-plasma glucose, and low HDL) had less regression of ECG LV hypertrophy for the same reduction of blood pressure (122). In view of the evidence of less reduction of LV mass for the same blood pressure reduction in the presence of diabetes, it is possible that treatment to lower BP targets will be needed to achieve LV hypertrophy regression in diabetic patients, as has been shown recently in the SANDS study (75). Conversely, it has recently been shown in this population that regression of electrocardiographic LV hypertrophy was associated with a 26% lower incidence of new diabetes, after adjustment for multiple risk factors for diabetes (123).

Left Ventricular Function

Diabetes is associated with systolic and diastolic dysfunction, independent of coronary artery disease or hypertension. Hemodynamic, biochemical, and histological studies in dogs with alloxan-induced diabetes demonstrated a lower stroke volume despite normal LV end diastolic pressure. Chamber stiffness was increased in diabetic dogs compared to control dogs (124). Isolated papillary muscle studies in diabetic rats indicate prolongation of contraction, prolonged relaxation, and a reduced rate of shortening (111). A wide range of abnormal biochemical changes have been described in the hearts of diabetic rats including alterations in ATPase, impaired calcium ion transport, and alterations in carbohydrate, lipid, and adenine nucleotide metabolism.

In a clinical study, Jain et al. found increased LV chamber stiffness in diabetic as compared with nondiabetic patients (125). In addition, epidemiological studies have found that adults with diabetes have lower LV fractional shortening (by a mean of 0.7%) and LV midwall fractional shortening, an index of myocardial contractility, by a mean of 0.9%. Hildebrandt et al. (126) showed in a large series of hypertensive patients with ECG LV hypertrophy that participants who also had diabetes had lower LV systolic chamber and myocardial function, as well as lower mean stroke volume than their nondiabetic counterparts. Of note, LV mass was similar in diabetic and nondiabetic patients, indicating that the observed functional abnormalities are independent of the degree of hypertrophy. Impaired LV systolic function is the strongest predictor of morbid cardiac events in CAD (127).

Diabetes is also associated with diastolic dysfunction, which appears to predate the onset of systolic dysfunction. The severity of diabetes-associated abnormal LV relaxation is similar to the well-known impaired relaxation associated with hypertension (128). The combination of both diabetes and hypertension induces more severe abnormal LV relaxation than does either condition alone. In addition, abnormal relaxation in subjects with diabetes is associated with worse glycemic control and positively associated with duration of diabetes. Evidence of impaired LV relaxation is associated with higher CV and all-cause mortality in diabetes (129). Evidence of diabetic cardiomyopathy is seen early in the course of the disease, often at the onset of diabetes (108).

In a recent analysis of the Strong Heart Study population that was free of CHD (130), incident heart failure was predicted by a cluster of morphological and functional abnormalities, including higher LV mass and left atrial dimensions, lower LV chamber function, and prolonged LV relaxation, independent of age, sex, and other potential confounders. However, even accounting for these direct predictors, diabetes still remained a potent risk factor for myocardial infarction-independent heart failure, possibly due to increased myocardial stiffness, which characterizes the last (passive) part of diastole, a portion of cardiac cycle that cannot be accurately determined by conventional transthoracic echocardiography.

Potential Mechanisms

The etiology of diabetic cardiomyopathy, which is characterized by increased LV mass, left atrial enlargement, concentric LV geometry, systolic dysfunction and impaired LV relaxation, is not entirely clear. One hemodynamic mechanism that has been identified in several studies is an increase in arterial stiffness, which may augment central arterial pressure and thus the load placed on the LV and also on the coronary and cerebral arterial trees (114). It has been proposed that additional pathogenic mechanisms may include myocardial impacts of metabolic alterations due to hyperglycemia. Interstitial accumulation of AGES, collagen deposition, and fibrosis in the myocardium have been reported in human diabetic hearts (112,131–132). Animal studies have found p-aminosalicyclic acid–positive material among the muscle fibers and cholesterol and triglyceride deposition in the myocardium (111), but the evidence that AGEs also accumulate in the myocardium, in addition to the arterial wall, is still weak (133). These tissue alterations can increase end-diastolic myocardial stiffness as well as LV mass, and impair systolic function.

The pathogenic mechanisms underlying diabetes-associated changes in myocardial tissue composition are unclear. We have reported that albuminuria, a strong predictor of CV mortality and morbidity, is independently associated with increased LV mass and systolic and diastolic dysfunction among diabetic patients (134). Albuminuria has been proposed to represent a marker of a generalized vascular dysfunction (135) and has been associated with renal alterations, proliferative retinopathy, and CV disease in diabetic and nondiabetic adults. Albuminuria reflects a renal and systemic transvascular albumin leakage that is perhaps due to low vessel wall content of heparin sulfate, which has been shown not only in the glomerular basement membrane but also in the atherosclerotic aorta and coronary arteries (136). This generalized increase of vascular permeability can also cause leaking of collagen, cholesterol, and AGEs that have been reported in the myocardium of human hearts (124). Furthermore, this change in permeability causes insudation of lipoproteins into the intima of large vessels, which can contribute to atherosclerosis of the epicardial coronary arteries as well as small arterioles of the heart. Small vessel disease can lead to subendocardial ischemia causing systolic and diastolic myocardial dysfunction. The microvascular changes in the heart are the same as those throughout the rest of the body, including interstitial fibrosis, perivascular thickening, and fibrosis and micro-aneurysm formation.

■ CONCLUSION

The increasing prevalence of overweight and obesity are leading to a virtual epidemic of type 2 diabetes in the United States and other industrialized nations, which will lead to a rising tide of complications of diabetes after a lag phase of 10 or more years. The high rates of morbidity and especially mortality associated with diabetes are predominately due to CV disease. The risk of developing new CHD is high in diabetes, as are risks for cerebrovascular and peripheral arterial disease, in part because of the frequent association of diabetes with other risk factors for atherosclerosis. In addition, diabetes is associated with higher morbidity and mortality after myocardial infarction, and with increased rates of stroke and other manifestations of arterial disease beyond the coronary circulation. Diabetes is also often associated with a distinct cardiomyopathy—characterized by LV hypertrophy, reduced myocardial function, and impaired LV filling—which may partially mediate the high mortality associated with CHD and the increased frequency of congestive heart failure in diabetic individuals. Management goals for the diabetic patient should focus on optimal glucose control and intense modification of coronary disease risk factors, especially optimal control of arterial pressure, in general using combination antihypertensive therapies, and of lipids, using statins and other interventions as indicated. In addition, evaluation to detect subclinical or early clinical evidence of atherosclerosis and diabetic cardiomyopathy may be warranted to target especially intensive intervention most accurately.

■ REFERENCES

1. Centers for Disease Control and Prevention, National Center for Health Statistics, *Health, United States, 2007*. Data from the National Health Interview Survey, Youth Risk Behavior Survey, National Vital Statistics System.

2. Burt VL, Cutler JA, Higgins M, et al. Trends in prevalence, awareness, treatment and control of hypertension in the adult United States population: Data from the Health Examination Surveys 1960–1991. *Hypertension* 1995;26:60–69.

3. Cutler JA, Sorlie PD, Wolz M, et al. Trends in hypertension prevalence, awareness, treatment and control rates in United States adults between 1988–1994 and 1999–2004. *Hypertension* 2008;52:818–827.

4. Centers for Disease Control and Prevention, National Center for Health Statistics, *Health, United States, 2007*. Data from the National Vital Statistics System.

5. Centers for Disease Control and Prevention, National Center for Health Statistics. *Health, United States, 2007*. Data from the Vital Statistics System.

6. Lloyd-Jones D, Adams R, Carnethon M, et al. American Heart Association Statistics Committee and Stroke Statistics Subcommittee. Heart Disease and Stroke Statistics 2009 update. A Report from the American Heart Association Statistics Committee and Stroke Statistics Subcommittee. *Circulation* 2009;119:e1-e161 (online).

7. Centers for Disease Control and Prevention, National Center for Health Statistics, *Health, United States, 2007*. Data from the National Health and Nutrition Examination Survey.

8. Ogden CL, Carroll MD, Curtin LR, et al. Prevalence of overweight and obesity in the United States, 1999–2004. *JAMA* 2006;295:1549–1555.

9. Gregg EW, Cheng YJ, Narayan KM, Thompson TJ, Williamson DF. The relative contributions of different levels of overweight and obesity to the increased prevalence of diabetes in the United States:1976–2004. *Prev Med* 2007;45:348–352.

10. Centers for Disease Control and Prevention, National Center for Health Statistics. National Health and Nutrition Survey, 2007. National Diabetes Fact Sheet.

11. Garcia MJ, McNamara M, Gordon T, Kannel WB. 16-year follow-up study. Morbidity and mortality in diabetics in the Framingham population. *Diabetes* 1974;23:105–111.

12. Kannel WB, McGee DL. Diabetes and cardiovascular disease: The Framingham Study, *JAMA* 1979;241:2035–2038.

13. Roglic G, Unwin N, Bennett PH, et al. The burden of mortality attributable to diabetes: Realistic estimates for the year 2000. *Diabetes Care* 2005;28:2130–2135.

14. Grundy SM, Benjamin IJ, Burke GL, et al. Diabetes and cardiovascular disease: A statement for healthcare professionals from the American Heart Association. *Circulation* 1999;100:1134–1146.

15. Laakso M, Lehto S. Epidemiology of macrovascular disease in diabetes. *Diabetes Rev* 1997;5:294–315.

16. Brezinka V, Padmos I. Coronary heart disease risk factors in women. *Eur Heart J*, 1994; 15, 1571–1584.

17. Haffner SM, Lehto S, Ronnemaa T, et al. Mortality from coronary heart disease in subjects with type 2 diabetes and in nondiabetic subjects with and without prior myocardial infarction. *N Engl J Med* 1998;339:229–234.

18. Donahoe SM, Stewart GC, McCabe CH, et al. Diabetes and mortality following acute coronary syndromes. *JAMA* 2007;298:765–775.

19. Gu K, Cowie CC, Harris MI. Diabetes and decline in heart disease mortality in US adults. *JAMA* 1999;281:1291–1297.

20. Jemal A, Ward E, Hao Y, et al. Trends in the leading causes of death in the United States, 1970–2002. *JAMA* 2005;294:1255–1259.

21. McGuire DK, Granger CB. Diabetes and ischemic heart disease. *Am Heart J* 1999;138:S366–S375.

22. Greenland P, Reicher-Reiss H, Goldbourt U, Behar S. In-hospital and 1-year mortality in 1,524 women after myocardial infarction. Comparison with 4,315 men. *Circulation* 1991;83:484–491.

23. Miettinen H, Lehto S, Salomaa V, et al. Impact of diabetes on mortality after the first myocardial infarction. *Diabetes Care* 1998;21:69–75.

24. Gottlieb SO, Weisfeldt ML, Ouyang P, et al. Silent ischemia as a marker for early unfavorable outcomes in patients with unstable angina. *N Engl J Med* 1986;314:1214–1219.

25. Naka M, Hiramatsu K, Aizawa T, et al. Silent myocardial ischemia in non-insulin dependent diabetes mellitus as judged by treadmill exercise testing and coronary angiography. *Am Heart J* 1992;123:46–52.

26. Langer A, Freeman M, Josse R, et al. Detection of silent myocardial ischemia in diabetes mellitus. *Am J Cardiol* 1991;67:1073–1078.

27. Caracciolo EZ, Chaitman BR, Forman SR, et al. Diabetics with coronary disease have a prevalence of asymptomatic ischemia during exercise treadmill testing and ambulatory ischemia monitoring similar to that of non-diabetic patients. *Circulation* 1996;93:2097–2105.

28. Goraya TY, Leibson CL, Palumbo PJ, et al. Coronary atherosclerosis in diabetes mellitus: a population-based autopsy study. *J Am Coll Cardiol* 2002;40:946–953.

29. Airaksinen KE, Koistinen MJ. Association between silent coronary artery disease, diabetes, and autonomic neuropathy. Fact or fallacy? *Diabetes Care* 1992;15:288–292.

30. Koistinen MJ, Airaksinen KE, Huikuri HV, et al. Asymptomatic coronary artery disease in diabetes: associated with autonomic neuropathy? *Acta Diabetol* 1992;28:199–202.

31. Scholte AJ, Schuijf JD, Kharagjitsingh AV, et al. Different manifestations of coronary artery disease by stress SPECT myocardial perfusion imaging, coronary calcium scoring, and multislice CT coronary angiography in asymptomatic patients with type 2 diabetes mellitus. *J Nucl Cardiol* 2008;15:503–509.

32. Wackers FJ, Young LH, Inzucchi SE, et al. Detection of silent myocardial ischemia in asymptomatic diabetic subjects: the DIAD study. *Diabetes Care* 2004;27:1954–1961.

33. Wackers FJ, Chyun DA, Young LH, et al. Detection of Ischemia in Asymptomatic Diabetics (DIAD) Investigators. Resolution of asymptomatic myocardial ischemia in patients with type 2 diabetes in the Detection of Ischemia in Asymptomatic Diabetics (DIAD) study. *Diabetes Care* 2007;30:2892–2898.

34. Scognamiglio R, Negut C, Ramondo A, et al. Detection of coronary artery disease in asymptomatic patients with type 2 diabetes mellitus. *J Am Coll Cardiol* 2006;47:65–71.

35. Stamler J, Vaccaro O, Neaton JD, et al. Diabetes, other risk factors and 12-year cardiovascular mortality in men screened in the Multiple Risk Factor Intervention Trial (MRFIT). *Diabetes Care* 1993;16:434–444.

36. WHO. Definition of metabolic syndrome in definition, diagnosis and classification of diabetes and its complications. Report of a WHO consultation. Part 1: Diagnosis and classification of diabetes mellitus. WHO/NCD/NCS/99.2. Geneva: World Health Organization Department of Noncommunicable Disease Surveillance, 1999.

37. Third Report of the National Cholesterol Education Program (NCEP) Expert Panel on Detection, Evaluation, and Treatment of High Blood Cholesterol in Adults (Adult Treatment Panel III) final report. *Circulation* 2002;106:3143–3421.

38. Balkau B, Charles MA, Drivsholm T, et al. Frequency of the WHO metabolic syndrome in European cohorts, and an alternative definition of an insulin resistance syndrome. *Diabetes Metab* 2002;28:364–376.

39. Einhorn D, Reaven GM, Cobin RH, et al. American College of Endocrinology position statement on the insulin resistance syndrome. *Endocr Pract* 2003;9:237–252.

40. Alberti G. Introduction to the metabolic syndrome. *Eur Heart J* 2005;7 (Suppl):3–5.

41. Wilson PW. Insulin resistance syndrome and the prothrombotic state: a Framingham perspective. *Endocr Pract* 2003;9(Suppl 2):50–52.

42. Kim JA, Montagnani M, Koh KK, Quon MJ. Reciprocal relationships between insulin resistance and endothelial dysfunction: molecular and pathophysiological mechanisms. *Circulation* 2006;113:1888–1904.

43. Howard BV, Best LG, Galloway JM, et al. Coronary heart disease risk equivalence in diabetes depends on concomitant risk factors. *Diabetes Care* 2006;29:391–397.

44. Folsom AR, Chambless LE, Duncan BB, et al. Atherosclerosis Risk in Communities Study Investigators. Prediction of coronary heart disease in middle-aged adults with diabetes. *Diabetes Care* 2003;26:2777–2784.

45. Almgren P, Tuomi T, Forsen B, et al. Cardiovascular morbidity and mortality associated with the metabolic syndrome. *Diabetes Care* 2001;24:683–689.

46. Alexander CM, Landsman PB, Teutsch SM, Haffner SM. NCEP-defined metabolic syndrome, diabetes, and prevalence of coronary heart disease among NHANES III participants age 50 years and older. *Diabetes* 2003;52:1210–1214.

47. Goldberg RB. Cardiovascular disease in diabetic patients. *Med Clin North Am* 2000;84(1):81–93.

48. Koskinen P, Manttari M, Manninen V, et al. Coronary heart disease incidence in NIDDM patients in the Helsinki Heart Study. *Diabetes Care* 1992;15:820–825.

49. Keech A, Simes RJ, Barter P, et al. Effects of long-term fenofibrate therapy on cardiovascular events in 9795 people with type 2 diabetes mellitus (the FIELD study): randomised controlled trial. *Lancet* 2005;366:1849–1861.

50. Pyprala K, Pedersen TR, Kjekshus J, et al. Cholesterol lowering with simvastatin improves prognosis of diabetic patients with coronary heart disease. A subgroup analysis of the Scandinavian Simvastatin Survival Study (4S). *Diabetes Care* 1997;20:614–620.

51. Goldberg RB, Mellies MJ, Sacks FM, et al. for the CARE Investigators: Cardiovascular events and their reduction with pravastatin in diabetic and glucose intolerant myocardial infarction survivors with average cholesterol levels: subgroup analyses in the Cholesterol and Recurrent Events (CARE) trial. *Circulation* 1998;98:2513–2519.

52. Shepherd J, Barter P, Carmena R, et al. Effect of lowering LDL cholesterol substantially below currently recommended levels in patients with coronary heart disease and diabetes: the Treating to New Targets (TNT) study. *Diabetes Care* 2006;29:1220–1226.

53. Kearney PM, Blackwell L, Collins R, et al. Efficacy of cholesterol lowering therapy in 18,686 people with diabetes in 14 randomised trials of statins: a meta-analysis. Cholesterol Treatment Trialists' (CTT) Collaborators. *Lancet* 2008;371:117–125.

54. Canner PL, Furberg CD, Terrin ML, et al. Benefits of niacin by glycemic status in patients with healed myocardial infarction (from the Coronary Drug Project). *Am J Cardiol* 2005;95:254–257.

55. de Simone G, Devereux RB, Chinali M, et al. Risk factors for arterial hypertension in adults with initial optimal blood pressure: the Strong Heart Study. *Hypertension* 2006;47:162–167.

56. Salomaa V, Riley W, Kark JD, et al. Non-insulin-dependent diabetes mellitus and fasting glucose and insulin concentrations are associated with arterial stiffness indexes. The ARIC

Study. Atherosclerosis Risk in Communities Study. *Circulation* 1995;91:1432–1443.

57. Meisinger C, Doring A, Heier M. Blood pressure and risk of type 2 diabetes mellitus in men and women from the general population: the Monitoring Trends and Determinants on Cardiovascular Diseases/Cooperative Health Research in the Region of Augsburg Cohort Study. *J Hypertens* 2008;26:1809–1815.

58. UK Prospective Diabetes Study Group. Efficacy of atenolol and captopril in reducing risk of macrovascular and microvascular complications in type 2 diabetes: UKPDS 39. *B Med J* 1998;317(7160):713–720.

59. Heart Outcomes Prevention Evaluation study investigators. Effects of ramipril on cardiovascular and microvascular outcomes in people with diabetes mellitus: results of the HOPE study and MICRO-HOPE substudy. *Lancet* 2000;355:253–259.

60. Ostergren J, Poulter NR, Sever PS, et al. for the ASCOT investigators: The Anglo-Scandinavian Cardiac Outcomes Trial: blood pressure-lowering limb: effects in patients with type II diabetes. *J Hypertens* 2008;26:2103–2011.

61. Dahlöf B, Devereux RB, Kjeldsen SE, et al. for the LIFE study group: Cardiovascular morbidity and mortality in the Losartan Intervention for Endpoint reduction in hypertension study (LIFE): a randomised trial against atenolol. *Lancet* 2002;359:995–1003.

62. Barzilay JI, Davis BR, Cutler JA et al. Fasting glucose levels and incident diabetes mellitus in older nondiabetic adults randomized to receive 3 different classes of antihypertensive treatment: A report from the Antihypertensive and Lipid-Lowering Treatment to Prevent Heart Attack Trial (ALLHAT). *Arch Intern Med* 2006;166:2191–2201.

63. Dahlöf B, Sever PS, Pulter NR, et al. Prevention of cardiovascular events with an antihypertensive regimen of amlodipine adding perindopril as required versus atenolol adding bendroflumethiazide as required, in the Anglo-Scandinavian Cardiac Outcomes Trial-Blood Pressure Lowering Arm (ASCOT-BPLA): a multicentre randomized controlled trial. *Lancet* 2005;366:895–906.

64. Rapoport Mi, Hurd Hf. Thiazide-induced glucose intolerance treated with potassium. *Arch Intern Med* 1964;113:405–408.

65. Fossum E, Gleim GW, Kjeldsen SE, et al. The effect of baseline physical activity on cardiovascular outcomes and new-onset diabetes in patients treated for hypertension and left ventricular hypertrophy: the LIFE study. *J Intern Med* 2007;262:439–448.

66. Hansson L, Zanchetti A, Carruthers SG, et al. Effects of intensive blood-pressure lowering and low-dose aspirin in patients with hypertension: principal results of the Hypertension Optimal Treatment (HOT) randomized trial. Hot Study Group. *Lancet* 1998;351:1755–1762.

67. Curb JD, Pressel SL, Cutler JA, et al. For the Systolic Hypertension in the Elderly Program Cooperative Research Group. Effect of diuretic-based antihypertensive treatment on cardiovascular disease risk in older diabetic patients with isolated systolic hypertension. *JAMA* 1996;276:1886–1892.

68. Estacio RO, Jeffers BW, Hiatt WR et al. The effect of nisoldipine as compared with enalapril on cardiovascular outcomes in patients with non-insulin dependent diabetes and hypertension. *N Engl J Med* 1998;338:645–652.

69. Tatti P, Pahor M, Byrington RB, et al. Outcome results of the Fosinopril versus Amlodipine Cardiovascular Events Randomized Trial (FACET) in patients with hypertension and NIDDM. *Diabetes Care* 1998;21:597–603.

70. Lindholm LH, Ibsen H, Dahlöf B, et al., for the LIFE study group: Cardiovascular morbidity and mortality in hypertensive patients with diabetes: The LIFE Study. *Lancet* 2002;359:1004–1010.

71. Patel A, ADVANCE Collaborative Group, MacMahon S, Chalmers J, et al. Effects of a fixed combination of perindopril and indapamide on macrovascular and microvascular outcomes in patients with type 2 diabetes mellitus (the ADVANCE trial): a randomised controlled trial. *Lancet* 2007;370:829–840.

72. Mogensen CE. Microalbuminuria predicts clinical proteinuria and early mortality in maturity-onset diabetes. *N Engl J Med* 1994;310:356–360.

73. Brenner BM, Cooper ME, de Zeeuw D, et al. Effects of losartan on renal and cardiovascular outcomes in maturity-onset diabetes. *N Engl J Med* 2001;345:861–869.

74. Parving H-H, Lehnert H, Brochner-Mortensen J et al. The effect of irbesartan on the development of diabetic nephropathy in patients with type 2 diabetes. *N Engl J Med* 2001;345:870–878.

75. Howard BV, Roman MJ, Devereux RB, et al. Effect of lower targets for blood pressure and LDL cholesterol on atherosclerosis in diabetes: the SANDS randomized trial. *JAMA* 2008;299:1678–1689.

76. Brownlee M: Glycation and diabetic complications. *Diabetes* 1994;43:836–841.

77. Capaldo B, Galderisi M, Turco AA, et al. Acute hyperglycemia does not affect the reactivity of coronary microcirculation in humans. *J Clin Endocrinol Metab* 2005;90:3871–3876.

78. West KM, Ahuja MM, Bennet PH, et al. The role of circulating glucose and triglyceride concentrations and their interactions with other "risk factors" as determinants of arterial disease in nine diabetic population samples from the WHO Multinational Study. *Diabetes Care* 1983;6:361–369.

79. Wilson PW, Cupples LA, Kannel WB. Is hyperglycemia associated with cardiovascular disease? The Framingham Study. *Am Heart J* 1991;121(2; Pt 1):586–590.

80. Jarrett RJ, Shipley MJ. Type 2 (non-insulin dependent) diabetes mellitus and cardiovascular disease. Putative associations via common antecedents. Further evidence from the Whitehall Study. *Diabetologia* 1988;31:737–740.

81. Kuusisto J, Mykkänen L, Pyorala K, et al. NIDDM and its metabolic control predict coronary heart disease in elderly subjects. *Diabetes* 1994;43:960–967.

82. Klein R. Kelly West Lecture 1994. Hyperglycemia and microvascular and macrovascular disease in diabetes. *Diabetes Care* 1995;18:258–268.

83. Diabetes Control and Complications Trial Research Group (DCCT). The effect of intensive treatment of diabetes on the development and progression of long-term complications in insulin-dependent diabetes mellitus. *N Engl J Med* 1993;329:977–986.

84. UK Prospective Diabetes Study (UKPDS) Group. Intensive blood-glucose control with sulfonylureas or insulin compared with conventional treatment and risk of complications in patients with type 2 diabetes (UKPDS33). *Lancet* 1998;352:837–852.

85. Duckworth W, Abraira C, Moritz T, et al. for the VADT Investigators. Glucose control and vascular complications in veterans with type 2 diabetes. *N Engl J Med* 2008;360:129–139.

86. Action to Control Cardiovascular Risk in Diabetes (ACCORD) Study Group, Gerstein HC, Miller ME, Byington RP, et al. Effects of intensive glucose lowering in type 2 diabetes. *N Engl J Med* 2008;358:2545–2559.

87. ADVANCE Collaborative Group, Patel A, MacMahon S, Chalmers J, et al. Intensive blood glucose control and vascular outcomes in patients with type 2 diabetes. *N Engl J Med* 2008;358:2560–2572.

88. Wilcox R, Kupfer S, Erdmann E; PROactive Study investigators. Effects of pioglitazone on major adverse cardiovascular events in high-risk patients with type 2 diabetes: results from PROspective pioglitAzone Clinical Trial In macro Vascular Events (PROACTIVE 10). *Am Heart J* 2008;155:712–717.

89. Soylemez Wiener R, Wiener DC, Larson RJ. Benefits and risks of tight glucose control in critically ill adults: a meta-analysis. *JAMA* 2008;300:933–944.

90. Colwell JA: Aspirin therapy in diabetes. *Diabetes Care* 1997;20:1767–1771.

91. Cederholm J, Eeg-Olofsson K, Eliasson B, et al. on behalf of the Swedish National Diabetes Register. Risk prediction of cardiovascular disease in type 2 diabetes: A risk equation from the Swedish National Diabetes Register (NDR). *Diabetes Care* 2008;31:2038–2043.

92. Malmberg K, Ryden L, Efendic S, et al. Randomized trial of insulin-glucose infusion followed by subcutaneous insulin treatment in diabetic patients with acute myocardial infarction (DIGAMI Study): effects on mortality at 1 year. *J Am Coll Cardiol* 1995;26:57–65.

93. Kendall MJ, Lynch KP, Hjalmarson A, et al. Beta-blockers and sudden cardiac death. *Ann Intern Med* 1995;123:358–367.

94. Komowski R, Mintz GS, Kent KM, et al. Increased restenosis in diabetes mellitus after coronary interventions is due to exaggerated intimal hyperplasia. *Circulation* 1997;95:1366–1369.

95. The Bypass Angioplasty Revascularization Investigation (BARI) Investigators. Comparison of coronary bypass surgery with angioplasty in patients with multivessel disease. *N Engl J Med* 1996;335:217–225.

96. BARI Investigators. The final 10-year follow-up results from the BARI randomized trial. *J Am Coll Cardiol* 2007;49:1600–1606.

97. Brooks MM, Grye RL, Genuth S, et al. Hypotheses, design and methods for the Bypass Angioplasty Revascularization Investigation 2 Diabetes (BARI 2D) Trial. *Am J Cardiol* 2006;12(Suppl 1):9–19.

98. Lee TT, Feinberg L, Baim DS. Effect of diabetes mellitus on five-year clinical outcomes after single-vessel coronary stenting (a pooled analysis of coronary stent clinical trials). *Am J Cardiol* 2006;98:718–721.

99. King SB, Lembo NJ, Weintraub WS, et al. For the Emory Angioplasty versus Surgery Trial (EAST). A randomized trial comparing coronary angioplasty with coronary bypass surgery. *N Engl J Med* 1994;331:1044–1050.

100. Mahmud E, Bromberg-Marin G, Palakodeti V, et al. Clinical efficacy of drug-eluting stents in diabetic patients: a meta-analysis. *J Am Coll Cardiol* 2007;49:1600–1606.

101. Kissela BM, Khoury J, Kleindorfer D. Epidemiology of ischemic stroke in patients with diabetes: the greater Cincinnati/Northern Kentucky Stroke Study. *Diabetes Care* 2005;28:355–359.

102. Ohira T, Shahar E, Chambless LE, et al. Risk factors for ischemic stroke subtypes: the Atherosclerosis Risk in Communities study. *Stroke* 2006;37:2493–2498.

103. Zhang Y, Galloway JM, Welty TK, et al. Incidence and risk factors for stroke in American Indians: The Strong Heart Study. *Circulation* 2008;118:1577–1584.

104. Jamerson K, Weber MA, Bakris GL, et al.; ACCOMPLISH Trial Investigators: Benazepril plus amlodipine or hydrochlorothiazide for hypertension in high-risk patients. *N Engl J Med* 2008;359:2417–2428.

105. Abbott RD, Donahue RP, Kannel WB, et al. The impact of diabetes on survival following myocardial infarction men vs. women. The Framingham Study. *JAMA* 1988;260:3456–3460.

106. Gottdiener JS, Arnold AM, Aurigemma GP, et al. Predictors of congestive heart failure in the elderly: the Cardiovascular Health Study. *J Am Coll Cardiol* 2000;35:1628–1637.

107. de Simone G, Devereux RB, Chinali M, et al. Diabetes and incident congestive heart failure: The Strong Heart Study. *Circulation* 2007;116(Suppl II).

108. Liu JE, Robbins DC, Sosenko J, et al. Abnormal left ventricular structure and function are associated with recent conversion from normal glucose tolerance to diabetes mellitus—the Strong Heart Study. *Diabetes* 2001;50(Suppl 2):s147.

109. Levy D, Garrison RJ, Savage DD, et al. Prognostic implications of echocardiographically determined left ventricular mass in the Framingham Heart Study. *N Engl J Med* 1990;322:1561–1566.

110. Liao Y, Cooper RS, McGee DL, et al. The relative effects of left ventricular hypertrophy, coronary artery disease, and ventricular dysfunction on survival among black adults. *JAMA* 1995;273:1592–1597.

111. Fein FS, Sonnenblick EH. Diabetic cardiomyopathy. *Cardiovasc Drugs Ther* 1994;8:65–73.

112. Van Hoeven KH, Factor SM. A comparison of the pathological spectrum of hypertensive, diabetic and hypertensive-diabetic heart disease. *Circulation* 1990;82:848–855.

113. Galderisi M, Anderson KM, Wilson PW, et al. Echocardiographic evidence for the existence of a distinct diabetic cardiomyopathy (The Framingham Heart Study). *Am J Cardiol* 1991;68:85–89.

114. Devereux RB, Roman MJ, Paranicas M, et al. Impact of diabetes on cardiac structure and function: The Strong Heart Study. *Circulation* 2000;101:2271–2276.

115. Bella JN, Devereux RB, Roman MJ, et al. Separate and joint cardiovascular effects of hypertension and diabetes: The Strong Heart Study. *Am J Cardiol* 2001;87:1260–1265.

116. Palmieri V, Bella JN, Arnett DK, et al. Impact of type II diabetes on left ventricular geometry and function: The Hypertension Genetic Epidemiology Network (HyperGEN) Study. *Circulation* 2001;103:102–107.

117. De Marco M, de Simone G, Roman MJ, Chinali M, Lee ET, Russell M, Howard BV, Devereux RB: Cardiovascular and metabolic predictors of progression of prehypertension into hypertension: The Strong Heart Study. *Hypertension* 2009;54:974–980.

118. Liu JE, Palmieri V, Roman MJ, et al. Cardiovascular disease and prognosis in adults with glucose disorders: The Strong Heart Study. *J Am Coll Cardiol* 2000;35:263A.

119. Okin PM, Devereux RB, Lee ET, et al. Electrocardiographic repolarization complexity and abnormality predict all-cause and cardiovascular mortality in diabetes: The Strong Heart Study. *Diabetes* 2004;53:434–440.

120. Okin PM, Gerdts E, Snapinn SM, et al. The impact of diabetes on regression of electrocardiographic left ventricular hypertrophy

and the prediction of outcome during antihypertensive therapy: The LIFE Study. *Circulation* 2006;113:1588–1596.

121. Gerdts E, Okin PM, Omvik P, Wachtell K, Dahlöf B, Nieminen MS, Devereux RB: Impact of concomitant diabetes on changes in left ventricular structure and systolic function during long-term antihypertensive treatment in hypertensive patients with left ventricular hypertrophy (the LIFE study). *Nutr Metab Cardiovasc Dis* 2009;19:306-312. Epub 18 March 2009.

122. de Simone G, Okin PM, Gerdts E, Olsen MH, Wachtell K, Hille DA, Dahlöf B, Kjeldsen SE, Devereux RB: Clustered metabolic abnormalities blunt regression of hypertensive left ventricular hypertrophy: the LIFE study. *Nutr Metab Cardiovasc Dis* 2009;(in press). Epub 2009 April 8.

123. Okin PM, Harris KE, Jern S, et al. In-treatment resolution or absence of electrocardiographic left ventricular hypertrophy is associated with decreased incidence of new-onset diabetes mellitus in hypertensive patients: The LIFE Study. *Hypertension* 2007;50:984–990.

124. Regan TJ, Wu CF, Yeh CK, et al. Myocardial composition and function in diabetes: the effect of chronic insulin use. *Circ Res* 1981;49:1268–1277.

125. Jain A, Avendano G, Dharamsey S, et al. Left ventricular diastolic function in hypertension and role of plasma glucose and insulin. Comparison with diabetic heart. *Circulation* 1996;93:1396–1402.

126. Hildebrandt P, Wachtell K, Dahlöf B, et al. Impairment of cardiac function in hypertensive patients with type 2 diabetes. A LIFE study. *Diabet Med* 2005;22:1005–1011.

127. Mock MB, Ringqvist I, Fischer LD, and Participants in the Coronary Artery Surgery Study (CASS) Registry. Survival of medically treated patients in the Coronary Artery Study (CASS) registry. *Circulation* 1982;66:562–571.

128. Liu JE, Palmieri V, Roman MJ, et al. The impact of glycemia and diabetes on left ventricular filling pattern: The Strong Heart Study. *J Am Coll Cardiol* 2001;37:1943–1949.

129. Bella JN, Palmieri V, Liu JE, et al. Mitral E/A ratio as a predictor of mortality in middle-aged and elderly adults: The Strong Heart Study. *Circulation* 2002;105:1928–1933.

130. de Simone G, Devereux RB, Chinali M, Lee ET, Galloway JM, Howard BV. Cardiovascular Phenotype Predicting Incident Heart Failure in Diabetes: The Strong Heart Study. *J Am Coll Cardiol* 2008;51(suppl A):A359.

131. van Heerebeek L, Hamdani N, Handoko ML, et al. Diastolic stiffness of the failing diabetic heart: importance of fibrosis, advanced glycation end products, and myocyte resting tension. *Circulation* 2008;117:43–51.

132. *Rojas A, Mercadal E, Figueroa H, Morales MA. Advanced Glycation and ROS: a link between diabetes and heart failure.* Curr Vasc Pharmacol 2008;6:44–51.

133. *Shapiro BP, Owan TE, Mohammed SF, et al. Advanced glycation end products accumulate in vascular smooth muscle and modify vascular but not ventricular properties in elderly hypertensive canines.* Circulation 2008;118:1002–1010.

134. *Liu JE, Robbins DC, Palmieri V, et al. Association of albuminuria with systolic and diastolic left ventricular dysfunction in type 2 diabetes: The Strong Heart Study.* J Am Coll Cardiol 2003;41:2022–2028.

135. Deckert T, Feldt-Rasmussen B, Borch-Johnsen K, et al. Albuminuria reflects widespread vascular damage—The Steno Hypothesis. *Diabetologia* 1989;32:219–226.

136. Yla-Herrtuala S, Sumuvuori H, Karkola K, et al. Glycosoaminoglycans in normal and atherosclerotic human coronary arteries. *Lab Invest* 1986;61:231–236.

137. Frye RL, August P, Brooks MM, et al. BARI 2D Study Group. A randomized trial of therapies for type 2 diabetes and coronary artery disease. *N Engl J Med.* 2009;360:2503–2315.

6

The Noninvasive Vascular Laboratory: Physiologic Testing and Vascular Ultrasonography for the Assessment of Peripheral Arterial Disease

GEORGE BELL

INGRID HRILJAC

OUTLINE

Lower Extremity PAD   89

Ankle-Brachial Index   91

Physiologic Testing for PAD   94

Arterial Duplex Ultrasound   96

Future Directions   111

References   111

Peripheral arterial disease (PAD) encompasses a range of noncoronary arterial syndromes that are caused by altered structure and function of the arteries that supply the brain, visceral organs, and the extremities. Atherosclerosis remains the most common disease process affecting the aorta and its branch arteries. However, numerous diverse pathophysiological processes can contribute to the creation of stenoses or aneurysms in noncoronary arteries. These include degenerative diseases, dysplastic disorders, vascular inflammation, and both in situ thrombosis and thromboembolism. Recognizing this pathogenic diversity permits creation of an inclusive differential diagnosis and a comprehensive long-term treatment plan for patients presenting with symptoms of peripheral arterial disease.

The noninvasive vascular laboratory offers a number of safe, cost-effective and reliable tests to accurately diagnose peripheral arterial disease and establish a treatment plan. This chapter will review the principles of physiologic testing and arterial Duplex ultrasonography, and their utility in the diagnosis of lower extremity peripheral arterial disease, extracranial cerebrovascular disease, renal artery disease, mesenteric artery disease, and diseases of the aorta and iliac arteries.

■ LOWER EXTREMITY PAD

Typically, lower extremity PAD is secondary to atherosclerotic occlusive disease of the aortoiliac, femoral, popliteal and/or the infrapopliteal arteries. It affects between 8 and 12 million Americans and is often a chronic lifestyle-limiting disease that leads to impaired mobility and quality of life, and potential limb loss (1,2). As a manifestation of the systemic atherosclerotic disease process, it is associated with classic cardiovascular risk factors and carries with it a high incidence of adverse cardiovascular events and high cardiovascular mortality. Patients with PAD have a 6.6-fold greater risk of death from coronary disease compared to patients without PAD, and a 3.1-fold greater mortality from any cause (3). Cardiovascular ischemic events are more frequent than ischemic limb events in any PAD population studied (Figure 6.1) (4).

The clinical manifestations of lower extremity PAD depend in part on the level of disease and its severity, as well as concomitant morbidities that affect limb function. The most well-known clinical manifestation of PAD is intermittent claudication, defined as pain in the calf, thigh, or buttock that is brought on by exertion, limits walking distance, and is relieved by rest. This classic syndrome, however, is found in a minority of patients with PAD, as documented by large epidemiologic studies. In the PARTNERS study of 6,979 primary care patients, 29% of those who were either older than 70 years or between the ages of 50 and 69 years with a history of tobacco smoking or diabetes mellitus, had PAD, as diagnosed by a low ankle-brachial index (ABI).

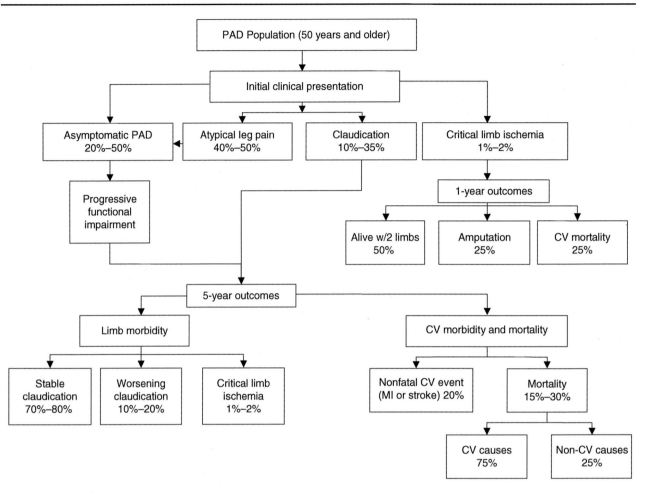

FIGURE 6.1   Natural history of atherosclerotic lower extremity PAD. (From Ref. 4, with permission.)

Despite its known association with coronary artery disease, PAD is typically unrecognized or under-treated because many patients with PAD are asymptomatic or have atypical symptoms, and findings on physical examination may be subtle or misleading (5,6).

Diagnosis of lower extremity PAD begins in the physicians' office with a detailed history of vascular symptoms, including a history of claudication, exertional leg symptoms, and walking impairment, as well as leg pain at rest. A vascular examination, which includes auscultation for arterial bruits, palpation of the abdominal aorta as well as assessment of peripheral pulses may raise the suspicion for PAD. The ABI, an assessment of limb perfusion at rest, can be performed in the office setting, and establishes the diagnosis in a majority of patients. Symptomatic patients, however, should be referred to the vascular laboratory for further evaluation. The noninvasive vascular lab offers several tests that not only establish the diagnosis of PAD, but also assess the functional significance of occlusive arterial disease. These include segmental limb pressures, pulse volume recordings, toe-brachial indices and treadmill exercise testing. If an interventional treatment strategy is planned, further anatomic imaging may be achieved with arterial Duplex ultrasound, computerized tomographic angiography (CTA) and/or magnetic resonance angiography (MRA). Thus, a step-wise approach utilizing noninvasive physiologic and imaging techniques allows for a full evaluation of location, severity, and functional significance of arterial occlusive disease and for the establishment of an appropriate treatment strategy for the patient with ischemic limb symptoms.

■ ANKLE-BRACHIAL INDEX

The ABI is the most studied and best validated method for the assessment of lower extremity PAD. It is a convenient and cost-effective tool available for diagnosing PAD in office practice, in vascular laboratories, and in epidemiological surveys. It can be performed quickly, and has high validity, and good reproducibility. The ABI can be used both as a screening tool in at-risk or symptomatic patients or for monitoring the results of therapeutic interventions.

When compared to lower extremity invasive contrast angiography, the sensitivity and specificity of ABI recordings to diagnose PAD (defined as a stenosis of at least 50% reduction in lumen diameter) has been measured to be 79% and 96%, respectively (7). Fowkes found a similar sensitivity (95%) and specificity (100%) when comparing ABI measurements to angiography for the diagnosis of PAD (8). While these two studies used an ABI cutoff of 0.91 and 0.90, respectively, another study used only posterior tibial measurements and a threshold of 0.8 for the diagnosis of PAD. Compared to angiography, the sensitivity was 89% and specificity was 99% (9).

Measurement Technique

ABI measurements can be performed with relatively little equipment in about 15 minutes. After the patient has been supine for about 10 minutes, the systolic blood pressure is obtained from the brachial and ankle (lower calf immediately above the ankle) positions using a handheld 5- or 10-mHz Doppler instrument and appropriately sized blood pressure cuffs (10). The left and right dorsalis pedis and posterior tibial artery pulses should both be measured in assessing ankle systolic blood pressures. The higher of the right or left brachial artery systolic blood pressure should be used when calculating the ABI. There is usually less than a 12 mm Hg difference between the right and left brachial artery systolic blood pressures. However, a subclavian or axillary artery atherosclerotic stenosis may be present, falsely lowering one of the pressure readings, and subclavian or axillary artery stenoses are more likely in patients with lower extremity PAD. The right ABI is calculated by dividing the higher of the right dorsalis pedis or posterior tibial pressure by the greater of the right or left brachial arm pressure. Conversely, the left ABI is calculated by dividing the higher of the left dorsalis pedis or posterior tibial pressure by the greater of the right or

left brachial arm pressure (Figure 6.2). In the absence of PAD, the ankle pressure should be between 10 and 15 mm Hg higher than the brachial systolic pressure. This is due to pulse wave reflection and its affect on pressure augmentation. As a result, the ABI is greater than 1.00 in healthy individuals. The normal range of ABI values is from 1.00 to 1.29, and PAD should be suspected when the ABI is 0.90 or lower. An ABI of ≤0.4 reflects severe disease, and ischemic rest pain is more likely to occur in this range. ABI values of 1.30 or higher represent noncompressible arteries, and therefore PAD cannot be excluded (Table 6.1).

The ABI should be calculated to two decimal places, and it is said to be reproducible within 0.10. Two studies found a standard deviation of 0.07 when serially measuring ABI readings, which prompted the authors to declare a significant change in ABI measurements to be at least two standard deviations or 0.15 (11,12). Whether ABI measurements were obtained serially in volunteers on different days or were obtained using different observers, the ABI standard deviation has been measured to be between 0.05 and 0.08. Such variation is inherent in the measurement method and is not based on the observer (13,14).

Prognostic Utility of the ABI

The ABI offers important prognostic information, both in terms of limb outcomes as well as cardiovascular ischemic events and mortality. Patients with ABI values greater than 0.50 are unlikely to develop critical leg ischemia over the subsequent 6.5 years, while patients with severe PAD by ABI are at high risk for gangrene, ischemic ulceration, and rest pain (11,15). The ABI has also shown to be useful for monitoring PAD progression after lower extremity surgical intervention (16). An ABI decrease of 0.15 has correlated well with disease progression when compared to angiography or duplex scanning.

The diagnosis of lower extremity PAD indicates a higher systemic atherosclerotic disease risk, and the prevalence of atherosclerotic risk factors, cardiovascular disease, and cerebrovascular disease have all been shown to increase with a worsening ABI (17). All-cause and cardiovascular mortality is increased with low ABI values, and this is seen along a continuum (Figure 6.3) (18). An ABI value of 0.70 or lower has been associated with 30% mortality at 5 years, and an ABI value of 0.40 or lower has been associated with a 50% 5-year mortality (19). In addition, Sikkink et al. demonstrated

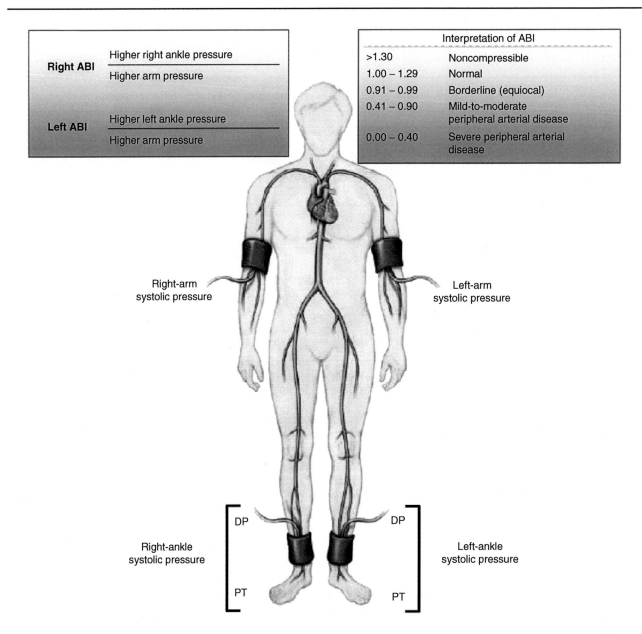

Right ABI	Higher right ankle pressure
	Higher arm pressure

Left ABI	Higher left ankle pressure
	Higher arm pressure

Interpretation of ABI	
>1.30	Noncompressible
1.00 – 1.29	Normal
0.91 – 0.99	Borderline (equiocal)
0.41 – 0.90	Mild-to-moderate peripheral arterial disease
0.00 – 0.40	Severe peripheral arterial disease

Right-arm systolic pressure

Left-arm systolic pressure

Right-ankle systolic pressure

Left-ankle systolic pressure

DP

PT

DP

PT

FIGURE 6.2 Ankle-brachial index. DP indicates dorsalis pedis and PT posterior tibial artery. (From Hiatt WR. Medical treatment of peripheral arterial disease and claudication. *N Engl J Med* 2001;344:1608-21 (158a). Copyright © 2001 Massachusetts Medical Society. All rights reserved.)

that the 5-year survival rate for patients with a resting ABI between 0.70 and 0.89 is 91%, but decreases to 71% for those with an ABI between 0.50 and 0.69, and further decreases to 63% for patients with an ABI less than 0.50 (20). Furthermore, Criqui et al. showed that progressive PAD, defined as a decrease in ABI of more than 0.15, was significantly and independently associated with increased risk of cardiovascular events (21).

Measurement of the ABI may improve the accuracy of cardiovascular risk prediction beyond the Framingham risk score (FRS). In a recent systematic review of 27 studies using the Framingham risk equation, an ABI less than or equal to 0.90 when combined with the FRS approximately doubled the risk of total mortality, cardiovascular mortality, and major coronary events across all Framingham risk categories. In addition, in

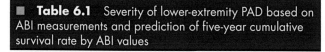

Table 6.1 Severity of lower-extremity PAD based on ABI measurements and prediction of five-year cumulative survival rate by ABI values

ABI and PAD Severity
>1.30 Noncompressible
1.00–1.29 Normal
0.91–0.99 Equivocal
0.41–0.90 Mild-to-Moderate
0.00–0.40 Severe

ABI and Five-Year Cumulative Survival Rate
0.70–0.89: 91% Survival
0.50–0.69: 71% Survival
<0.50: 63% Survival

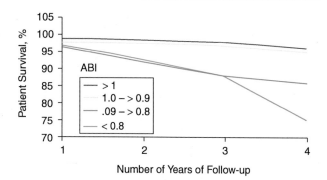

FIGURE 6.3 All-cause and cardiovascular mortality based on ABI value. From Newman AB, Sutton-Tyrrell K, Vogt MT, et al. Morbidity and mortality in hypertensive adults with a low ankle/arm blood pressure index. JAMA 1993;270:487–9, with permission.

predicting the 10-year risk of total CHD, one in three women at low risk with the FRS (<10%) would be restratified to a higher risk level with inclusion of the ABI (22). Approximately one of five men would have their category of risk changed from higher to lower upon inclusion of the ABI in addition to the FRS. This would likely have an effect on decisions to commence preventive treatment, such as lipid-lowering therapy.

Elderly individuals and patients with long-standing diabetes and chronic renal failure can have densely calcified vessels that are poorly compressible and have falsely elevated ankle pressures and ABI values. However, these individuals may have underlying arterial disease. The Strong Heart Study demonstrated the value of identifying subjects with abnormally high as well as low ABI measurements. Cardiovascular and all-cause mortality were lowest in patients with ABI values between 1.0 and 1.39. Risk-adjusted odds ratios for all-cause mortality were 1.69 and 1.77 for those with an ABI ≤0.90 and ≥1.40, respectively. Similar risk ratios for cardiovascular mortality were 2.52 for those in the low- and 2.09 for the high-ABI categories (23).

Indications for ABI Measurement

The ABI should be determined in patients suspected of having lower extremity PAD, including patients with exertional leg symptoms, ischemic rest pain, or nonhealing wounds (7). The ACC/AHA also recommends resting ABI measurements for screening at-risk patients to better identify those who may benefit from more stringent cardiovascular risk factor modifications. Based on the epidemiologic evidence, an "at risk" population for

PAD can be objectively defined by (a) age 70 and older, (b) age 50 to 69 with a history of smoking or diabetes mellitus, or (c) age less than 50 with at least one other atherosclerotic risk factor. In addition, the American Diabetes Association suggests ABI measurements in those who have had diabetes for at least 10 years (24). Other at-risk individuals who could benefit from ABI measurements include patients with an abnormal lower extremity pulse by exam and those with other known atherosclerotic disease, including carotid, coronary, aortic, or renal artery disease.

Limitations of the ABI

One limitation of the ABI is the inability to detect the systolic blood pressure due to noncompressible lower extremity arteries (7). If an air-filled blood pressure cuff cannot obliterate the systolic blood pressure, the ABI will be falsely elevated. This most commonly occurs in diabetic or elderly patients and is thought to be due to medial arterial calcification. Pulse volume recordings and determination of toe-brachial indices in the vascular laboratory overcome this limitation of ABI measurement, with greater sensitivity for the diagnosis of PAD. PAD of moderate severity may be undetected with a resting ABI measurement. Older studies have evaluated the accuracy of the ABI for diagnosis of PAD and were limited to cases with relatively advanced PAD. In a study of 146 limbs with angiographically documented atherosclerosis, the predictive value of reduced ABI measurements for the detection of PAD of lesser severity was found to be limited, with no significant difference in ABI between asymptomatic patients with angiographically normal-appearing arteries and those with nonobstructive PAD (25). Another population at risk for inaccurate ABI measurements is the group of patients with significant (severely stenotic or totally occluded) iliofemoral arterial disease (7). These patients may have enough collateral flow present for normal limb perfusion and to yield a normal ABI value at rest. Exercise testing and measurement of postexercise ABI may enhance the detection of PAD in these situations.

of the physiologic consequences of specific arterial stenoses. Physiologic testing for lower extremity PAD includes techniques that utilize sphygmomanometric cuffs, Doppler instruments, and plethysmographic recording devices. These tests are cost-effective and can be performed at minimal risk to the patient (25).

Segmental Pressures

Segmental pressure measurements of the lower extremities can accurately localize stenoses to specific arterial segments of the limb. Segmental pressure measurements are obtained by placing blood-pressure cuffs along the limbs, usually at the upper thigh, lower thigh, upper calf, and lower calf just above the ankle (Figure 6.4)

■ PHYSIOLOGIC TESTING FOR PAD

The noninvasive vascular laboratory provides tools to establish the anatomic localization and quantification

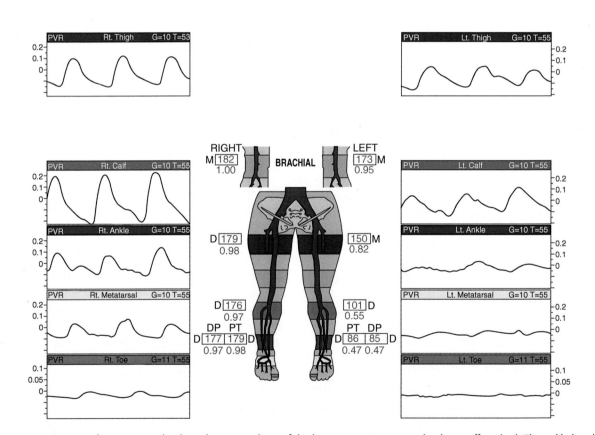

FIGURE 6.4 Segmental pressures and pulse volume recordings of the lower extremities using the three-cuff method. The ankle-brachial index is normal in the right lower extremity at rest. On the left, there is a 23 mm Hg drop from brachial to thigh pressure, consistent with possible iliofemoral artery disease. In addition, there is a 49 mm Hg pressure gradient at the level of the calf, consistent with superficial femoral artery and/or popliteal artery disease. Pulse volume recordings on the right are normal: there is a rapid systolic upstroke, a sharp peak, the downslope of the tracing bows toward the baseline and there is a dicrotic notch in diastole. On the left, pulse volume recordings are abnormal: there is a delay in systolic upstroke with a dampened peak, the downslope bows away from the baseline and the dicrotic notch is lost.

(26,27). Most vascular laboratories define a pressure gradient between adjacent segments as being significant when it is 20 mm Hg or higher (10). An aortoiliac stenosis would create a gradient between the brachial and upper thigh systolic pressures, while a superficial femoral artery (SFA) stenosis would decrease the systolic pressure recordings between the upper and lower thigh cuffs. A distal SFA or popliteal artery stenosis would cause a gradient between the lower thigh and upper calf pressures, while an infrapopliteal stenosis would decrease the lower calf pressure compared to the upper calf. Some laboratories use one thigh cuff instead of two, and some laboratories will index the pressure measurements relative to the brachial artery pressure, similar to the ABI.

Toe-Brachial Index

The toe-brachial index can be used to overcome falsely elevated or uninterpretable ABI or pressure recordings (10). Digital arteries do not undergo the same medial calcification as more proximal lower extremity arteries, thus allowing the toe-brachial index to be used for diagnosing PAD (28–33). The toe-brachial index is calculated by dividing the toe systolic pressure by the brachial artery systolic pressure. The toe systolic pressure is obtained by occluding the proximal portion of the great or second toe with a small cuff and then using a plethysmographic measuring device to record the pressure at which pulsatility returns. A toe-brachial index less than 0.7 generally leads to the diagnostic of lower extremity PAD.

Pulse Volume Recordings

Lower extremity PAD can also be diagnosed by pulse volume recordings (PVRs). The pulsatile nature of the cardiac cycle leads to an increase in blood flow during systole. Since blood vessels have an elastic wall, this pulsatility is translated into a change of volume of the lower limbs. Volume changes with each cardiac cycle can be measured by either a pneumoplethysmograph or a mercury-in-silastic strain gauge (34). The pneumoplethysmograph is the most commonly used method for PVR (Figure 6.4). When utilizing a pneumoplethysmograph for PVR, volume sensing cuffs are placed on the upper thigh, calf, and upper ankle. Pulsatility of arterial flow is transformed into a pulse volume measurement, and the pneumoplethysmograph can record the

magnitude of the pulse upstroke and its amplitude. A significant stenosis will cause dampening of the pulse volume (35,36). Decreased amplitude of PVR has been correlated with a pressure gradient of 10 mm Hg at rest and a gradient of 20 mm Hg after vasodilator exposure with papaverine (37). PVR is more accurate for assessing iliac and superficial femoral artery stenoses than for assessing distal lesions in PAD (38). PVR is useful for assessing efficacy of aortofemoral surgery in the postoperative setting, and is also useful in the preoperative setting (39,40). PVR tracings have correlated with limb salvage surgery and revascularization in patients with jeopardized limbs and flat pulse recordings. The PVR overcomes the limitations of ABI and segmental pressure recordings caused by noncompressible arteries in elderly, diabetic, or other patients.

Treadmill Exercise Testing

Exercise testing provides an important complement to the evaluation of patients with lower extremity PAD. It is useful for objectively assessing the functional severity of claudication. It can unmask PAD when the resting ABI is normal and the suspicion for lower extremity PAD is high. It aids in differentiating claudication from other nonarterial causes of leg pain ("pseudoclaudication") such as degenerative disc disease of the lumbosacral spine, spinal stenosis, hip and knee arthritis, and venous claudication. In addition, the impact of interventional and medical interventions on functional improvement can be demonstrated.

Walking ability is tested utilizing a motorized treadmill programmed for workloads that are significantly less intensive than those used for patients with coronary artery disease. Constant protocols, such as the Carter, are set at a specific speed (1.5 to 2.0 miles/hour) and treadmill grade (0% to 12%), while graded protocols, such as the Hiatt or Gardner, utilize adjustable parameters as the speed and/or treadmill grade may increase (41,42,43). First, the rest brachial and ankle pressures are measured. Second, patients exercise until they are unable to continue. During the first minute of recovery, the brachial and ankle pressures are remeasured. Patients whose exercise is limited by PAD will have a fall in ankle pressure, thus lowering the ABI. This ABI decreases because flow cannot increase during exercise beyond the zone of significant stenosis despite the reduction of resistance resulting from arteriolar dilatation, so blood pressure drops distally. A decrease in ABI of more than 20% postexercise is diagnostic for PAD. The fall in ankle pressure is directly related to the severity of arterial occlusive disease. Length of recovery to baseline ankle pressure is also directly related to severity of disease. In addition to the ABI, two parameters are recorded: the time the claudication begins (initial claudication time) and the time until cessation (absolute claudication time) (33).

Available data support the value of exercise assessment in patients with exertional limb symptoms who have normal ABI at rest. Stein et al. assessed the added value of postexercise studies in patients referred to the noninvasive vascular laboratory. Of 84 symptomatic patients who had normal ABI measurements at rest, 31% had abnormal readings after exercise (44). A study of 218 patients showed an incremental yield of 22% for the diagnosis of PAD when patients with intermittent claudication and normal resting ABI values were subjected to exercise testing (45). The limitations to the use of treadmill testing relate to patient characteristics including comorbid conditions that prevent treadmill walking. Furthermore, access to motorized devices may be limited. A six-minute walk test may serve as a reasonable alternative to treadmill testing and provide an objective assessment of the functional limitation of claudication and response to therapy in elderly individuals or others not amenable to treadmill testing (46–48).

■ ARTERIAL DUPLEX ULTRASOUND

For patients with lower extremity PAD in whom revascularization is considered, the location and severity of disease should be evaluated by additional imaging. Contrast angiography has been generally regarded as the definitive examination of lower extremity arterial disease, but this approach is invasive, expensive, and unsuitable for screening and follow-up testing. Due to technological advances in ultrasonography, CTA, and MRA in the past decade, imaging of the vascular system can be achieved noninvasively. Arterial duplex ultrasonography obtains anatomic and physiologic information directly from sites of arterial disease.

Duplex ultrasound instruments are real-time brightness mode (B-mode) scanners with built-in Doppler capabilities. A real-time B-mode imager and a Doppler instrument provide complementary information; the scanner can best outline anatomic structures, whereas a Doppler instrument yields information regarding flow and movement patterns (49). The primary clinically relevant information derived from duplex studies has been validated from analysis of the velocity of blood flow (50–58).

Hemodynamics of Blood Flow

The measurement of velocity by ultrasound requires a fundamental understanding of normal blood flow through a vessel and the hemodynamic consequences of occlusive disease. Flow is normally laminar as long as there are no curves or bends in the vessel segment (34,49). Friction occurs where blood flow comes into contact with the vessel wall, and this friction leads to a loss of kinetic energy from the flowing blood inside the vessel. Therefore, blood flow velocity decreases closer to the vessel wall. Blood flowing through the luminal center of the vessel does not experience the same friction and subsequent loss of kinetic energy, so velocities are greatest at the center of the lumen. This type of laminar flow occurs in the straight segment of a vessel. Because the vessel is not an inanimate conduit, there are variations in blood flow based on the cardiac cycle. As expected, blood flow velocity increases during systole and decreases during diastole. When there are perturbations of the vessel conduit, such as a normal branch point or an atherosclerotic plaque, laminar flow is disturbed. There is a greater pressure decrease in the presence of nonlaminar or turbulent flow compared to laminar flow.

Flow through a conduit is driven by a change in pressure across the length of the conduit. A higher pressure head at the proximal segment of a vessel drives flow through the vessel to the lower pressure distal segment of the vessel. As such, blood flow follows Poiseuille's law, which states that flow through a conduit is proportional to the change in pressure between the proximal and distal ends of the conduit. The blood vessel radius is the most influential variable affecting flow. Flow is proportional to the radius of the vessel to the fourth power and therefore small increases or decreases in vessel diameter can greatly impact blood flow velocity. For example, a 25% narrowing of a blood vessel leads to a 70% decrease in blood flow. Blood flow is inversely proportional to the viscosity of the liquid and length of the segment. The viscosity of blood and the pressure and length of the vessel do not vary greatly in the cardiovascular system (34,49). Since flow through a vessel is constant, flow at the segment proximal to a stenosis must equal flow through the stenosis, as well as flow distal to the stenosis. Following the continuity equation, which states that flow can be calculated by the product of velocity and cross-sectional area of a vessel, velocity must increase through a stenotic area in order to preserve constant flow through a vessel. The increase in "stenotic zone" velocity is directly proportional to the severity of luminal narrowing (45). Measuring velocity of blood flow by Doppler ultrasound can be used to determine the presence of a stenosis, and it is the most validated method for grading stenosis severity.

Doppler Ultrasound

Vascular ultrasonography can measure blood flow velocity by way of the Doppler affect, which relies on the change in ultrasound frequency associated with movement of a reflective surface towards or away from the ultrasound source. The reflective surface in the vasculature is the red blood cell. As blood flow moves away from the observer and the ultrasound source the ultrasound wave is reflected off of red blood cells that are moving away from the ultrasound source. This causes a decrease in the frequency of the ultrasound waves as they travel back from the reflective surface to the ultrasound source. Conversely, as blood flow moves toward the ultrasound source, the ultrasound waves reflected off of red blood cells have an increase in frequency. The Doppler shift frequency compares the frequency of emitted ultrasound waves to the frequency of the reflected waves as they return to the ultrasound source. The Doppler shift depends on the source ultrasound wave frequency, the velocity of the reflecting surface, and the angle between the emitted ultrasound beam and the direction of the moving reflective surface, or Doppler angle (Figure 6.5).

The Doppler equation can be used to convert the frequency shift to velocity of blood flow once the Doppler beam-to-vessel angle is determined. The maximum measurement of frequency shift is at a Doppler angle of 0 degrees; however, as blood vessels run parallel to the body's surface, this angle cannot be reliably obtained in vascular imaging. Thus the ultrasound beam will be incident at angle other than 0 degrees and the detected Doppler frequency will be reduced by the cosine of this angle for blood flow velocity measurements. The ideal angle of measurement between the emitted ultrasound

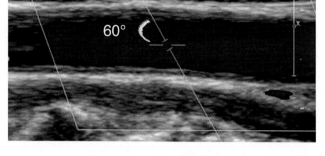

FIGURE 6.5 The Doppler angle is the angle between the emitted ultrasound beam and sample cursor aligned with flow. Blood flow velocity measurements are corrected by the cosine of the Doppler angle. In the vascular laboratory a Doppler angle of 60 degrees is optimal.

wave and blood flow in the vascular laboratory is 60°. Small errors in determining the Doppler angle when the angle of insonation is 60° or less have little overall effect on the velocity calculation, and Doppler angles between 45° and 60° are acceptable for most clinical studies (49).

Spectral Doppler Analysis

Doppler velocity measurements are the main tools used for evaluation of stenosis severity (Table 6.2). The increase in stenotic zone flow velocity is directly proportional to the severity of arterial luminal narrowing. Peak systole is the first Doppler measurement to increase in the area of a stenosis. The region of maximal velocity may be small and therefore the sonographer must carefully interrogate the stenotic lumen with the sample volume in order to detect the area of highest flow velocity. If the vessel diameter reduction is generally less that 50%, a pressure gradient will not present during diastole. With moderate stenoses (50%–70%), however, a pressure gradient exists throughout diastole and end diastolic velocity (EDV) increases. Diastolic velocities are high in the presence of severe stenoses (70%–90%). The systolic velocity ratio, which is a ratio of the peak systolic velocity within the stenosis compared with that of a proximal normal arterial segment, is commonly used. This parameter is used to compensate for patient-to-patient hemodynamic variables such as cardiac function, heart rate, blood pressure, and arterial compliance (49).

■ **Table 6.2**	Doppler characteristics and stenosis severity		
Stenosis	Velocity	Waveform	Spectral Broadening
0% to 19%	Normal	Triphasic	–
20% to 49%	< double the proximal segment; plaque present	Triphasic or biphasic	+
50% to 99%	> double the proximal segment and >200 cm/s	Monophasic	+
Occlusion	No flow	Monophasic Occlusive thump	NA

Source: Zierler RE, Zierler BK. Duplex sonography of lower extremity arteries. *Semin Ultrasound CT MR* 1997;18:43, with permission.

Peak systolic velocity (PSV) rises with progressive narrowing of the arterial lumen; however, in high-grade stenoses (>80% diameter reduction) the flow resistance becomes so high that PSV falls to normal or low levels (49). In the presence of a complete occlusion, a low velocity monophasic signal or "thump" is visualized and often heard (Figure 6.6). It is important to differentiate low velocity flow in a high-grade occlusion from a complete occlusion. Power Doppler flow imaging, or power Doppler, is an additional way to detect blood flow and has utility in this situation (Figure 6.7). Unlike standard Doppler, in which the Doppler frequency shift is mapped, power Doppler displays the whole amplitude of the returning Doppler signal. This provides a more sensitive way to detect blood flow and is less influenced by the Doppler angle (49). Sensitivity for the detection of blood flow is increased 3 to 5 times (60).

Additional information about blood flow can be obtained by analyzing the Doppler velocity waveform. There are distinctive characteristics of blood flow in the normal vessel and in the diseased state that can be used in the evaluation of atherosclerotic vessels. PSV varies according to the location of the artery, and the Doppler velocity waveform may also vary according to the segment being examined. Healthy peripheral arteries will have a triphasic waveform, and they are said to be of high resistance (Figure 6.8). Ventricular systole causes an initial high-velocity forward flow, which gives a PSV measurement. As the ventricle relaxes during diastole, the aortic pressure is briefly greater than the ventricular

pressure while the aortic valve is still open. This results in early diastolic flow reversal, which is the second part of the triphasic waveform. Healthy blood vessels will then propel blood forward as they recoil due to their vessel wall elasticity. This represents the third phase of the triphasic waveform. When peripheral arteries are atherosclerotic, they often lose their ability for elastic recoil, and the third phase of the triphasic waveform is absent. Contrasting the high resistance waveform of normal peripheral arteries, the Doppler velocity waveform recorded from low resistance vessels will have continuous flow during diastole. The resistance is low in these vessels due to either dilation of distal arterioles or continuation with a low-resistant circuit. One example of a low-resistance vessel is the normal internal carotid artery (ICA) (Figure 6.9).

As previously described, blood flow through a vessel should be laminar. When all blood cells are moving at the same speed through a vessel during the various times of a cardiac cycle, the Doppler waveform should be a narrow, sharply defined tracing (34,61). The tracing appears as an envelope with a hollow center (Figure 6.9). When a luminal irregularity, such as a bifurcation or stenosis, is present, turbulent flow replaces laminar flow. The Doppler waveform tracing broadens (termed "spectral broadening"), and the envelope with a hollow center is replaced by a waveform that is either almost or completely filled in (see Figure 6.12). A poststenotic waveform often has a delayed systolic upstroke and decreased amplitude in addition to spectral broadening and turbulence.

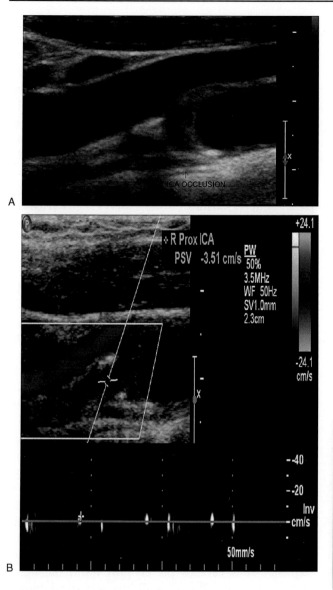

FIGURE 6.6 Grayscale image (A) of a totally occluded internal carotid artery. (B): the typical preocclusive Doppler signal or "thump" at the sight of a total occlusion.

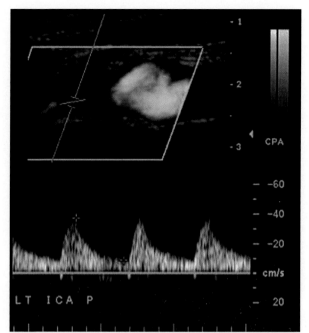

FIGURE 6.7 Power Doppler image displaying the "string sign," indicating a near-total occlusion of the internal carotid artery. Spectral Doppler shows low velocity flow within the near-total occlusion.

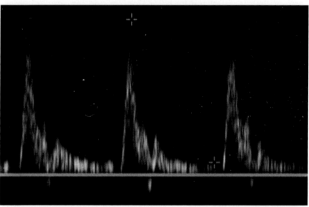

FIGURE 6.8 Normal, triphasic waveform of high-resistance vessels.

Grayscale Imaging

Pairing ultrasound grayscale technology with Doppler waveform analysis further enhances the evaluation of atherosclerotic disease. Grayscale imaging enables visualization and characterization of plaque, calcification and aneurysmal disease. However, it is not possible to accurately define the degree of arterial luminal narrowing based on the grayscale imaging alone. Ultrasound

waves emitted from a probe are reflected by tissue just as they are reflected by red blood cells. Tissue structure, such as density and size, determine the proportion of reflected ultrasound waves. Tissue depth determines the time between sound wave emission, reflection, and detection. A grayscale, or B-mode, image reconstructs an image of the tissue based on the number of reflected waves and the time required for their return to the ultrasound probe. Each emitted and detected

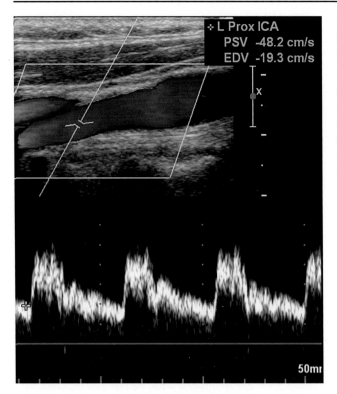

FIGURE 6.9 Duplex ultrasound of a normal internal carotid artery. Laminar flow is visualized by color Doppler and the spectral waveform appears as an envelope with a hollow center. The waveform of the internal carotid artery demonstrates continuous diastolic flow seen in low resistance vessels. The peak systolic velocity is 48 cm/sec, which is normal.

pulse is displayed as a gray dot on a video screen, with the strength of the reflected wave correlating with the brightness mode. The transmitting frequency of Doppler probes used for peripheral arterial examinations ranges from 2 to 10 MHz. Ultrasound probes with higher frequencies are better suited to image superficial structures, while probes with lower frequencies are able to image structures at greater depth without attenuation. Harmonic algorithms provide greater clarity with B-mode imaging. This elimination of artifacts such as speckle and reverberation is due to the wider bandwidth of ultrasound transducers that allows the detection of the fundamental frequency and its harmonics.

Color Doppler

Color Doppler is another important tool available for vascular imaging. Color Doppler entails processing the frequency shift of each reflected ultrasound wave

that returns to the ultrasound probe and reconstructing a velocity map from this information. The velocity map provides velocity information for each point in the Doppler field. When superimposed on the grayscale anatomic image, real-time flow can be seen in relation to the vessel walls. This serves as a "road map" for the imager and has been shown to improve detection of arterial stenoses (62). A two-color system is used, with one color representing flow toward the probe, and the second color representing flow away from the probe. Assigning the color to an increasing or decreasing frequency shift is arbitrary, but most users assign red to flow within arteries and blue to flow within veins. Within the two color system, there is a color spectrum representing frequency shifts or velocities (Figure 6.10A). At each end of the spectrum white represents the highest velocity, including both velocities towards the probe and velocities away from the probe. The hue of the color becomes more saturated as the velocity of blood flow decreases and desaturated as velocity increases. The pulse repetition frequency should be adjusted so that laminar flow is represented as a homogeneous color in the color map.

Incorporating the principles of the Doppler shift and laminar blood flow, the observer can delineate areas of stenosis within a vessel. When the flow velocity increases in the area of a stenosis, flow color will desaturate. Similarly, when a stenosis causes turbulent flow, the flow velocity increases, and a sudden color change is seen on the color Doppler velocity map (Figure 6.10B). The Nyquist limit can be reached due to the higher velocities of flow through a stenosis, resulting in aliasing at the site of an arterial stenosis. Once the Doppler frequency shift exceeds the Nyquist limit, the signal appears as a reversal in flow direction (termed "wraparound"). Wraparound is seen in poststenotic segments and can be visualized as a mosaic pattern in the area of turbulent flow. Whenever a significant flow disturbance is detected, the sonographer should search carefully for an adjacent stenosis or other arterial pathology such as an arterial dissection or an arteriovenous fistula. Occasionally acoustic shadowing from calcified plaque may obscure visualization of a stenosis and poststenotic flow disturbance may be the clue (49). Color Doppler images from a healthy peripheral artery should have an alternating color flow pattern due to the diastolic flow reversal seen during the second phase of the triphasic waveform. Severely stenosed vessels will not have early diastolic flow reversal, and the Doppler waveform will

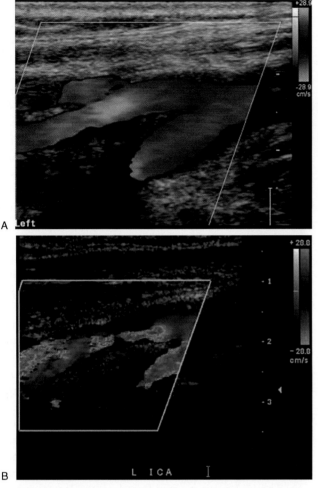

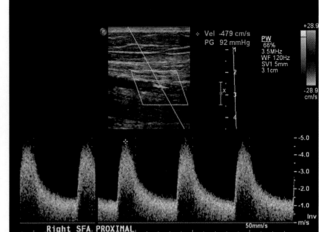

FIGURE 6.11 Stenosis of the superficial femoral artery. Peak systolic velocity is 479 cm/sec, consistent with a 50% to 99% stenosis.

FIGURE 6.10 (A) Color Doppler image of the carotid bifurcation and the internal and external carotid arteries. (B) Color Doppler image of an internal carotid artery stenosis, showing turbulent flow and color aliasing at the site of a severe stenosis. An echolucent plaque is visualized.

be a spectral monophasic waveform (63). This flow pattern results in color persistence, which is continuous flow in the forward direction only.

Peripheral Arterial Ultrasonography

Duplex ultrasound is extremely useful in determining the presence and severity of lower extremity PAD. Grayscale imaging, color Doppler imaging, and pulsed Doppler velocity analysis are used in combination to elucidate the location and severity of disease (Figure 6.11). Color Doppler displays abnormal flow patterns of turbulence and aliasing in areas of stenoses. Spectral Doppler is used to characterize stenoses through determination of elevated systolic velocity or EDV within the area of stenosis, together with visualization of spectral broadening of the Doppler waveform and changes in arterial pulsatility (see Table 6.2) (34). In general, the ratios of PSV within an area of stenosis compared with velocities in an adjacent upstream segment have been found to be the most accurate diagnostic criterion. A ratio greater than 2 is commonly used to diagnose a stenosis greater than 50% diameter (46,47,50,52).

The sensitivity and specificity for the diagnosis of stenoses greater than 50% diameter from the iliac arteries to the popliteal arteries are both 90% to 95%. One meta-analysis determined a sensitivity of 93% and a specificity of 95% for color-guided duplex (58). One pitfall of arterial ultrasound is the presence of serial or "tandem" stenoses. Because of dissipation of flow distally to the site of a significant stenosis, the severity of stenoses located distally to the first lesion may be underestimated (48,64). Accuracy is diminished in examinations of the iliac arteries if the vessels are suboptimally visualized due to bowel gas or body habitus. Dense calcification can also obscure flow due to acoustic shadowing.

Duplex ultrasound is used following endovascular procedures of the lower extremities to detect restenosis. Duplex surveillance after percutaneous transluminal angioplasty (PTA) and stenting procedures is performed immediately following intervention, at one, three, and six months postintervention, then annually. Color Doppler, pulsed-wave Doppler velocity measurements, and Doppler waveform analysis are utilized for evaluation of restenosis at the site of intervention. A doubling of the PSV is consistent with a hemodynamically significant stenosis. Immediately after angioplasty, several studies suggested that velocities in the treated segment may be abnormally elevated and do not predict decreased subsequent patency rates (65–67). This may be due to vessel dissections produced by angioplasty that successfully remodel over time. Two contradictory studies suggest that elevated velocities immediately after PTA do predict early PTA failure (68,69). It is generally assumed that early detection of lesions and identification of the need for reintervention may improve long-term arterial patency. However, there are no published studies that have evaluated this hypothesis.

Peripheral arterial bypass grafts fail when stenoses develop within the body of the graft, at the anastomosis, or upstream or downstream from the graft. These stenoses may thrombose and threaten the graft patency even if the patient is asymptomatic and the ABI is unchanged. Duplex ultrasound surveillance studies of grafts allow detection of these stenoses before graft thrombosis with greater sensitivity than evaluation by clinical history, physical examination, or use of the resting ABI (70–76). Case series have indicated that revision of such asymptomatic stenoses improves long-term patency of vein grafts. Recommended surveillance intervals for vein grafts are usually one, three, six and 12 months after surgery and annually thereafter. Duplex ultrasound surveillance of synthetic grafts is of unclear value. Studies have reported conflicting results regarding improvement in patency of synthetic grafts when clinician decisions were guided by results of duplex studies (77–79).

Duplex ultrasound is also employed for the evaluation of aneurysms and pseudoaneurysms of the lower extremities, arteriovenous fistulae, arterial dissection, popliteal artery entrapment syndrome, as well as evaluation of the upper extremities in individuals with vascular disease.

Carotid Duplex Ultrasonography

Stroke is the third leading cause of death in the United States where over 350,000 strokes per year are due to extracranial carotid artery disease (10,80). When symptoms occur due to extracranial carotid artery disease, embolic events are usually the precursor, not thrombotic events. The risk of ischemic stroke is directly related to the severity of stenosis.

Carotid duplex ultrasound is a noninvasive, safe, reliable and reproducible diagnostic test that combines grayscale imaging color Doppler and pulsed Doppler analysis to localize a stenosis and assess its severity. The positive predictive value for carotid duplex ultrasonography to detect a hemodynamically significant stenosis is more than 95% (82). In many centers carotid ultrasonography, often combined with computerized tomographic angiography (CTA) and magnetic resonance angiography (MRA), has replaced the need for most contrast angiograms in patients with carotid artery disease. Indications for extracranial carotid artery imaging include stroke, transient ischemic attack, amaurosis fugax, carotid bruit in an asymptomatic individual, as well as follow-up of known carotid artery stenosis and surveillance after carotid endarterectomy or carotid stenting (34,80). A comprehensive duplex examination of the extracranial arteries includes imaging of the brachiocephalic, carotid, subclavian, and vertebral arteries.

It is important to remember that the common carotid artery (CCA) usually lies medial to the internal jugular vein, and it bifurcates into the ICA and external carotid artery (ECA) at the level of the cricoid cartilage. The ICA is most often found posterolateral to the anteromedially located ECA, and usually has a larger diameter at its origin (Figure 6.10A). The ECA is further distinguished by its branches found in the cervical region, which are not found in the ICA in this region. For ultrasound interrogation of the extracranial carotid arteries, transverse and longitudinal images using grayscale technique are acquired first, starting at the clavicle and then moving cephalad to the angle of the jaw using both the anterolateral and posterolateral views (81). Atherosclerosis is most often found at the ostia of the ICA, while fibromuscular dysplasia is usually more distally located.

When evaluating for carotid artery stenosis, color Doppler is very useful in identifying abnormal flow patterns of turbulence and aliasing in areas of stenoses (Figure 6.10B). Interpretation of disease severity and quantification of stenosis by Doppler spectral waveform evaluation remains the most accurate method of quantifying disease. Pulse-wave Doppler sample volumes should be taken sequentially along the entire length of the stenotic lumen in order to obtain the maximal Doppler velocity. Each sample should be taken immediately adjacent to the previous sample, providing a thorough evaluation of the entire vessel segment. Flow patterns can normalize shortly after a focal carotid artery stenosis. Without such an approach, a significant stenosis can be easily missed or underestimated. Proximal, mid, and distal velocity measurements should be taken from the CCA, and PSV and EDV measurements should be taken from the proximal, mid, and distal segments of the ICA.

PSV, EDV, and velocity ratios are used to estimate the severity of ICA stenoses (Table 6.3). An ICA PSV less than 125 cm/sec with no visible plaque or intimal thickening is indicative of a normal artery, while an ICA PSV less than 125 cm/sec with visual evidence of plaque or intimal thickening suggests stenosis less than 50% (82). An ICA PSV between 125–230 cm/sec with visual evidence of plaque suggests a 50% to 69% stenosis, and an ICA PSV greater than 230 cm/sec with evidence of plaque and lumen narrowing suggests a stenosis of at least 70%. As previously discussed, flow through a severe stenosis

(>90% obstruction) may be impaired to the extent that the velocities are actually decreased instead of increased. Near occlusion is suggested by a markedly narrowed lumen seen by color Doppler ultrasound, and total occlusion is suggested by the absence of a patent lumen on grayscale imaging and no flow visualized by spectral, power, and color Doppler (Figures 6.6, 6.7).

The EDV is also useful for the evaluation of ICA stenoses, particularly high-grade stenoses. EDV is usually less than 40 cm/sec until a 60% stenosis is encountered. The EDV velocity increases to between 40 and 110 cm/sec for a 60% to 69 % stenosis, 110 and 140 cm/sec for a 70% to 79% stenosis, and more than 140 cm/sec for an 80% to 95% stenosis (Figure 6.12). Decreased cardiac output or aortic valve disease can limit the usual velocity increases expected in the presence of a stenosis. To compensate for such hemodynamic variables, the PSV of the ICA is compared to the PSV of the distal CCA as a ratio. An ICA/CCA PSV ratio >2 is consistent with significant narrowing, while a ratio >4 is consistent with high-grade stenosis.

Analysis of the spectral Doppler waveform is also useful in the evaluation of carotid artery stenosis. The CCA waveform can provide clues to stenoses located

■ Table 6.3 Doppler criteria for carotid artery stenosis

| Degree of Stenosis, % | Primary Parameters | | Additional Parameters | |
	ICA PSV, cm/sec	Plaque Estimate, %	ICA/CCA PSV Ratio	ICA EDV, cm/sec
Normal	<125	None	<2.0	<40
<50	<125	<50	<2.0	<40
50–69	125–230	≥50	2.0–4.0	40–100
≥ but less than near occlusion	>230	≥50	<4.0	>100
Near occlusion	High, low, or undetectable	Vissible	Variable	Variable
Total occlusion	Undetectable	Visible, no detectable lumen	Not applicable	Not applicable

Plaque estimate (diameter reduction) with grayscale and color Doppler ultrasound.
CCA, common carotid artery; ICA, internal carotid artery; EDV, end diastolic velocity; PSV, peak systolic velocity.
Source: From Ref. 82, with permission.

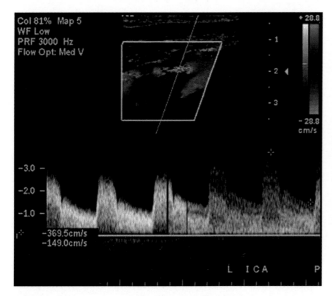

FIGURE 6.12 Internal carotid artery stenosis. The peak systolic velocity is 369 cm/s and the end diastolic velocity is 149 cm/s, consistent with a 80% to 99% stenosis. Filling of the Doppler spectral window or "spectral broadening" is displayed.

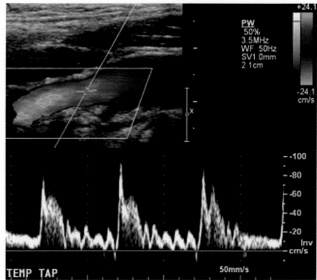

FIGURE 6.13 External carotid artery with "temporal tap" reflected in the Doppler waveform.

proximally or distally. If the brachiocephalic artery is severely stenosed, the attached CCA waveform will be dampened with a delayed upstroke and low PSV. The CCA waveform can provide a clue for a total ICA occlusion. The CCA spectral waveform should have greater diastolic flow than the ECA, but less diastolic flow than the ICA. When the ipsilateral ICA is totally occluded, the CCA waveform will display impaired (or even absent) diastolic flow.

One practical pitfall in carotid duplex ultrasonography is confusing the ICA and ECA. In addition to recognizing distinguishing anatomic features, analysis of the spectral Doppler waveforms is helpful. The ICA, being a low-resistance vessel, has more diastolic flow than the ECA. However in the setting of a near or total ICA occlusion, the ECA waveform may demonstrate more diastolic flow or diminished "pulsatility," as it supplies collateral flow to the low-resistance cerebral circulation. Tapping on the preauricular branch of the temporal artery ("temporal tap") will cause oscillation in the diastolic portion of the ECA Doppler waveform but not in the diastolic portion of the ICA waveform (Figure 6.13).

After the carotid arteries are evaluated, the vertebral artery is imaged in a similar fashion. The vertebral artery lies posterior to the carotid artery between the spinous processes. Because of this course, assessment of the vertebral artery with duplex ultrasound is incomplete, with lower sensitivity for the detection of stenoses. Spectral Doppler sampling should be performed along the length of the vertebral artery as cephalad as anatomy allows. Vertebral artery stenosis is suggested when velocities are greater than 125 cm/sec (34). Due to limited visualization of the vessel, the Doppler waveform may serve as a particularly valuable clue to the presence of a significant stenosis. A dampened waveform is suggestive of a more proximal stenosis, whereas a highly resistive waveform with loss of diastolic flow raises suspicion for a high-grade distal vertebral artery stenosis. When subclavian steal occurs, vertebral artery flow is reversed. This can be confirmed by comparing the retrograde vertebral artery flow to the antegrade CCA flow. The subclavian artery is a high resistance vessel, so diastolic flow is decreased during subclavian steal. If subclavian steal is suspected by antegrade vertebral artery flow paired with decreased or reversed diastolic flow, maneuvers can be performed to elicit retrograde systolic vertebral artery flow (34). Arm exercise or inflation and then deflation of a blood pressure cuff (both on the ipsilateral side of the vertebral artery being examined) will increase blood flow requirements in the subclavian artery. If a stenosis is present proximal to the takeoff of the vertebral artery, this increased circulatory demand will cause retrograde systolic vertebral artery flow.

Imaging of the subclavian artery follows. Because the subclavian artery lies beneath the clavicle, the ultrasound probe should be placed longitudinally over the clavicle and positioned so that images can be obtained under the clavicle. The artery should be scanned from its most proximal portion to its most distal point. Color Doppler should be used to detect turbulence suggestive of stenosis. A marked increase in PSV suggests stenosis. A doubling of the PSV coincides with at least a 50% stenosis.

In addition to Doppler waveform analysis and velocity measurements, grayscale or B-mode images of the carotid arteries add to the evaluation of plaque (Figure 6.14). The presence, characteristic, and volume of carotid artery plaque can be described. The presence of carotid plaque is noted when matter thickens the intima and extends into the vessel lumen. Two examples of plaque characteristics are ulceration and echolucency. An ulceration is presumed present when an indentation containing flow is seen in the plaque, and echolucency is defined as plaque that is less echogenic than the adjacent muscle (Figure 6.10B). Volume is best measured with the transducer probe slicing a cross-sectional view through the artery. Besides plaque, B-mode imaging can also detect dissection. If a dissection flap is not noticed by B-mode imaging, color Doppler may be helpful by displaying flow in the true and false lumina. Once a dissection is detected, luminal velocities should be measured, and the extent of the dissection should be determined.

Carotid Ultrasound and Cardiovascular Risk Assessment

Measurement of carotid intima-media thickness (C-IMT) with B-mode ultrasound is a noninvasive, sensitive, and reproducible technique for identifying and quantifying subclinical vascular disease and for evaluating cardiovascular disease (CVD) risk (83). Intimal thickening of the carotid arteries has correlated well with systemic atherosclerosis, but since the intima alone is difficult to image, intima-media thickness (IMT) has substituted the measurement of the intima. IMT is the measurement from the lumen-intima interface to the media-adventitia interface (Figure 6.15), and is a useful marker of systemic atherosclerosis since the carotid artery media is relatively thin and does not significantly alter the measurement of intimal thickening. IMT increases with age, correlates well with other coronary artery disease risk factors, and predicts future cardiovascular events (84). Increases in C-IMT, whether measured as an absolute value or as the rate of progression, have correlated with myocardial infarcton and stroke (85–87). Plaque should be differentiated from IMT. Carotid plaque is defined as the presence of focal wall thickening that is at least 50% greater than that of the surrounding vessel wall. A number of large epidemiologic studies have demonstrated similar or greater predictive power for carotid plaque and CVD (88).

C-IMT measurements should be limited to the far wall of the CCA and acquired at end diastole. The

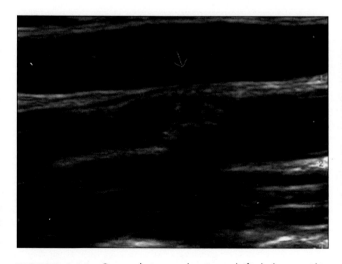

FIGURE 6.14 Grayscale image showing calcified plaque within the internal carotid artery.

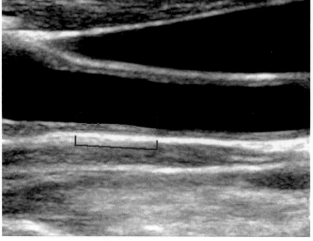

FIGURE 6.15 Measurement of carotid intimal medial thickness. Semiautomated edge detection software is used to measure mean far wall IMT of the common carotid artery.

exam should be supplemented by a thorough scan of the extracranial carotid arteries for the presence of carotid plaque to increase sensitivity for identifying subclinical vascular disease. There are ways of improving the quality of IMT ultrasound images (89,90). Utilizing harmonic frequencies improves clarity by increasing the signal-to-noise ratio as well as spatial resolution, while contrast agents provide a better estimation of the intima-lumen border. Eliminating manual measurement techniques with computerized edge-tracking methods also improves reproducibility.

Measuring C-IMT and identifying carotid plaque can be useful for refining CVD risk assessment in patients at intermediate CVD risk according to the Framingham risk score (i.e., patients with a 6%–20% 10-year risk of myocardial infarction or coronary heart disease death who do not have established coronary heart disease or coronary disease risk equivalent conditions). Patients with the following clinical circumstances also might be considered for testing: (a) family history of premature CVD in a first-degree relative, (b) individuals younger than 60 years old with severe abnormalities in a single risk factor who otherwise would not be candidates for pharmacotherapy, or (c) women younger than 60 years old with at least two CVD risk factors (83). Normal IMT measurements have been reported in the range of 0.4–1.0 mm, and 1.2 mm has been used as the cutoff between normal and abnormal (90,91). However, age, gender, ethnicity, and timing with respect to the cardiac cycle all influence IMT measurement. For CVD risk assessment, CIMT values should be reported in percentiles by age, sex, and race/ethnicity, as determined by the Atherosclerosis Risk in Communities Study, a large epidemiologic study (85). The presence of carotid plaque or C-IMT greater than or equal to 75th percentile for the patient's age, sex, and race/ethnicity are indicative of increased CVD risk and may signify the need for more aggressive risk-reduction interventions.

Abdominal Aortic Aneurysm

Atherosclerosis can manifest as diseases of the aorta and iliac arteries, leading to stenosis or the formation of aneurysm. Aneurysmal dilatation most commonly affects the abdominal aorta below the renal arteries (92). When the diameter of a segment of the abdominal aorta is greater than 1.5 times the nearest normal segment, it is considered aneurysmal. Dilatation of the distal abdominal aorta to more than 3.0 cm also qualifies

as an aneurysm. Abdominal aneurysms are more often fusiform and less often saccular (Figure 6.16).

The prevalence of abdominal aortic aneurysms (AAA) in Western nations is 4.5% at age 65 and 10.8% at 80 (93,94). The risk of developing an AAA increases with a family history of AAA (95). The same risk factors that lead to atherosclerosis contribute to the formation of abdominal aneurysms, including tobacco use, male gender, age, hypertension, and hyperlipidemia. For unknown reasons, men are at greater risk for developing an aneurysm, while women are at greater risk for aneurysm rupture. Most individuals with an aneurysm are asymptomatic, and are diagnosed incidentally on imaging studies or physical examination. Notably, physical exam is only 58% sensitive and 75% specific for the detection of AAA of 3 cm and larger (97–99). The risk of rupture increases directly with aneurysm size, and the death rate associated with rupture approaches 90%. A large, prospective study in men 65 to 74 years of age has demonstrated the utility and cost-effectiveness of ultrasound screening in reducing aneurysm-related deaths (100). Most aortic aneurysms evolve between ages 60 and 70; if the abdominal aorta is normal in size by age 70, the likelihood of developing a significant aneurysm is very low (80,101–103). Current ACC/AHA guidelines recommend ultrasound screening of AAAs for men ≥60 years of age who are siblings or offspring of patients with AAAs (class 1), and men 65 to 75 years of age who have ever smoked (class 2a) (10).

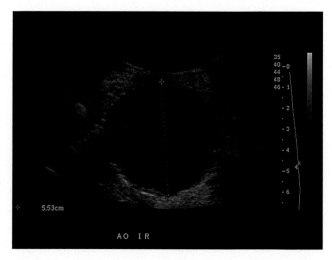

FIGURE 6.16 Grayscale image of a 5.5-cm infrarenal abdominal aortic aneurysm.

Whether performed for diagnostic or screening purposes, abdominal duplex ultrasound is an efficient, reliable imaging modality for the evaluation of abdominal aortic aneurysms. Since the aorta is located deep to the body surface, a low frequency probe should be used—2.5 MHz, for example (34). Bowel gas can obscure imaging, so the patient should fast prior to the exam. It is recommended that the aorta be visualized in the transverse, sagittal, and coronal plains from the diaphragm to the aortic bifurcation, and that the iliac arteries (to the level of the iliac bifurcation) also be examined. Diameter measurements are taken from outer wall to outer wall at end diastole. Aneurysms can be measured to within 0.3 cm, and the sensitivity ranges from 87% to 99% (79). While scanning the abdominal aorta, the celiac artery, superior mesenteric artery, and then right and left renal arteries should be visualized and examined for stenoses. The inferior mesenteric artery should be seen just proximal to the iliac bifurcation. The celiac, superior mesenteric, and inferior mesenteric arteries exhibit high-resistance Doppler waveforms in the fasting state and low-resistance waveforms postprandially.

Renal Artery Duplex Ultrasonography

Atherosclerotic renal artery stenosis can cause flash pulmonary edema, refractory hypertension, renal insufficiency, and unstable angina (104). It is an important cause of renal failure, leading to nearly 20% of end-stage renal disease in patients over the age of 50.

Renovascular disease most commonly occurs as one of two types (105): Atherosclerotic disease, which usually affects the proximal third of the main renal artery in older men, and fibromuscular dysplasia (FMD), which more often affects the distal two thirds of the main renal artery or its side branches in younger women. Fibromuscular dysplasia is a dysplastic disorder of unknown etiology that involves overgrowth of smooth muscle cells and fibrous tissue within the arterial wall. In its most common form, the media is primarily involved and has a characteristic "beads on a string" angiographic appearance cause by alternating areas of medial fibroplasia and focal aneurysmal dilatation (49). It is preferentially seen in young Caucasian women, and it is eight times more common in women than men (106). Although the renal arteries are the most common site for FMD, atherosclerotic etiologies for renovascular disease are more common. Significant renal artery stenosis, defined as at least 60% narrowing of renal artery diameter by duplex ultrasonography, has been found in nearly 7% of elderly people, and renal artery narrowing by 70% or greater has been found in 7% of hypertensive patients undergoing invasive coronary angiography. When a renal artery is stenosed by at least 60%, there is a greater likelihood of developing total occlusion over time (at a rate of 10%–20% per year) (107).

Screening for renal artery stenosis is appropriate when clinical features that increase suspicion are present (Table 6.4). Both invasive and noninvasive modalities can be used to evaluate renal arterial anatomy. If a patient suspected of having renal artery stenosis will be undergoing an invasive arterial procedure for a different purpose, it may be reasonable to perform a low-volume digital subtraction aortogram (DSA) during the invasive arterial procedure. Additionally, if an invasive evaluation will be performed regardless of the results of

Table 6.4 Clinical predictors of renal artery stenosis	
Risk Factors	**Renal Markers**
Smoker	Renal impairment of unknown etiology
Other atherosclerotic disease (coronary, peripheral)	Azotemia or decline in renal function after ACEI or ARB therapy
	Size discrepancy between kidneys greater than 1.5 cm by ultrasound
Patient History	Atrophic kidney
Onset of hypertension before age 30 or after age 55	
Abrupt, severe, or resistant hypertension	**Physical Exam**
Pulmonary edema	Abdominal or other bruits

Note: Increasing number of clinical predictors should heighten the suspicion of renal artery stenosis.
ACEI, angiotensin-converting enzyme inhibitor; ARB, angiotensin receptor blocker.

noninvasive testing, imaging should be bypassed in favor of DSA aortogram. However, in the absence of indications for direct renal artery angiography, noninvasive imaging of the renal arteries with renal artery duplex ultrasound, CTA, and MRA are preferred (108).

Renal artery duplex ultrasonography is accurate and reliable in detecting hemodynamically significant renal artery stenosis, and its use is an ACC/AHA Class Ib recommendation for screening patients for renal artery stenosis (10,109,110). When compared to invasive angiography, Duplex ultrasound has a sensitivity of 84% to 98% and a specificity of 62% to 99% for detecting renal artery stenosis (111–117) Additionally, unlike other procedures that require contrast dye, there is no risk of exacerbating renal dysfunction with ultrasonography. As with other sonographic studies of the abdomen, patients should fast overnight prior to imaging to minimize bowel gas. When renal artery disease is suspected as a cause of renal insufficiency, a negative renal duplex ultrasound examination is sufficient to exclude obstructive disease (usually bilateral stenosis of the main renal arteries) as the etiology (118). However, renovascular hypertension may still be present despite a negative renal artery duplex scan; it can arise from a stenotic lesion of an accessory or branch renal artery, and only 40% of accessory renal arteries are identified by this examination (34,96). Renal artery duplex ultrasonography involves systematic spectral Doppler evaluation of the aorta, renal arteries, and renal parenchyma (34). Renal artery flow is compared to aortic flow at the level of the renal arteries when characterizing the severity of a renal arterial stenosis (renal/aortic ratio). Additionally, B-mode images of the kidneys are obtained for measurement and comparison of kidney size.

To ensure that a stenosis is not missed, the renal arteries should be evaluated from two views. Imaging begins with the patient in the supine position. By imaging the aorta along its longitudinal axis the renal arteries are visualized just caudal to the celiac artery and superior mesenteric artery. The right renal artery can also be visualized with the patient in the left lateral decubitis position. Similarly, the left renal artery should be imaged with the patient in the right lateral position and the operator using a posterolateral transducer position (119). A diligent search should be made for duplicate main renal arteries. B-mode measurements for kidney length should be measured with the patient in the decubitus position. This is important since an affected kidney is often less than 9 cm in length in the presence of an occluded renal artery, and there is often a 1.5 cm or greater size discrepancy between kidney lengths in the presence of significant renal artery stenosis. The right renal artery is often evaluated first; it is more readily visualized compared to the left. Once the ostium of the right renal artery has been identified, the Doppler cursor should be repositioned from the aorta to the origin of the right renal artery. Color and spectral Doppler images should be obtained from the ostium to the hilum of the kidney (Fig. 6.17). When evaluating the segmental renal arteries and the hilum, low velocity range and low wall filter settings should be used.

There are a number of ways to evaluate a renal artery segment for stenosis. Nonstenosed renal arteries have a low resistance waveform. Systolic waveforms are broad, and forward flow is present throughout diastole. The PSV in normal renal arteries ranges from 74 to 127 cm/sec (120–123). In the presence of renal artery stenosis, velocity of blood flow through a stenosed arterial segment is increased, and systolic and diastolic velocities are increased (Figures 6.18A and B). The most universally accepted Doppler criteria that correlate to a ≥60% renal artery stenosis are a PSV greater than 180–200 cm/sec and a renal-to-aortic PSV ratio greater than 3.5. An EDV greater than 150 cm/sec predicts severe (>80% narrowing) renal artery stenosis (124). Subtotal renal artery occlusion is suspected in the presence of

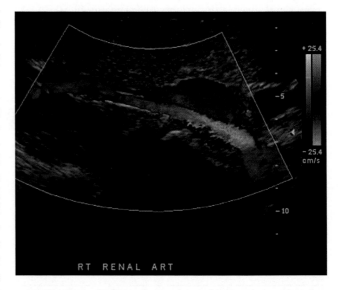

FIGURE 6.17 Right renal artery imaged in its entirety with patient in the left lateral decubitus position.

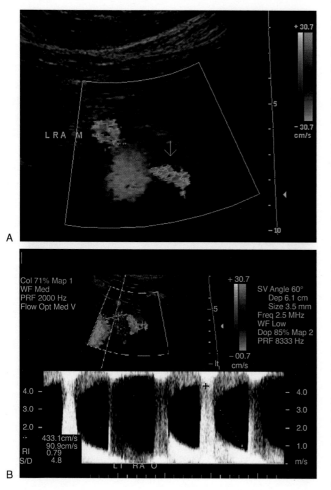

A

B

FIGURE 6.18 (A) Bilateral renal artery stenosis. A mosaic color Doppler flow pattern is displayed in the proximal renal arteries, indicative of turbulent flow and suggesting the presence of stenosis. (B) Renal artery stenosis. Peak systolic velocity in the proximal left renal artery is 433 cm/sec, consistent with a 60% to 99% stenosis.

low systolic flow velocity, post-stenotic turbulence, or a color mosaic pattern (96). Total renal artery occlusion is suspected by the combination of no renal artery flow and low parenchymal Doppler velocities.

In addition to detecting main renal artery or side branch artery stenosis, renal artery Duplex ultrasound can detect small-vessel or renal parenchymal disease. Doppler interrogation of the segmental and interlobar arteries of the kidney permits calculation of the renal artery resistive index (RI). The renal artery RI is defined by the formula, RI = [1 − (V$_{min}$ ÷ V$_{max}$)] × 100, where V$_{min}$ represents EDV and V$_{max}$ represents PSV (96). When measuring velocities for RI, at least three areas

of the kidney should be imaged. In normal kidneys, a large amount of diastolic blood flow is evident on visual inspection of the intrarenal Doppler signals and the RI does not exceed 0.7. A greater RI is caused by increased microvascular resistance, which indicates generalized renal parenchymal disease (125). Currently, the RI's role in guiding renal artery revascularization is unclear. One retrospective study (126) found no improvement in blood pressure or renal function from revascularization when the RI was 0.80 or higher, while another prospective study did find improved blood pressure control following revascularization in patients with an RI of 0.7 or higher (127).

Limitations of duplex ultrasonography for the evaluation of renal artery stenosis include operator experience, patient cooperation, and body habitus. Since mortality risk increases with degree of stenosis, the accurate diagnosis and grading of renal artery stenosis has clinical significance (128). As discussed earlier, the sensitivity for detection of duplicate or accessory renal arteries is reduced. Contrast agents can be useful in patients in whom accessory renal arteries are present (96). Currently, the U.S. Food and Drug Administration recommends that high-risk patients with pulmonary hypertension or unstable cardiopulmonary conditions should be monitored closely during and after microbubble contrast agent injection. Monitoring is advised due to the risk of serious cardiopulmonary reactions during or within 30 min of injection in high-risk patients.

Mesenteric Artery Disease

Just as atherosclerosis can lead to lower extremity PAD, carotid artery disease, and renal artery stenosis, atherosclerotic disease can lead to either acute or chronic mesenteric ischemia. Other causes of mesenteric ischemia include fibromuscular disease and hypoperfusion.

Acute and chronic mesenteric ischemia have different etiologies, presentations, diagnostic techniques, and therapeutic options. Acute mesenteric ischemia results from either acute obstruction or hypoperfusion of nonobstructed arteries. Embolism or arterial thrombosis are the most likely causes of acute obstruction, and thrombosis may occur in the setting of underlying atherosclerotic disease or in the presence of a hypercoagulable state (129–131). Aneurysm, dissection, and vasculitis can also cause acute obstruction (132,133). Acute mesenteric ischemia is a highly fatal condition, and its rapid diagnosis and treatment are crucial. Acute intestinal ischemia is often accompanied by dilated loops of bowel, abdominal distention, and abdominal fluid. These findings preclude an adequate duplex abdominal ultrasound, imaging that relies on minimal bowel gas. Therefore, abdominal duplex ultrasound is contraindicated for the evaluation of patients suspected of having acute mesenteric ischemia (ACC/AHA class 3 recommendation) (10). Abdominal computed tomography scans are often performed on patients with acute abdominal pain, however it is not the best test for evaluating acute mesenteric ischemia. Arteriography is the best diagnostic imaging tool available for the evaluation of patients suspected of having acute mesenteric ischemia, but its role is not clearly defined, partly owing to the small number of patients presenting it.

In contrast, duplex ultrasound is recommended for the evaluation of patients suspected of having chronic mesenteric ischemia. Patients with chronic ischemia are often women (3:1 female to male ratio), aged 40 to 70 years, who experience pain after eating and present weight loss. The pain is usually midabdominal or epigastric, colicky or dull, and may radiate to the back. The onset of pain usually starts 15 to 30 minutes after ingestion and may last up to 4 hours. Although atherosclerosis of the mesenteric vasculature (celiac artery [CA], superior mesenteric artery [SMA], and inferior mesenteric arteries [IMA]) is common, chronic mesenteric ischemia is rare. Chronic ischemia may be rare due to collaterals between the SMA and IMA circulation. When ischemia is not due to occlusion of multiple vessels (combination of either the CA, SMA, or IMA), the SMA is most often the culprit vessel in single-vessel chronic mesenteric ischemia.

Duplex ultrasound for the evaluation of mesenteric ischemia is technically difficult. Bowel gas interferes with the imaging of the deeper arterial vasculature of the celiac artery, SMA, and IMA, so patients should fast overnight prior to an early morning exam. Duplex ultrasound should be done to evaluate for obstructing plaques, which often arise from the aorta and obscure the proximal ostia of the mesenteric vessels (Figure 6.19) (134). Duplex ultrasound is 90% accurate for detecting 70% or greater stenoses of the celiac artery and SMA (135–137). Since the celiac artery perfuses the liver and spleen with their high metabolic requirements, the CA is a low-resistance vessel. Therefore, peak systolic flow is followed by an increased end diastolic velocity. Because there is no flow reversal at the end of systole, the Doppler waveform is biphasic. In contrast,

the intestines do not have a high metabolic demand in the fasting state, and the SMA subsequently has a high resistance waveform by Doppler ultrasound. The fasting SMA Doppler waveform is triphasic with peak systolic flow followed by end systolic reversal and then minimal diastolic flow. The postprandial SMA Doppler waveform loses its end systolic flow reversal reflecting the decreased resistance from the more metabolically active intestines.

Understanding the physiology of healthy CA and SMA flow led to the determination of flow in diseased states (Figure 6.20). A CA PSV of at least 200 cm/sec has been associated with a 70% or greater stenosis in

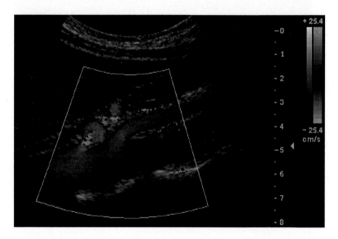

FIGURE 6.19 Color Doppler image of the abdominal aorta with the origin of the celiac artery and the superior mesenteric artery displayed.

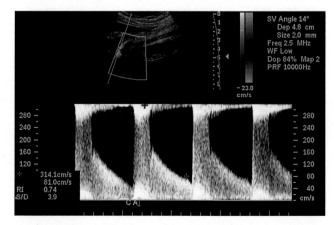

FIGURE 6.20 Celiac artery stenosis. Peak systolic velocity at the origin of the celiac artery is 314 cm/sec, consistent with a 50% to 99% stenosis.

that vessel, while an SMA PSV of at least 275 cm/sec has been associated with a 70% or greater stenosis in the same vessel (138). The sensitivities were 87% and 92%, and the specificities were 80% and 96%, respectively, for the findings of CA and SMA when compared to angiography. A CA EDV of 55 cm/sec or greater suggests at least a 50% stenosis with a sensitivity of 93% and a specificity of 100%, while an SMA end diastolic velocity of at least 45 cm/sec suggests a 50% or greater SMA stenosis with a sensitivity of 100% and a specificity of 92% (139,140). Postprandial duplex scanning has not proven beneficial in the evaluation of suspected chronic mesenteric ischemia, and when duplex ultrasound suggests mesenteric ischemia, angiography is needed to solidify the diagnosis.

■ **FUTURE DIRECTIONS**

There are subgroups of patients with symptomatic and asymptomatic carotid artery stenosis for whom the benefit of revascularization is uncertain. Several studies have suggested that, for these subgroups, the targeting of potentially unstable plaques may help to identify those most at risk of cerebrovascular accidents, and thus most likely to benefit from surgery. Plaque characterization, which will allow identification of features of clinically unstable plaques, is an area of active clinical research. Further advances in ultrasound technology, ranging from continued improvements in grayscale resolution to use of contrast agents, promises to make advances in this area. Currently, 3-dimensional imaging is under development, and promises to improve visualization of vessel geometry and plaque characteristics.

Controversy exists about the appropriateness and efficacy of screening programs to detect atherosclerotic vascular diseases. The ABI and carotid duplex ultrasound for assessment of carotid intimal-medial thickness, plaque, and stenosis, are potentially useful tools for identification of atherosclerotic disease of the leg and carotid arteries, and for prediction of cardiovascular risk in targeted populations. Randomized trial data on the effect of using these studies on long-term clinical outcomes, however, does not exist at this time. Cost-effectiveness modeling for these studies is of great interest. Ultrasound for AAA detection has strong clinical trial support in appropriate populations, and is currently recommended by the American

College of Cardiology/AHA for men ≥60 years of age with a family history of AAAs, and for men 65 to 75 years of age who have ever smoked. Its use is likely to become more widespread. Finally, duplex ultrasound for renal artery disease has the weakest evidence base among the screening tests and thus is problematic for use in screening; however, an ongoing treatment trial of patients with renal artery stenosis (the CORAL trial) should provide additional insight (141).

■ **REFERENCES**

1. Belch JJ, Topol EJ, Agnelli G, et al. Critical issues in peripheral disease detection and management: A call to action. *Arch Int Med* 2003;163:884.
2. Selvin E, Erlinger TP. Prevalence of and risk factrors for peripheral arterial disease in the United States: Results from the National Health and Nutrition Examination Survey, 1999–2000. *Circulation* 2004;110:738.
3. Criqui MH, Langer RD, Fronek A, et al. Mortality over a period of 10 years in patients with peripheral arterial disease. *N Engl J Med* 1992;326:381–86.
4. Hirsch AT, Haskal, ZJ, Hertzer NR, et al.; ACC/AHA Task Force on ·Practice Guidelines for the Management of Patients With Peripheral Arterial Disease. *J Am Coll Cardiol* 2006;47:1239.
5. McDermott MM, Kerwin DR, Liu K, et al. Prevalence and significance of unrecognized lower extremity peripheral arterial disease in general medicine practice. *J Gen Intern Med* 2001;16:384–90.
6. Criqui MH, Fronek A, Klauber MR, et al. The sensitivity, specificity, and predictive value of traditional clinical evaluation of peripheral arterial disease: results from noninvasive testing in a defined population. *Circulation* 1985;71:516–22.
7. Lijmer JG, Hunink MG, van den Dungen JJ, et al. ROC analysis of noninvasive tests for peripheral arterial disease. *Ultrasound Med Biol* 1996;22:391–8.
8. Fowkes FG. The measurement of atherosclerotic peripheral arterial disease in epidemiological surveys. *Int J Epidemiol* 1988;17:248–54.
9. Feigelson HS, Criqui MH, Fronek A, et al. Screening for peripheral arterial disease: the sensitivity, specificity, and predictive value of noninvasive tests in a defined population. *Am J Epidemiol* 1994;140:526–34.
10. Hirsch AT, Haskal, ZJ, Hertzer NR, et al.; ACC/AHA Task Force on Practice Guidelines for the Management of Patients With Peripheral Arterial Disease. *J Am Coll Cardiol* 2006;47:1239.
11. Baker JD, Dix DE. Variability of Doppler ankle pressures with arterial occlusive disease: an evaluation of ankle index and brachial-ankle pressure gradient. *Surgery* 1981;89:134–137.
12. Carter SA. Clinical measurement of systolic pressures in limbs with arterial occlusive disease. *JAMA* 1969;207(10):1869–1874.
13. Strandness DE Jr., Dalman RL, Panian S, et al. Effect of cilostazol in patients with intermittent claudication: a randomized,

double-blind, placebo-controlled study. *Vasc Endovascular Surg* 2002;36:83–91.

14. Yao ST. Haemodynamic studies inperipheral arterial disease. *Br J Surg* 1970;57:761–766.

15. Jelnes R, Gaardsting O, Hougaard Jensen K, et al. Fate in intermittent claudication: outcome and risk factors. *Br Med J (Clin Res Ed)* 1986;293:1137–1140.

16. McLafferty RB, Moneta GL, Taylor LM Jr., et al. Ability of ankle-brachial index to detect lower-extremity atherosclerotic disease progression. *Arch Surg* 1997;132:836–840.

17. Newman AB, Siscovick DS, Manolio TA, et al. Ankle-arm index as a marker of atherosclerosis in the Cardiovascular Health Study. Cardiovascular Heart Study (CHS) Collaborative Research Group. *Circulation* 1993;88:837–845.

18. Newman AB, Sutton-Tyrrell K, Vogt MT, et al. Morbidity and mortality in hypertensive adults with a low ankle/arm blood pressure index. *JAMA* 1993;270:487–489.

19. McKenna M, Wolfson S, Kuller L. The ratio of ankle and arm arterial pressure as an independent predictor of mortality. *Atherosclerosis* 1991;87:119–128.

20. Sikkink CJ, van Asten WN, van't Hof MA, et al. Decreased ankle/brachial indices in relation to morbidity and mortality in patients with peripheral arterial disease. *Vasc Med* 1997;2:169–173.

21. Criqui M, Ninomiya J, Wingard D. Progression of peripheral arterial disease predicts cardiovascular disease morbidity and mortality. *JACC* 2008; 52:1736–1742.

22. Fowkes G. Ankle brachial index combined with Framingham Risk Score to predict cardiovascular events and mortality A Meta-analysis. *JAMA* 2008;300:197–208.

23. Resnick HE, Lindsay RS, McDermott MM, et al. Relationship of high and low ankle brachial index to all-cause and cardiovascular disease mortality: the Strong Heart Study. *Circulation* 2004;109(6):733–739.

24. American Diabetes Association. Peripheral arterial disease in people with diabetes. *Diabetes Care* 2003;26:3333–41.

25. Jager K. Non-invasive mapping gof lower limb arterial lesions. *Ultrasound Med Biol* 1985;11:515.

26. Heintz SE, Bone GE, Slaymaker EE, et al. Value of arterial pressure measurements in the proximal and distal part of the thigh in arterial occlusive disease. *Surg Gynecol Obstet* 1978;146:337–343.

27. Rutherford RB, Lowenstein DH, Klein MF. Combining segmental systolic pressures and plethysmography to diagnose arterial occlusive disease of the legs. *Am J Surg* 1979;138:211–218.

28. Carter SA. Indirect systolic pressures and pulse waves in arterial occlusive diseases of the lower extremities. *Circulation* 1968;37:624–637.

29. Carter SA. Clinical measurement of systolic pressures in limbs with arterial occlusive disease. *JAMA* 1969;207:1869–1874.

30. Carter SA, Tate RB. Value of toe pulse waves in addition to systolic pressures in the assessment of the severity of peripheral arterial disease and critical limb ischemia. *J Vasc Surg* 1996;24:258–265.

31. Carter SA, Tate RB. The value of toe pulse waves in determination of risks for limb amputation and death in patients with peripheral arterial disease and skin ulcers or gangrene. *J Vasc Surg* 2001;33:708–714.

32. Brooks B, Dean R, Patel S, et al. TBI or not TBI: that is the question. Is it better to measure toe pressure than ankle pressure in diabetic patients? *Diabet Med* 2001;18:528–532.

33. Ramsey DE, Manke DA, Sumner DS. Toe blood pressure: a valuable adjunct to ankle pressure measurement for assessing peripheral arterial disease. *J Cardiovasc Surg* (Torino) 1983;24:43–48.

34. Gerhard-Herman M, Beckman JA, Creager MA, Vascular Laboratory Testing. In: Creager MA, Loscalzo J, Dzau VJ, eds. *Vascular Medicine: A Companion to Braunwald's Heart Disease*. Philadelphia: Saunders Elsevier, 2006, pp. 146–65.

35. Rutherford RB, Lowenstein DH, Klein MF. Combining segmental systolic pressures and plethysmography to diagnose arterial occlusive disease of the legs. *Am J Surg* 1979;138:211–218.

36. Raines JK. The pulse volume recorder in peripheral arterial disease. In: Bernstein EF, ed. *Noninvasive Diagnostic Techniques in Vascular Disease*. St Louis, MO: Mosby, 1985, pp. 513–44.

37. Jorgensen JJ, Stranden E, Gjolberg T. Measurements of common femoral artery flow velocity in the evaluation of aortoiliac atherosclerosis: comparisons between pulsatility index, pressure measurements and pulse-volume recordings. *Acta Chir Scand* 1988;154:261–6.

38. Symes JF, Graham AM, Mousseau M. Doppler waveform analysis versus segmental pressure and pulse-volume recording: assessment of occlusive disease in the lower extremity. *Can J Surg* 1984;27:345–7.

39. Clifford PC, Morgan AP, Thomas WE, et al. Monitoring arterial surgery: a comparison of pulse volume recording and electromagnetic flowmetering in aortofemoral reconstruction. *J Cardiovasc Surg* 1986;27:262–7.

40. Kaufman JL, Fitzgerald KM, Shah DM, et al. The fate of extremities with flat lower calf pulse volume recordings. *J Cardiovasc Surg* 1989;30:216–9.

41. Gardner AW, Skinner JS, Cantwell BW, et al. Progressive vs single-stage treadmill tests for evaluation of claudication. *Med Sci Sports Exerc* 1991;23:402–8.

42. Hiatt WR, Nawaz, D, Regensteiner JG, et al. The evaluation of exercise performance in patients with peripheral vascular disease. *J Cardiopulm Rehabil* 1988;8:525–32.

43. Nagle FJ, Balke B, Naughton JP. Gradational step tests for assessing work capacity. *J Appl Physiol* 1965;20:745–8.

44. Stein R, Hrljac I, Halperin J, Limitation of the resting ankle–brachial index in symptomatic patients with peripheral arterial disease. *Vascu Med* 2006;11:1–5.

45. Ouriel K, McDonnell AE, Metz CE, et al. Critical evaluation of stress testing in the diagnosis of peripheral vascular disease. *Surgery* 1982;91:686–93.

46. Greig C, Butler F, Skelton D, et al. Treadmill walking in old age may not reproduce the real life situation. *J Am Geriatr Soc* 1993;41:15–8.

47. Gardner AW, Katzel LI, Sorkin JD, et al. Exercise rehabilitation improves functional outcomes and peripheral circulation in patients with intermittent claudication: a randomized controlled trial. *J Am Geriatr Soc* 2001;49:755–62.

48. Simonsick EM, Gardner AW, Poehlman ET. Assessment of physical function and exercise tolerance in older adults: reproducibility and comparability of five measures. *Aging* (Milano) 2000;12:274–80.

49. Zwiebel W, Pellerito J. *Introduction to Vascular Ultrasonography*. 5th Ed. Philadelphia: Elsevier Saunders, 2005.

50. Moneta GL, Yeager RA, Lee RW, et al. Noninvasive localization of arterial occlusive disease: a comparison of segmental

Doppler pressures and arterial duplex mapping. *J Vasc Surg* 1993;17:578–82.

51. Pinto F, Lencioni R, Napoli V, et al. Peripheral ischemic occlusive arterial disease: comparison of color Doppler sonography and angiography. *J Ultrasound Med* 1996;15:697–704.

52. Sacks D, Robinson ML, Marinelli DL, et al. Peripheral arterial Doppler ultrasonography: diagnostic criteria. *J Ultrasound Med* 1992;11:95–103.

53. de Smet AA, Ermers EJ, Kitslaar PJ. Duplex velocity characteristics of aortoiliac stenoses. *J Vasc Surg* 1996;23:628–36.

54. Fletcher JP, Kershaw LZ, Chan A, et al. Noninvasive imaging of the superficial femoral artery using ultrasound Duplex scanning. *J Cardiovasc Surg* (Torino) 1990;31:364–7.

55. Ranke C, Creutzig A, Alexander K. Duplex scanning of the peripheral arteries: correlation of the peak velocity ratio with angiographic diameter reduction. *Ultrasound Med Biol* 1992;18:433–40.

56. Whelan JF, Barry MH, Moir JD. Color flow Doppler ultrasonography: comparison with peripheral arteriography for the investigation of peripheral vascular disease. *J Clin Ultrasound* 1992;20:369–74.

57. Davies AH, Wilcox JH, Magee TR, et al. Colour duplex in assessing the infrainguinal arteries in patients with claudication. *Cardiovasc Surg* 1995;3:211–2.

58. Currie IC, Jones AJ, Wakeley CJ, et al. Non-invasive aortoiliac assessment. *Eur J Vasc Endovasc Surg* 1995;9:24–8.

59. Oh JK, Seward JB, Tajik AJ. *The Echo Manual.* 3rd Ed. New York: Lippincott Williams & Wilkins, 2007, pp. 59–66.

60. Rubin J.Power Doppler US: A potentially useful alternative to mean frequency-based color Doppler US. *Radiology* 1994;190:853.

61. Strandness DE, Jr., Schultz RD, Sumner DS, et al. Ultrasonic flow detection. A useful technique in the evaluation of peripheral vascular disease. *Am J Surg* 1967;113:311.

62. De Vries SO, Hunink MG, Polak JF. Summary receiver operating characteristic curves as a technique for meta-analysis of the diagnostic performance of duplex ultrasonography in peripheral arterial disease. *Acad Radiol* 1996;3:361–9.

63. Pellerito J. Color persistence: Indicator of hemodynamically significant peripheral arterial stenosis. *Radiology* 1991;181:89.

64. Allard L, Cloutier G, Durand LG, et al. Limitations of ultrasonic duplex scanning for diagnosing lower limb arterial stenoses in the presence of adjacent segment disease. *J Vasc Surg* 1994;19:650–7.

65. Sacks D, Robinson ML, Marinelli DL, et al. Evaluation of the peripheral arteries with duplex US after angioplasty. *Radiology* 1990;176:39–44.

66. Sacks D, Robinson ML, Summers TA, et al. The value of duplex sonography after peripheral artery angioplasty in predicting subacute restenosis. *Am J Roentgenol* 1994;162:179–83.

67. Spijkerboer AM, Nass PC, de Valois JC, et al. Iliac artery stenoses after percutaneous transluminal angioplasty: follow-up with duplex ultrasonography. *J Vasc Surg* 1996;23:691–7.

68. Spijkerboer AM, Nass PC, de Valois JC, et al. Evaluation of femoropopliteal arteries with duplex ultrasound after angioplasty. Can we predict results at one year? *Eur J Vasc Endovasc Surg* 1996;12:418–23.

69. Mewissen MW, Kinney EV, Bandyk DF, et al. The role of duplex scanning versus angiography in predicting outcome after balloon angioplasty in the femoropopliteal artery. *J Vasc Surg* 1992;15:860–5.

70. Idu MM, Blankenstein JD, de Gier P, et al. Impact of a color-flow duplex surveillance program on infrainguinal vein graft patency: a five-year experience. *J Vasc Surg* 1993;17:42–52.

71. Mattos MA, van Bemmelen PS, Hodgson KJ, et al. Does correction of stenoses identified with color duplex scanning improve infrainguinal graft patency? *J Vasc Surg* 1993;17:54–64.

72. Mills JL, Harris EJ, Taylor LM Jr., et al. The importance of routine surveillance of distal bypass grafts with duplex scanning: a study of 379 reversed vein grafts. *J Vasc Surg* 1990;12:379–86.

73. Laborde AL, Synn AY, Worsey MJ, et al. A prospective comparison of ankle/brachial indices and color duplex imaging in surveillance of the in situ saphenous vein bypass. *J Cardiovasc Surg* (Torino) 1992;33:420–5.

74. Taylor PR, Tyrrell MR, Crofton M, et al. Colour flow imaging in the detection of femoro-distal graft and native artery stenosis: improved criteria. *Eur J Vasc Surg* 1992;6:232–6.

75. Bandyk DF, Schmitt DD, Seabrook GR, et al. Monitoring functional patency of in situ saphenous vein bypasses: the impact of a surveillance protocol and elective revision. *J Vasc Surg* 1989;9:286–96.

76. Golledge J, Beattie DK, Greenhalgh RM, et al. Have the results of infrainguinal bypass improved with the widespread utilization of postoperative surveillance? *Eur J Vasc Endovasc Surg* 1996;11:388–92.

77. Lundell A, Lindblad B, Bergqvist D, et al. Femoropopliteal-crural graft patency is improved by an intensive surveillance program: a prospective randomized study. *J Vasc Surg* 1995;21:26–33.

78. Lalak NJ, Hanel KC, Hunt J, et al. Duplex scan surveillance of infrainguinal prosthetic bypass grafts. *J Vasc Surg* 1994;20:637–41.

79. Dunlop P, Sayers RD, Naylor AR, et al. The effect fo a surveillance programme on the patency of synthetic infrainguinal bypass grafts. *Eur J Vasc Endovasc Surg* 1996;11:441–5.

80. Eisenhauer AC, White CJ. Endovascular treatment of noncoronary obstructive vascular disease. In: Libby P, Bonow R, Mann D, Zipes D. *Braunwald's Heart Disease. A Textbook of Cardiovascular Medicine.* 8th Ed. Philadelphia: Saunders, 2008, pp. 1523–39.

81. Langlois Y, Roederer G, Strandness DJ: Ultrasonic evaluation of carotid bifurcation. *Echocardiography* 4:141, 1987.

82. Grant EG, Benson CB, Moneta GL, et al. Carotid artery stenosis: gray-scale and Doppler US diagnosis- Society of Radiologists in Ultrasound Consensus Conference. *Radiology* 2003;229:340.

83. Stein J, Korcarz C, Hurst, R. T. ASE Consensus Statement. Use of Carotid Ultrasound to Identify Subclinical Vascular Disease and Evaluate Cardiovascular Disease Risk: A Consensus Statement from the American Society of Echocardiography Carotid Intima-Media Thickness Task Force. *J Am Soc Echocardiogr* 2008;21(2):93–111.

84. Crouse JR, Goldbourt U, Evans G, et al. Risk factors and segment-specific carotid arterial enlargement in the Atherosclerosis Risk in Communities (ARIC) cohort. *Stroke* 1996;27:69–75.

85. Chambless LE, Heiss G, Folsom AR, et al. Association of coronary heart disease incidence with carotid arterial wall thickness and major risk factors: The Atherosclerosis Risk in Communities (ARIC) Study. *Am J Epidemiol* 1997;146:483–494.

86. O'Leary DH, Polak JF, Kronmal RA, et al. Cardiovascular Health Study Collaborative Research Group. Carotid-artery

intima and media thickness as a risk factor for myocardial infarction and stroke in older adults. *NEJM* 1999;340:14–22.

87. Salonen JT, Salonen R. Ultrasonographically assessed carotid morphology and the risk of coronary heart disease. *Atheroscler Thrombo* 1991;11:1245–1249.

88. Chambless LE, Heiss G, Folsom AR, Rosamond W, Szklo M, Sharrett AR, et al. Association of coronary heart disease incidence with carotid arterial wall thickness and major risk factors: the Atherosclerosis Risk in Communities (ARIC) study, 1987–1993. *Am J Epidemiol* 1997;146:483–94.

89. Patel SN, Rajaram V, Pandya S, et al. Emerging, noninvasive surrogate markers of atherosclerosis. *Curr Atheroscler Rep* 2004;6:60–8.

90. Kanters SD, Algra A, van Leeuwen MS, et al. Reproducibility of in vivo carotid intima-media thickness measurements: a review. *Stroke* 1997;28:665–71.

91. Jacoby DS, Mohler ER III, Rader DJ. Noninvasive atherosclerosis imaging for predicting cardiovascular events and assessing therapeutic interventions. Curr Atheroscler Rep 2004;6:20–26.

92. Isselbacher EM. Diseases of the Aorta. In: Libby P, Bonow R, Mann D, Zipes D. *Braunwald's Heart Disease. A Textbook of Cardiovascular Medicine.* 8th Ed. Philadelphia: Saunders, 2008, pp. 1457–61.

93. Lawrence-Brown MM, Norman PE, Jamrozik K, et al. Initial results of ultrasound screening for aneurysm of the abdominal aorta in Western Australia: Relevance for endoluminal treatment of aneurysm disease. *Cardiovasc Surg* 2001;9:234–40.

94. Scott RAP, Ashton HA, Kay DN. Abdominal aortic aneurysm in 4237 screened patients: prevalence, development and management over 6 years. *Br J Surg* 1991;78:1122–4.

95. Verloes A, Sakalihasan N, Koulischer L, et al. Aneurysms of the abdominal aorta: familial and genetic aspects in three hundred thirteen pedigrees. *J Vasc Surg* 1995;21:646–55.

96. Hallett JW. Abdominal aortic aneurysm: natural history and treatment. *Heart Dis Stroke* 1992;1:303–8.

97. Blau SA, Kerstein MD, Deterling RA. Abdominal aortic aneurysm. In Kerstein MD, Moulder MD, Webb WR (eds). *Aneurysms.* Baltimore: Williams & Wilkins, 1983, pp. 127–96.

98. Fink HA, Lederle FA, Roth CS, et al. The accuracy of physical examination to detect abdominal aortic aneurysm. *Arch Intern Med* 2000;160:833–836.

99. Chervu A, Clagett GP, Valentine RJ, et al. Role of physical examination in detection of abdominal aortic aneurysms. *Surgery* 1995;117:454–457.

100. Multicentre Aneurysm Screening Study Group. Multicentre Aneurysm Screening Study (MASS): cost effectiveness analysis of screening for abdominal aortic aneurysms based on four year results from a randomized controlled trial. *BMJ* 2002;325:1135–1138.

101. Kyriakides C, Byrne J, Green S, Hulton NR. Screening of abdominal aortic aneurysm: a pragmatic approach. *Ann R Coll Surg Engl* 2000;82:59–63.

102. Crow P, Shaw E, Earnshaw JJ, et al. A single normal ultrasonographic scan at age 65 years rules out significant aneurysm disease for life in men. *Br J Surg* 2001;88:941–942.

103. Wilmink AB, Hubbard CS, Day NE, Quick CR. The incidence of small abdominal aortic aneurysms and the change in

normal infrarenal aortic diameter: implications for screening. *Eur J Vasc Endovasc Surg* 2001;21:165–170.

104. Eisenhauer AC, White CJ. Endovascular Treatment of Noncoronary Obstructive Vascular Disease. In: Libby P, Bonow R, Mann D, Zipes D. *Braunwald's Heart Disease. A Textbook of Cardiovascular Medicine.* 8th Ed. Philadelphia: Saunders, 2008, pp. 1523–46.

105. Victor RG, Kaplan NM. Systemic Hypertension: Mechanisms and Diagnosis. In: Libby P, Bonow R, Mann D, Zipes D. *Braunwald's Heart Disease. A Textbook of Cardiovascular Medicine.* 8th Ed. Philadelphia: Saunders, 2008, pp. 1027–48.

106. Fauci, Braunwald, Kasper, et al. *Harrison's Principles of Internal Medicine.* 17th edition. New York: McGraw-Hill, pp. 1554–1555.

107. Safian RD, Textor SC: Renal-artery stenosis. *N Engl J Med* 344:431, 2001.

108. Hirsch AT, Haskal, ZJ, Hertzer NR, et al.; ACC/AHA Task Force on Practice Guidelines for the Management of Patients With Peripheral Arterial Disease. *J Am Coll Cardiol* 47:1239, 2006.

109. Motew SJ, Cherr GS, Craven TE, et al.: Renal duplex sonography: Main renal artery versus hilar analysis. *J Vasc Surg* 32:462, 2000.

110. Hansen KJ, Tribble RW, Reavis SW, et al.: Renal duplex sonography: Evaluation of clinical utility. *J Vasc Surg* 12:227, 1990.

111. Carman TL, Olin JW. Diagnosis of renal artery stenosis: what is the optimal diagnostic test? *Curr Interv Cardiol Rep* 2000;2:111–8.

112. Olin JW. Role of duplex ultrasonography in screening for significant renal artery disease. *Curr Interv Cardiol Rep* 1994;215–26.

113. Hoffmann U, Edwards JM, Carter S, et al. Role of duplex scanning for the detection of atherosclerotic renal artery disease. *Kidney Int* 1991;39:1232–9.

114. Kohler TR, Zierler RE, Martin RL, et al. Noninvasive diagnosis of renal artery stenosis by ultrasonic duplex scanning. *J Vasc Surg* 1986;4:450–6.

115. Taylor DC, Kettler MD, Moneta GL, et al. Duplex ultrasound scanning in the diagnosis of renal artery stenosis: a prospective evaluation. *J Vasc Surg* 1988;7:363–9.

116. Wilcox CS. Ischemic nephropathy: noninvasive testing. *Semin Nephrol* 1996;16:43–52.

117. Carman TL, Olin JW, Czum J. Noninvasive imaging of the renal arteries. *Curr Interv Cardiol Rep* 2001;28:815–26.

118. Wilson DB, Edwards MS, Ayerdi J, Hansen KJ. Surgical Management of Atherosclerotic Renal Artery Disease. In: Creager MA, Loscalzo J, Dzau VJ, eds. *Vascular Medicine: A Companion to Braunwald's Heart Disease.* Philadelphia: Saunders Elsevier, 2006, pp. 359–360.

119. Langholz J, Schlief R, Schurmann R, et al. Contrast enhancement in leg vessels. *Clin Radiol* 1996;51 Suppl 1: 31.

120. Strandenss DE Jr. Duplex scanning in diagnosis of renovascular hypertension. *Surg Clin North Am* 1990;70:109–117.

121. Brun P, Kchouk H, Mouchet B, et al. Value of Doppler ultrasound for the diagnosis of renal artery stenosis in children. *Pediatr Nephrol* 1997;11:27–30.

122. Stanley JC. Renal vascular disease and renovascular hypertension in children. *Curr Interv Cardiol Rep* 1984;11:451–463.

123. Strandness DE Jr. *Duplex scanning in vascular disorders.* New York, Lippincott-Raven, 1990, p. 240.

124. Olin JW, Piedmonte MR, Young JR, et al. The utility of duplex ultrasound scanning of the renal arteries for diagnosing significant renal artery stenosis. *Ann Intern Med* 1995;122:833–8.

125. Keating MA, Althausen AF. The clinical spectrum of renal vein thrombosis. *J Urol* 1985;133:938–945.

126. Radermacher J, Chavan A, Bleck J, et al. Use of Doppler ultrasonography to predict the outcome of therapy for renal-artery stenosis. *N Engl J Med* 2001;344:410–7.

127. Zeller T, Muller C, Frank U, et al. Stent angioplasty of severe atherosclerotic ostial renal artery stenosis in patients with diabetes mellitus and nephrosclerosis. *Catheter Cardiovasc Interv* 2003;58:510–5.

128. Conlon PJ, Little MA, Pieper K, Mark DB: Severity of renal vascular disease predicts mortality in patients undergoing coronary angiography. *Kidney Int* 60:1490, 2001.

129. Ottinger LW, Austen WG. A study of 136 patients with mesenteric infarction. *Surg Gynecol Obstet* 1967;124:251–61.

130. Hertzer NR, Beven EG, Humphries AW. Acute intestinal ischemia. *Am Surg* 1978;44:744–9.

131. Bergan JJ. Recognition and treatment of intestinal ischemia. *Surg Clin North Am* 1967;47:109–26.

132. Krupski WC, Effeney DJ, Ehrenfeld WK. Spontaneous dissection of the superior mesenteric artery. *J Vasc Surg* 1985;2:731–4.

133. Wolf EA Jr., Sumner DS, Strandness DE Jr. Disease of the mesenteric circulation in patients with thromboangiitis obliterans. *Vasc Surg* 1972;6:218–23.

134. Mikkelsen WP. Intestinal angina: its surgical significance. *Surg Gynecol Obstet* 1957;94:262–7.

135. Moneta GL, Yeager RA, Dalman R, et al. Duplex ultrasound criteria for diagnosis of splanchnic artery stenosis or occlusion. *J Vasc Surg* 1991;14:511–8.

136. GL, Lee RW, Yeager RA, et al. Mesenteric duplex scanning: a blinded prospective study. *J Vasc Surg* 1993;17:79–84.

137. RM, Fillinger MF, Walsh DB, et al. Mesenteric and celiac duplex scanning: a validation study. *J Vasc Surg* 1998;27:1078–87.

138. WD, McCarthy WJ, Bresticker M, et al. Mesenteric artery bypass: Objective patency determination. *J Vasc Surg* 1995;21:729.

139. GL. Screening for mesenteric vascular insufficiency and follow-up of mesenteric bypass procedures. *Semin Vasc Surg* 2001;14:186.

140. JE, Stemmer EA. Intestinal gangrene as the result of mesenteric arterial steal. *Am J Surg* 1973;126:197.

141. Creager MA, White CJ, Hiatt WR Criqui MH, Atherosclerotic Peripheral Vascular Disease Symposium II: Executive Summary. *Circulation* 2008;118; 2811–2825.

7 Cardiac and Aortic Causes of Stroke

MARIA G. KARAS

JORGE R. KIZER

OUTLINE

High-Risk Cardioaortic Sources
   of Embolism   118

Sources of Embolism of Medium or
   Uncertain Risk   125

Conclusion   132

References   132

Stroke is the third leading cause of death and a major cause of long-term disability in the United States (1). Almost 90% of strokes are ischemic in nature, as opposed to hemorrhagic (2). Ischemic strokes can be classified pathophysiologically as arising from large-vessel disease (atherosclerotic), small-vessel disease (fibrinoid degeneration or lipohyalinosis), cardiac embolism, or miscellaneous disorders (e.g., fibromuscular dysplasia, dissection, vasculitis) (3).

Cardiogenic cerebral embolism accounts for approximately 20% of ischemic strokes (3,4). Typically, cardioembolic stroke presents with neurologic symptoms that are of maximal intensity at onset, marking a sudden disruption in blood flow (5,6). In contrast, atherothrombotic stroke tends to manifest with a more prolonged onset of symptoms, reflecting the more dynamic process of *in situ* thrombogenesis (7). The clinical presentation , however, is not an accurate tool for differentiating cardioembolic from noncardioembolic stroke. Cardiogenic emboli can fragment or dislodge

after initial impaction, leading to progressive onset of symptoms (4,6). In addition, artery-to-artery embolism from a large-artery atherothrombotic source can lead to abrupt vessel occlusion, mimicking a classic cardioembolic picture (6,7).

Accordingly, the diagnosis of cardioembolic stroke principally depends on identification of the proximal emboligenic culprit—either of the residual material remaining in the heart or aorta, or of conditions that predispose to cardiac formation or transit of such material when its site of origin is not identifiable (6). Appropriate imaging of the cervicocranial circulation, together with directed laboratory testing, allows exclusion of other etiologies. Different potential etiologies may coexist in the individual patient, however, making identification of the genuine culprit challenging, if not impossible (6).

Long-recognized cardioembolic sources consist of pathologic substrates that may travel from their sites of initial formation within the left-sided heart chambers or valves to occlude cerebral vessels. These include thrombi in the left atrium or ventricle, cardiac tumors and vegetations. When these high-risk embolic entities are detected by imaging, the etiology of the stroke is fairly certain. Other high-risk conditions, such as atrial fibrillation (AF) and severe left ventricular dysfunction, lead to the presumption of a cardioembolic etiology even if the embolic substrate (thrombus) is not detected (8). Table 7.1 lists high-risk cardiac and aortic conditions that have been recognized to lead to cerebral embolism.

In a substantial proportion of strokes—as many as 30%—the etiology is undetermined. However, many of these strokes, termed *cryptogenic*, have embolic features and may be attributed clinically to a cardiac or aortic origin (9,10). Several cardiac, pulmonary, and aortic findings that can act as a nidus for thrombosis or as a

■ **Table 7.1** High-risk cardioembolic sources

Atrial dysrhythmias
- Atrial fibrillation
- Atrial flutter
- Sick sinus syndrome

Left atrial thrombus
- Atrial dysrhythmias
- Mitral valve stenosis

Left ventricular thrombus
- Acute myocardial infarction
- Dilated cardiomyopathy

Primary cardiac tumors
- Myxoma
- Papillary fibroelastoma

Metastatic tumors to the heart

Vegetations
- Infective
- Noninfective

Prosthetic cardiac valve

Complex aortic atheroma

■ **Table 7.2** Medium-or uncertain-risk cardioembolic sources

Interatrial septal abnormalities
- Patent foramen ovale
- Atrial septal defect
- Atrial septal aneurysm

Pulmonary arteriovenous malformation

Spontaneous echo contrast ("smoke")

Mitral valve prolapse

Valvular calcification
- Mitral annular calcification
- Aortic valve sclerosis

Valvular strands

The text that follows covers elements of the pathophysiology, diagnosis, prognosis, and treatment of proximal sources of cerebral embolism considered individually. Approaches to primary and secondary prevention of ischemic stroke for each of these disorders are described, summarizing published guidelines from treatment societies, where available, and drawing from considered opinion when appropriate evidence is lacking. Discussion of complex congenital heart disease, forms of which are closely associated with ischemic stroke, is beyond the scope of this chapter, as is aortic dissection, which can similarly lead to cerebral infarction. The reader is referred elsewhere for focused discussion of these topics (16–18).

■ HIGH-RISK CARDIOAORTIC SOURCES OF EMBOLISM

Left Ventricular Thrombus

Left ventricular thrombus (Figure 7.1) forms as a consequence of stasis within the cavity, generally secondary to regional or global myocardial systolic dysfunction (19,20). Prior to the contemporary era of thrombolytic therapy and primary angioplasty, 60% of emboli of left ventricular origin were associated with acute transmural myocardial infarction (21). Such transmural infarcts lead not only to segmental akinesis or dyskinesis and stasis of blood, but also to activation of inflammatory and thrombotic pathways that may heighten the risk of cavitary thrombogenesis (22–25). Formerly, approximately

veno-arterial passageway for emboli have been associated with ischemic, and particularly cryptogenic, strokes (11). The strength, and even the nature, of the relationship of these conditions to ischemic stroke are less well defined than for high-risk sources, and the pathogenic significance of these findings in the individual patient with ischemic stroke can be difficult to determine (6). Still, nearly all of these findings have been implicated in the pathogenesis of ischemic stroke in clinical or autopsy case series or reports, and warrant consideration during stroke evaluation and management (12–15). A list of these entities conferring medium or uncertain-risk for ischemic stroke is presented in Table 7.2.

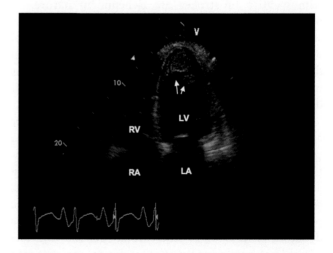

FIGURE 7.1 Transthoracic echocardiogram showing distinct thrombi in the left ventricular apex. Arrows indicate thrombus. (LV, left ventricle; LA, left atrium; RV, right ventricle; RA, right atrium.)

one-third of patients with anterior wall myocardial infarction were expected to develop a thrombus within two weeks of the event (25). In the contemporary setting of primary percutaneous coronary intervention, the occurrence of left ventricular thrombosis following ST-elevation myocardial infarction (STEMI) has declined, with an early incidence of 10% in patients with anterior STEMI undergoing timely intervention (26).

Greater than 75% of thrombi will form within the first week after a myocardial infarction. The risk of thrombus formation is associated with infarct size, clinical evidence of pump failure, akinetic or dyskinetic wall abnormalities, increased left ventricular volume and decreased global left ventricular systolic function (27). Thrombus typically forms in the apex of the ventricle and is most commonly associated with an anterior wall myocardial infarction, especially with involvement of the apex (22,28). The risk of thrombus embolization is dependent on its mobility and degree of protrusion into the left ventricular cavity. Approximately 55% of mobile thrombi and 45% of protruding thrombi will embolize, in contrast to 10% of nonmobile thrombi and 7% of flat thrombi (27).

In turn, recent studies show the incidence of stroke in the four weeks following acute myocardial infarction to range between 1 and 2.5%, with up to one-half occurring in the first five days (22,24,27–29). Although the majority of emboli occur in the first few weeks after the coronary event, patients with severe left ventricular systolic dysfunction remain at increased risk beyond this period (22,28,30). Dyskinetic segments that remodel into left ventricular aneurysms remain chronic potential foci for the formation of mural thrombi (31–33), but the risk of embolization in this setting appears to be much lower.

Ischemic and nonischemic dilated cardiomyopathies with generalized systolic dysfunction are also associated with the formation of left ventricular thrombus (20). In a retrospective cohort study, 16% of the 630 patients with incident heart failure suffered an ischemic stroke during a median follow-up of 4.3 years, although nearly 50% of incident stroke cases had atrial fibrillation (AF) at baseline (34). In other series, the annual risk of thromboembolism has ranged from 1% to 3.5% per year (35,36), but jumps to 9% once a stroke has occurred (35). Risk is directly related to the degree of left ventricular systolic dysfunction, both in the ischemic (37) and nonischemic settings (36,38).

Transthoracic echocardiography (TTE) is most commonly used to identify and follow left ventricular thrombi. Studies have shown that up to 46% of TTEs may be inconclusive in the diagnosis of thrombus (39). Techniques such as harmonic imaging (40) and intravenous contrast administration (41) improve diagnosis. More recently, contrast-enhanced magnetic resonance imaging (MRI) has been shown to have higher sensitivity and specificity in the detection of left ventricular thrombus (42,43).

Anticoagulation is typically instituted in patients with left ventricular thrombus. This therapy is started early in the poststroke period, provided that the risk of hemorrhagic conversion of the cerebral infarct is acceptable. Usually, anticoagulation is continued for at least three months for patients in sinus rhythm, with demonstration of interval thrombus resolution by echocardiography (2,44). For patients with cardiomyopathy (severe left ventricular systolic dysfunction with ejection fraction ≤35%) who have had a prior stroke or transient ischemic attack, either anticoagulation or antiplatelet therapy is recommended (2).

It is unclear if anticoagulation should be used in patients with a cardiomyopathy and sinus rhythm without a prior cerebrovascular ischemic event (2). A clinical trial bearing on this question was recently published (45). The study compared aspirin, clopidogrel and warfarin in patients with symptomatic systolic heart failure (left ventricular ejection fraction ≤35% and New York Heart Association Class II–IV) in normal sinus rhythm, but was terminated prematurely because of slow enrollment. There was no difference between treatment arms in incidence of the primary composite endpoint (death, nonfatal myocardial infarction, and nonfatal stroke) or all-cause mortality. The study did find a lower incidence of the secondary stroke endpoint in the warfarin group (0.6%) as compared with aspirin or clopidogrel (2.3% each, P = 0.016) after a mean follow-up of 1.9 years. This was offset, however, by a higher risk of major hemorrhage with warfarin (5.2%), which was significant as compared with clopidogrel (2.1%, P = 0.007) but not aspirin (3.6%, P = 0.218). There was also a greater incidence of minor hemorrhage with warfarin (28.7%) compared with aspirin (23.5%, P = 0.054) and clopidogrel (22.7%, P = 0.025). These findings support the view that antiplatelet therapy is reasonable for primary prevention in patients with heart failure in normal sinus rhythm (46), although findings from a larger, ongoing trial are expected to shed necessary additional light regarding the optimal approach (45).

Left Atrial Thrombus

Similar to left ventricular thrombus, left atrial thrombus formation is associated with stasis of blood in this chamber. Atrial dysrhythmias, particularly AF, lead to an absence of organized atrial contraction, with resultant stasis and increased risk of thrombus formation in the left atrium and left atrial appendage (47). Both persistent AF and paroxysmal AF are significant predictors of stroke; more than 10% of all ischemic strokes are attributed to this arrhythmia (2). Valvular AF carries a higher stroke risk than nonvalvular AF (48). In patients with AF and rheumatic mitral stenosis, there is a 17-fold increment in the risk of thromboembolism as compared with the five-fold increase seen in patients with the nonrheumatic variety of AF (49). Besides rheumatic valve disease, several atherosclerosis risk factors influence the risk of stroke associated with AF. The severity and duration of these factors are important in shaping changes in left ventricular function and left atrial size, increasing the likelihood of thrombus formation (50).

CHADS$_2$ has emerged as a useful instrument to stratify patients with AF with respect to thromboembolic risk. Patients are assigned one point each for Congestive heart failure, Hypertension, Age >75 years, and Diabetes, and two points for prior Stroke or transient ischemic attack (51). Prior cerebrovascular ischemia is in fact the foremost determinant of future stroke risk (52). While the annual risk of thromboembolism in lone AF is 0.5% per year, it increases to 12% per year in patients with AF and history of cerebral ischemia (48).

Atrial flutter and sick sinus syndrome are additional dysrhythmias that predispose to thrombus formation in the left atrium and stroke (53,54). Even though the embolic risk for these dysrhythmias alone is lower than for AF, they are often associated with AF and structural heart disease, which themselves heighten the risk of cerebral embolism (55–57).

In the absence of identified atrial dysrhythmias, structural heart disease can also lead to left atrial dilatation and thrombus formation. In a series of 20,643 transesophageal echocardiograms (TEEs) performed at a tertiary center during a 10-year period, 314 patients were found to have thrombus in the left atrium or left atrial appendage (58). Only 20 of these patients were in normal sinus rhythm at the time of TEE, but 19 had high-risk structural heart disease or prior AF. The remaining patient also had structural heart disease, but did not meet prespecified criteria for high-risk features.

In the absence of structural heart disease, AF or atrial flutter, thrombus occurrence in the left atrial appendage is a rare, but described phenomenon (59). Similar to left ventricular thrombi, size and mobility are important determinants of thromboembolic risk when left atrial thrombus is detected (60).

TTE is an insensitive tool for identifying left atrial thrombus (61). Because of superior imaging of the left atrium and, in particular, the left atrial appendage, TEE is the modality of choice for evaluation of left atrial thrombus (Figure 7.2) (62). Computed tomography (CT) (63) and MRI (64) have emerged as additional modalities for thrombus detection within the left atrium and appendage, but their diagnostic accuracy as compared with TEE requires investigation.

Treatment of left atrial thrombus is systemic anticoagulation with warfarin for a minimum of 4 weeks, with duration determined by associated rhythm or structural abnormalities (52,65). For patients with chronic or paroxysmal AF, randomized data has shown significant risk reduction for thromboembolism with the use of warfarin compared to aspirin (66). The decision to institute anticoagulation over antiplatelet therapy, however, must depend on balancing of the benefit of lowering thromboembolic risk against the associated hazard of major hemorrhage. Available guidelines therefore predicate their recommendation for adjusted-dose warfarin (target international normalized ratio [INR] of 2.0–3.0) on the presence of clinical factors documented to influence

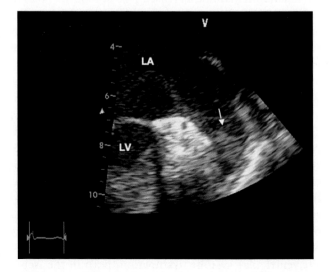

FIGURE 7.2 Transesophageal echocardiogram showing thrombus in the left atrial appendage. Arrow indicates thrombus. (LA, left atrium; LV, left ventricle.)

thromboembolic risk. The specific clinical risk factors considered by different professional societies in making their recommendations vary, although there is unanimity that, barring contraindications, previous stroke or transient ischemic attack (TIA) constitutes a compelling indication for anticoagulation. By contrast, in the absence of any $CHADS_2$-scheme risk factors, the risk of thromboembolism falls to 1% or less, which can be used to justify a decision favoring aspirin therapy (2,52,67).

Similar considerations apply to atrial flutter and sick sinus syndrome. Anticoagulation is generally advocated for primary thromboembolic prevention for isolated atrial flutter (68) and should likewise be considered for sick sinus syndrome, unless structural heart disease and, particularly, AF have been carefully excluded.

Cardiac Tumors

Primary tumors of the heart, three-quarters of which are benign, are rare, occurring in less than 0.2% of unselected autopsy reports (69). Myxomas make up almost 50% of primary heart tumors. Other primary heart tumors include lipomas, papillary fibroelastomas, rhabdomyomas, fibromas, hemangiomas, teratomas, and mesotheliomas of the atrioventricular node. Very rare tumors are granular-cell tumors, neurofibromas, and lymphangiomas (69).

Myxoma

Myxomas are heart neoplasms of endocardial origin, most frequently observed between the third and sixth decades of life with a 2:1 female preponderance (70). The majority of cardiac myxomas are sporadic, occurring as isolated tumors. As many as 10%, however, are part of a familial syndrome known as Carney Complex, which is associated with multiple or recurrent cardiac or cutaneous myxomas, lentigines, endocrinopathy, and both endocrine and nonendocrine tumors (71). Cardiac mxyomas have been rarely reported to be malignant (72,73), based on findings of myxomatous material growing in remote sites (74,75), but their malignant potential has been disputed, as such reports may have overlooked the multifocal nature of Carney Complex (71).

Myxomas are thought to arise from multipotential mesenchymal cells, which represent embryonal remnants of the process of cardiac septation. Approximately 75% of myxomas occur in the left atrium and 15% to 20% in the right atrium, most frequently originating in the interatrial septum. A small percentage are also detected in the right or left ventricle. Myxomas are usually polypoid, consisting of peduculated masses with a round or oval shape and smooth or mildly lobulated surface (Figure 7.3). Less commonly, the tumor has a villous or papillary morphology, with multiple extensions that are typically gelatinous and fragile. It is the papillary variety of myxoma that is particularly prone to fragmentation and embolism (69).

Among patients with myxoma, 30% to 40% suffer an embolic event, which results from tumor fragments or overlying thrombus breaking free into the circulation. A cerebral ischemic infarct is the most common neurologic manifestation, typically with pathologic evidence of myxomatous emboli (76). Intracranial metastases and myxoma-induced aneurysmal dilatation of cerebral arteries have also been reported (76). In addition, myxomas can become superinfected and vegetations can embolize (77,78). For all these reasons, myxoma must be considered in the differential diagnosis of an unexplained peripheral embolic event.

TTE is the primary mode of detection and diagnosis. TEE is a useful adjunct as is can further elucidate the tumor's attachment point and mobility, as well as its relationship to other cardiac structures (79). More accurate determination of anatomical relations can also be achieved with newer imaging modalities such as cardiac CT (80) or MRI (81). Anticoagulation is not deemed indicated for embolism prevention of cardiac myxoma. Surgical resection is the treatment of choice and should

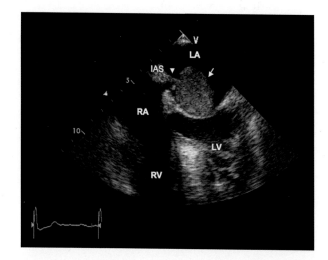

FIGURE 7.3 Transesophageal echocardiogram demonstrating a polypoid left atrial myxoma attached to the interatrial septum by a stalk. Arrow indicates myxoma; arrowhead indicates stalk. (LA, left atrium; LV, left ventricle; RA, right atrium; RV, right ventricle; IAS, interatrial septum.)

be performed promptly after diagnosis to prevent embolic complications. Resection is typically curative, except in the presence of Carney Complex (71).

Papillary Fibroelastoma

Papillary fibroelastoma (Figure 7.4) is a benign tumor of the heart usually found incidentally on echocardiography, at cardiac surgery or at autopsy. These masses contain multiple papillary fronds with a characteristic flower-like appearance, and are often attached to the endocardium by a short stalk. Histologically, the tumor is an avascular papilloma with a matrix consisting of proteoglycans, elastic fibers, and spindle cells covered by a single layer of endocardium. Their size can vary from 2 mm to 70 mm, with most tumors reaching 10 mm in their greatest dimension (82). Although they can arise anywhere within the heart, papillary fibroelastomas have a predilection for valvular endocardium, and are generally found on the atrial aspect of the atrioventricular valves or either surface of the semilunar valves (83). They can also appear on the atrial and ventricular walls, the atrial or ventricular septum, and the left atrial appendage (82).

Papillary fibroelastomas are associated with embolism, with case reports of cerebral (84), coronary (85), and pulmonary (86) involvement. In a review of a tertiary center's experience, 162 patients with pathologically confirmed papillary fibroelastomas were identified during a 16-year period (87). Mean age was 60 years;

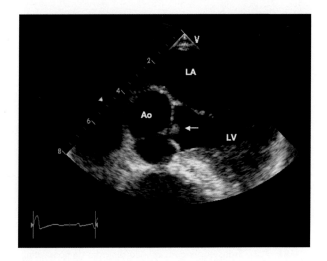

FIGURE 7.4 Transesophageal echocardiogram showing a globular echodensity on the ventricular surface of the aortic valve, consistent with a papillary fibroelastoma. Arrow indicates papillary fibroelastoma. (Ao, aortic root; LA, left atrium; LV, left ventricle.)

46.1% of patients were male. Most lesions (82.7%) were valvular, and more frequently located in the aortic than in the mitral position. They occurred singly in 91.4% of cases, and 43.6% were mobile.

Embolic events can occur when friable fibroelastoma tissue or thrombus deposits on the tumor surface break free into the circulation. However, it is unclear whether embolization more commonly reflects tumor fragments or associated thrombus (82). Transcranial Doppler-detected embolic signals have been reported in a patient with stroke in multiple territories and a metal valve papillary fibroelastoma, with documented resolution upon surgical resection of the tumor (88). TTE and TEE are able to detect and characterize these cardiac tumors. For symptomatic papillary fibroelastomas or large, mobile tumors, surgical excision is the treatment of choice and is usually curative. There is insufficient evidence to support anticoagulation for smaller tumors followed noninvasively, but antiplatelet therapy is a sensible option in this setting.

Other Benign Cardiac Tumors

Among other primary benign tumors of the heart, rhabdomyomas, and fibromas occur predominantly in children, where they involve the myocardium (89). Rhabdomyomas, the most common primary cardiac tumor in this population, tend to regress spontaneously (89). The clinical consequences of these tumors relate principally to obstruction or arrhythmia, and not to embolism (89). Lipomas principally arise in ventricular myocardium, but have also been reported to occur in heart valves (90), although there are no reports of embolism to date. In the setting of clinically important obstruction or serious arrhythmia, surgical resection is indicated for these primary benign cardiac tumors.

Primary Malignant Tumors

Twenty-five percent of primary cardiac tumors are malignant in nature (91). Sarcomas constitute 75% of all primary malignant tumors of the heart (92). Several types of sarcoma have been observed, including undifferentiated sarcoma, angiosarcoma, osteosarcoma, leiomyosarcoma, and myxoid sarcoma (93). Other types of malignant cardiac tumors include malignant fibrous histiocytoma and primary cardiac lymphoma. Sarcomas generally carry a dismal prognosis, and treatment involves a combination of surgical resection, chemotherapy, and radiation, depending on the subtype

(94,95). Cardiac autotransplation has also been used to treat difficult tumors (92,93). Lymphomas are primarily treated with chemotherapy (96).

Metastatic Tumors

Metastatic tumors to the heart occur far more frequently than primary tumors, yet their presence may not be recognized. As solitary metastases are exceedingly rare, cardiac metastases tend to present in patients with disseminated disease and signs of cardiac involvement are often clinically overlooked (97). Cardiac metastases rarely present as intracavitary lesions, but when they do occur, these are generally covered by thrombotic material. Metastatic cardiac tumors are most common in carcinomas of the lung, breast, and esophagus, as well as lymphoma, leukemia, and melanoma, occurring via hematogenous spread. Echocardiography is the foremost modality for intracavitary lesion detection (97), although additional characterization may be provided by cardiac CT (80) or MRI (98).

Valvular Vegetations

Infective and noninfective endocarditis leads to a significant risk of systemic embolization. The risk of ischemic stroke with infective endocarditis is 15% to 20%, with the first 7 to 10 days after presentation conferring the highest risk (99). Vegetations found on the mitral valve (Figure 7.5) carry a greater risk of stroke than vegetations on the aortic valve (100). Certain characteristics, in

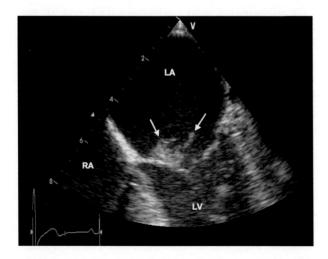

FIGURE 7.5 Transesophageal echocardiogram of mitral valve vegetation. Arrows indicate vegetation. (LA, left atrium; LV, left ventricle; RA, right atrium.)

particular, size, mobility, consistency, and extent, determine the embolic potential of the vegetations and the associated risk of stroke (100–102). Nonbacterial thrombotic (marantic) endocarditis consists of aseptic vegetations seen on the valve leaflets in patients with neoplastic disorders, acquired immunodeficiency syndrome, or autoimmune diseases such as systemic lupus erythematosus (Libman-Sachs endocarditis). These vegetations are also associated with a high risk of embolism (102–104).

Although TTE can be useful in the evaluation of endocarditis, TEE is more accurate for detection of vegetations (104,105) and can better characterize their size, location, and mobility. Treatment of endocarditis must be focused on the underlying cause. Infective endocarditis requires systemic antibiotics and, if clinically indicated, surgery (99). Noninfective endocarditis is treated with tumor-suppressive, antiretroviral, or immunosuppressive therapy. Professional-society guidelines also recommend systemic anticoagulation with unfractionated or low-molecular weight heparin, owing to their superior prophylaxis of thromboembolism as compared with warfarin anticoagulation (65).

Prosthetic Valves

Systemic embolization is a complication of both mechanical and bioprosthetic heart valves. Up to 80% of clinical thromboemboli associated with prosthetic valves involve the brain (6). Mechanical heart valves require lifelong anticoagulation to curtail the pronounced rates of thromboembolism—12% and 22% per year in aortic and mitral prostheses, respectively—observed in the absence of anithrombotic prophylaxis (65). Anticoagulation with vitamin K antagonists (e.g., warfarin) reduces yearly thromboembolism incidence to between 0.5% and 3.0% for aortic prostheses, and between 0.5% and 5.0% for mitral prostheses (106), with the lowest risk reported for late generation bileaflet prostheses (65). Target INR for contemporary mechanical prostheses is 2.5 to 3.5 for the mitral position, and 2.0 to 3.0 for the aortic position (65). Bioprosthetic valves do not require lifelong anticoagulation, but do carry the risk of thromboembolic disease. The risk is highest during the first three months after insertion, especially in the mitral position, in patients who do not undergo antithrombotic prophylaxis (107). Guidelines recommend unfractionated heparin or low molecular weight heparin in the early postoperative period with a transition to warfarin therapy (target INR 2.0–3.0) for the first three months after insertion (65).

Long-term risk of thromboembolism for bioprosthetic valves is reported to be 0.2% to 2.6% per year. The presence of AF or a pacemaker increases the rate of events (65). For patients in sinus rhythm, indefinite low-dose aspirin use is recommended after the first three months of insertion for bioprosthetic valves (65).

Complex Aortic Atheroma

With the capacity of TEE to image protruding atheromas of the thoracic aorta came recognition of the association of these lesions with stroke and systemic embolization (108). Pathologic correlations have contributed to our understanding of the relationship of aortic atheroma and cerebral infarction. In a series of 500 autopsies involving stroke and other neurologic diseases, ulcerated plaques in the aortic arch were more common in cases with cerebrovascular disease (26% of 239 patients) than nonvascular disorders (5% of 261 patients) (109). Moreover, cases with cryptogenic stroke were more likely to have ulcerated aortic arch plaques than cases with a known cause of stroke. Surgical pathology reports have also shown that mobile aortic plaque components imaged by TEE correspond to superimposed thrombi, likely secondary to plaque fissuring, rupture, or ulceration (110,111).

Identification of protruding aortic plaques, or plaques exhibiting ulceration or mobile components, as potentially important sources of atherothromboembolism led to their designation as "complex" aortic atheromas (CAA) (Figure 7.6). In fact, the thickness of such

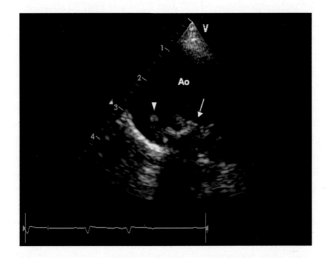

FIGURE 7.6 Transesophageal echocardiogram of complex atheroma in the aortic arch. Arrow indicates complex atheroma, arrowhead indicates mobile component (not appreciable in still image). (Ao, aorta.)

atheromas determines their associated risk. Among patients with cerebral infarction undergoing TEE, the presence of proximal thoracic aortic plaques of 4-mm or greater thickness conferred a heightened risk of incident cardiovascular events and recurrent stroke, as compared with plaques of lesser thickness or their absence (112). Furthermore, the odds ratio for stroke recurrence in patients with such severe atheromas of the ascending aorta and aortic arch was significantly higher than for severe atheromas of the descending aorta (112). These findings support the premise that atheromas in the proximal thoracic aorta can be the cause of stroke—presumably through atherothromboembolism—and not simply a marker for generalized atherosclerosis. In the same study, the absolute one-year risk for stroke recurrence associated with TEE-diagnosed complex atheroma of the proximal thoracic aorta was 12% (112).

The clinical significance of CAA also extends to the setting of AF. Analyses from the Stroke Prevention in Atrial Fibrillation (SPAF) III study showed that the risk of thromboembolism was four times greater for these high-risk patients with AF in the presence of CAA (atheroma ≥4 mm or containing ulceration or mobile components) as compared to its absence (113).

Data on the population prevalence of atheromas of the thoracic aorta come from the Stroke Prevention: Assessment of Risk in a Community (SPARC) study, a TEE survey of the frequency of cardiac sources of embolism among community dwelling stroke-free individuals (114). SPARC reported that 43.7% of the 588 older participants who underwent TEE had thoracic aortic plaque in any location. CAA was documented in 7.6% of subjects, but only 0.2% and 2.2% were found in the ascending aorta and aortic arch, respectively. By contrast, two large series of stroke patients have shown that the prevalence of severe aortic plaque (14%–21%) is substantially greater and similar in magnitude to other important etiologies of ischemic stroke, namely carotid artery disease (10%–13%) and AF (18%–30%) (115,116).

Several diagnostic imaging modalities can be used to aid the detection of aortic atheroma. The aortic root and proximal ascending aorta can be visualized frequently with TTE , and in some patients views of the aortic arch and descending aorta can be obtained (117). However, TEE offers higher resolution and is more accurate in overall detection, measurement of plaque thickness, and identifying the presence of mobile components. TEE allows evaluation of nearly the entire thoracic aorta, including plaque composition and burden, with good interobserver and intraobserver variability (118,119).

MRI has also been used to image aortic plaques. In 1999, a study comparing MRI to TEE in the evaluation of aortic plaque showed that MR angiography underestimated the plaque thickness in the aortic arch (120). Subsequently, in a study of 10 patients with known aortic plaque identified by TEE, MRI was used to assess the composition, extent, and size of the plaque. Its authors reported an 80% overall agreement between the two imaging modalities for the 25 cross-sectional aortic segments assessed (121). MRI has two important advantages. First, this modality can be used to differentiate components of the atheroma including calcification, fibrocellular tissue, lipid and thrombus, which in turn may help determine the overall stability of the plaque (122–124). Second, MRI is useful in monitoring changes in plaque thickness, both progression and regression over time (125). Indeed, early studies (126,127) in patients with cerebral ischemia suggest that this modality may have incremental utility for identification of aortic sources of thromboembolism, particularly when techniques that can detect associated intraplaque thrombus or hemorrhage are applied.

CT has also been utilized to evaluate the aorta and identify atherosclerotic lesions, especially in areas unable to be visualized by TEE. Prior studies have shown that noncontrast dual-helical CT can detect protruding aortic atheromas with similar rates to TEE (94% of plaques seen by TEE also detected by CT) (128). Contrast-enhanced spiral dual-helical CT has also been reported to identify atheromas and plaque thickness accurately (129). A recent study examining a cohort of stroke patients demonstrated similar rates of detection between cardiac-gated CT and TEE (130). It also reported that cardiac-gated CT was able to identify smaller plaques (130).

Anticoagulation and antiplatelet therapy for the prevention of thromboembolism associated with aortic atheroma has been studied. Two small observational nonrandomized studies showed a reduction in the number of embolic events in subjects treated with warfarin (131,132). The SPAF III study, which was a randomized trial of patients with nonvalvular AF, reported that adjusted-dose warfarin reduced the risk of thromboembolism associated with complex plaques (atheroma ≥4 mm or containing ulceration or mobile components) by 75%

relative to combination therapy with low-intensity warfarin and aspirin (113). However, current guidelines do not recommend routine anticoagulation of CAA for secondary stroke prevention (3,65), although either low-dose aspirin or adjusted-dose warfarin are deemed acceptable strategies in the presence of mobile aortic arch thrombi (65). For primary prevention, antiplatelet therapy is sensible, but anticoagulation may be considered for incidentally discovered plaque with mobile components, especially when located in the proximal thoracic aorta. Randomized clinical trials, however, are needed to determine the best antithrombotic therapy, particularly in the secondary prevention setting.

Beyond antithrombotic therapy, statins have been shown to reduce the risk of ischemic stroke (133–135). In addition, the use of statins has been associated with lower incidence of recurrent embolic events in patients found to have CAA by TEE (136), and aggressive therapy for LDL-cholesterol lowering has been associated with significant regression in plaque size as well as reverse remodeling (137–139). Thus, aggressive LDL lowering should be pursued in patients with CAA for both primary and secondary prevention.

■ SOURCES OF EMBOLISM OF MEDIUM OR UNCERTAIN RISK

Interatrial Septal Abnormalities

Patent Foramen Ovale

Patent foramen ovale (PFO) is a remnant of the fetal circulation that is present in 25% to 30% of adults (140). The interatrial septum arises from the septum primum, which grows caudally from the roof of the atrium, and septum secundum, which grows cephalad from the interventricular septum. In utero, oxygenated blood from the placenta, directed at the foramen ovale from the inferior vena cava by the Eustachian valve, Chiari network, or both, bypasses the unaerated fetal lungs through this interatrial pathway. The septum primum flap is thus maintained open by right atrial pressures that exceed left atrial pressures (141). After birth, the lungs are ventilated and pressures in the pulmonary circulation decrease, leading to a decline in right-heart pressures below those of the left heart. As a result, the septum primum flap is apposed against the septum secundum (141). These two structures fuse in a majority of infants to form a permanent seal, completely separating the left and right atria. However, this fusion does not occur in about a quarter of infants, and a potential conduit for right-to-left shunting remains (140).

Echocardiography is the primary imaging modality used to diagnose PFO. TEE can detect this structure by three different methods: abnormal flow across the PFO by color Doppler, direct B-mode visualization of the separation of the septum primum and septum secundum via multiplane transducers, and detection of microbubbles from intravenously injected agitated saline in left-sided chambers of the heart that would otherwise by filtered by the lung capillaries (142,143). TTE is also used, but the sensitivity of TTE with agitated saline contrast for right-to-left shunts has been inferior to TEE (144). The advent of second-harmonic imaging, however, with improved 2-dimensional cardiac visualization, and development of contrast-based transmitral Doppler techniques have improved the diagnostic accuracy of TTE (142,145–147).

Contrast transcranial Doppler is another sonographic alternative. Detecting right-to-left shunting of microbubbles in the middle cerebral arteries, this technique has been shown to have similar accuracy to TEE (142), but it does not allow visualization of the morphologic features of the interatrial septum and other cardiac structures.

More recently, gadolinium-based contrast-enhanced MRI has been used to detect PFO. The contrast signal is plotted on a signal-time curve for both the right and left atria and the diagnosis of PFO is made when the signal is demonstrated in both atria simultaneously (148). The spatial resolution of current MRI techniques does not allow for the size of the PFO to be assessed accurately (81). Multidetector CT scans have also been used to identify PFO. CT criteria for diagnosis include the identification of a channel in the interatrial septum or a left atrial flap in the location of the septum primum associated with a jet of contrast from the left atrium to the right atrium (requiring an incompetent septum primum valve) (149,150). Currently, CT is not as sensitive or specific in recognizing PFO in comparison to TEE (149,150), although reappraisal will be necessary in light of the rapid evolution of CT, as well as MRI, technology.

Several (151), but not all (152–154), studies have shown a significant association between PFO and ischemic stroke. Initially, the pathologic significance of this potential pathway between the atria was recognized in autopsy cases with systemic emboli wherein thrombi

were observed trapped in the foramen (155,156). This finding has since been documented in a number of case reports by echocardiography (155,156), demonstrating the pathophysiologic mechanism of paradoxical embolism as an etiology of stroke.

Additional support for the clinical relevance of PFO to ischemic stroke came when a case-control study found PFO to be substantially more prevalent in younger patients with cryptogenic stroke as compared with matched control subjects (54% versus 10%, respectively, by TTE) (157). A meta-analysis (158) of this and several case-control studies that followed confirmed the higher frequency of PFO among patients less than 55-years-old with cryptogenic stroke compared to stroke-free controls (odds ratio 5.01, 95% confidence interval [CI] 3.24–7.75). However, it found no difference among subjects 55-years-old or older (odds ratio 1.20, 95% CI 0.56–2.56) (158). Because many of these studies lacked blinded interpretation of echocardiograms, ascertainment bias may have skewed results. Still, a prospective clinical trial in which echocardiograms were interpreted without knowledge of subjects' clinical histories also reported an association between stroke and PFO (159). In addition, a subsequent prospective investigation reported a significantly higher prevalence of PFOs for patients with cryptogenic stroke than those with stroke of known cause, both in younger and older adults, supporting the potential pathogenic role of PFO in patients of more advanced age (160).

Despite the documented association of PFO and ischemic stroke, however, the validity of invoking paradoxical embolism as the underlying mechanism in the majority of such cases remains open to question. For thrombus to transit across a PFO, a pressure gradient leading to right-to-left shunting is necessary. Yet such a favorable gradient occurs only in early systole, and is very transient (161). Moreover, elevated right heart pressures secondary to pulmonary hypertension, or the performance of a Valsalva-type activity immediately prior to the clinical event, have been reported infrequently in stroke patients with PFO (162). In addition, a venous source of embolism is rarely detected in the evaluation of patients with cryptogenic stroke (162).

Accordingly, alternative explanations for the stroke-PFO relationship have been advanced, including in situ septal thrombosis and atrial dysrhythmias (163). However, these findings are rarely documented in patients with cryptogenic stroke (163). Furthermore, the infrequent detection of venous sources in cryptogenic stroke patients with PFO does not necessarily exclude their presence. Apart from the possibility that the proximal venous thrombus might have migrated in its entirety, leaving no trace, the consideration that standard sonographic assessment for deep venous thrombosis focuses solely on the femoral and popliteal veins merits notice. In fact, conventional venography (164) and MRI venography (165) have been reported to detect calf-vein and pelvic-vein thrombosis in sizable proportions of patients with unexplained systemic embolism and interatrial shunts (163).

In the general population, PFO can be estimated to confer, on average, a yearly risk of cryptogenic stroke as low as 0.1% (166). Yet certain PFO characteristics may act to influence the associated level of risk. These relate to the ease and magnitude of right-to-left shunting. Maximal anatomical separation between the primum and secundum septa during provocative maneuvers (Valsalva maneuver or coughing), as measured by 2-dimensional TEE imaging (Figure 7.7), has been linked with increased risk of stroke, particularly when such separation is of 4 mm or greater (167,168). PFOs have been categorized as small, medium or large based on separation distances of <2 mm, 2 to 4 mm, and ≥4 mm, respectively (167,168). The extent of microbubble passage across the foramen provides another measure of the magnitude of right-to-left shunting, and has also been reported to predict incidence of recurrent ischemic events (169). Although no standardized criteria exist, the magnitude of right-to-left interatrial shunting in the setting of provocative maneuvers can be defined as mild when less than 10 bubbles/frame are identified in the left heart, intermediate when the number ranges from 10 to 50, and large when it reaches or exceeds 50 bubbles/frame (170,171).

Shunting at rest and hypermobility of the septum primum have also been reported to amplify the embolic risk of PFO (172), as has the presence of an atrial septal aneurysm (ASA) (Fig. 7.7) (173). In addition, joint occurrence of a prominent Eustachian valve or a Chiari network, remnants of the sinus venosus that direct inferior vena caval flow toward the fossa ovale, have been associated with stroke risk in some, but not all, studies (174).

Beyond characteristics inherent to the foramen and associated cardiac structures, a second factor pivotal to the occurrence of paradoxical embolism is proclivity to the development of venous thrombosis. Whether as a result of immobility, trauma or malignancy, or as a consequence of a heritable or acquired hypercoagulable

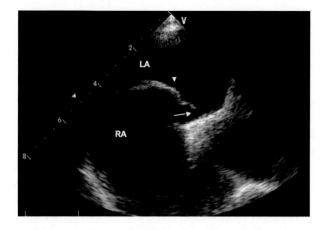

FIGURE 7.7 Transesophageal echocardiogram demonstrating separation (*arrow*) between the primum and secundum septa, as well as bulging of a redundant septum primum membrane (arrowhead) during Valsalva maneuver. These findings are consistent with a patent foramen ovale with associated atrial septal aneurysm. (RA, right atrium; LA, left atrium.)

disorder, propensity to venous thromboembolism is a determinant of PFO-associated stroke risk (156).

Atrial Septal Aneurysm

ASA is the bulging of a redundant interatrial septum at the level of fossa ovalis into the left or right atrium or both. The magnitude of excursion from the midline as a defining characteristic is inconsistent in the literature, with some authors citing a value of 11 mm or greater (172,175), while others use 15 mm or greater (170,176). The prevalence of ASA in the general population using a cutoff value of 15-mm excursion has been reported to be 2.2% (177), as compared with 1% in autopsy studies (178). However, among patients with ischemic stroke, this prevalence rises to 7.9% (173,177). Several other studies have shown a relationship between ASA and ischemic stroke (179–183), but the underlying pathophysiologic mechanism is unclear. Findings of thrombotic material in the redundant aneurysmal sac at autopsy or in surgical patients have shown that the hypermobile septum may be a nidus for thrombosis (183). ASA has also been associated with atrial dysrhythmias that predispose to thromboembolism (184). However, the ASA-stroke relationship has mostly been attributed to the high prevalence (as high as 90%) of a coexisting PFO or atrial septal defect (177,183), thus increasing the possibility of paradoxical embolism as an explanation. ASA are also associated with prominent

Eustachian valves or Chiari networks, which can direct flow of blood from the inferior vena cava toward the fossa ovalis and facilitate right-to-left shunting through a PFO or atrial septal defect (174).

Patent Foramen Ovale and Atrial Septal Aneurysm

Treatment strategies for PFO include antiplatelet therapy, anticoagulant therapy, percutaneous closure, and surgical closure. There is insufficient clinical evidence to guide therapy for primary prevention of ischemic stroke in asymptomatic patients with PFO. For secondary prevention, no randomized data are available, but guidance can be drawn from observational studies (143).

Antiplatelet and anticoagulant therapy both target thrombus formation, although the latter would be expected to have greater antithrombotic efficacy against fibrin-rich thrombi of venous origin—the principal substrate for paradoxical embolization. In the Patent Foramen Ovale in Cryptogenic Stroke Study (PICSS), which focused on the subgroup of patients referred for TEE in a randomized trial comparing aspirin versus warfarin for secondary prevention in noncardioembolic stroke, there was no difference in recurrent stroke or death, irrespective of PFO size or presence of ASA detected by this technique (159). Analysis restricted to the subgroup with cryptogenic stroke and PFO showed, however, that warfarin was associated with a nonsignificantly decreased risk of stroke or death (hazard ratio 0.52, 95% CI 0.16–1.67), with a similar result observed for cryptogenic stroke patients without PFO. Even though this subgroup analysis was underpowered, it does suggest that warfarin may be superior in preventing recurrent events in this patient population.

Another prospective study examined 581 cryptogenic stroke patients treated with 300 mg of aspirin daily followed over a four-year period (173). Of these patients, 25% had a PFO, 2% had an ASA, and 9% had both. There was no significant difference in the recurrent stroke risk between patients with PFO alone (0.6% per year) and those without a PFO (1.1% per year). However, patients with both interatrial findings had a significantly higher incidence of stroke (3.8% per year) during the four-year follow-up. The results of this study suggest that aspirin therapy alone may be insufficient to prevent recurrent strokes in young cryptogenic stroke patients with concomitant PFO and ASA.

By contrast, mechanical closure of PFO aims to eliminate the conduit for paradoxical embolism,

barring the way into the arterial circulation for thrombi of venous origin. Traditionally, closure of PFO has been performed surgically via open thoracotomy. Mortality rates for surgical closure of an uncomplicated atrial septal defect is less than 1.5% (185). Perioperative risks include AF, pericardial sequelae, wound infection, and the need for reoperation for bleeding (186–188). In small case series, the rate of postoperative stroke has been reported to be between 0% and 3.5% after two years (186–188). One study followed young cryptogenic stroke patients who underwent surgical closure of PFO if they presented with two of four high-risk features, defined as major shunt with >50 bubbles/frame, ASA, infarcts in multiple vascular territories, or Valsalva-provoking activity prior to the onset of stroke symptoms (187). The authors reported no recurrent ischemic events 23 months after PFO closure in these subjects, but the study did not include a control group.

Percutaneous endovascular closure of PFO was first reported in the early 1990s (189). Endovascular deployment of percutaneous devices eliminates right-to-left interatrial shunting while obviating the need for thoracotomy or sternotomy, although the procedure is not without its associated risks. Reported complications include transient ischemic attack, stroke, atrial dysrhythmias, device dislodgement and embolization, retroperitoneal hemorrhage, endocarditis, and thrombus formation on the device (143). Several PFO closure devices are available, each with its own technical and clinical success profile (176). Complete sealing of the foramen is achieved in 90% to 95% of cases at one year post-procedure (163).

Comparisons of medical treatment and percutaneous closure of PFO for prevention of recurrent ischemic stroke, to date, have only involved nonrandomized case series. The largest available report examined 308 cryptogenic stroke patients with PFO receiving either medical management (warfarin with INR 2–3, aspirin 233 ± 83 mg/day, or clopidogrel 75 mg/day per the discretion of the attending neurologist) or percutaneous PFO closure (190). At four years of follow up, there was a nonsignificant trend favoring percutaneous closure for the primary composite endpoint of death, stroke, and transient ischemic attack (8.5 versus 24.3%, $P = 0.05$). Yet lack of randomized treatment assignment, together with outcome adjudication by family practitioners who were not blinded to therapy, introduces potential biases that make the findings inconclusive. Several randomized clinical trials are currently underway to compare percutaneous PFO closure with medical management for the prevention of ischemic stroke (65).

Current guidelines conclude that available data do not allow for definitive treatment recommendations (2,3). In patients with a prior stroke or transient ischemic attack and a PFO, antiplatelet therapy is the favored treatment (2,3). Both the combination of extended-release dipyridamole and aspirin, and monotherapy with clopidogrel are deemed preferable to aspirin for secondary prevention of noncardioembolic stroke (191), although the relative merits of these agents in patients with cryptogenic brain embolism have not been directly tested. If concurrent venous thromboembolism (deep venous thrombosis or pulmonary embolism) is detected, however, anticoagulation is advised (65). Anticoagulation may also be indicated when a hypercoagulable state is present. Furthermore, long-term anticoagulation may be the preferred treatment strategy in young patients with cryptogenic stroke and PFO with the high-risk features mentioned previously (163).

In the absence of randomized evidence, use of percutaneous devices is not currently approved by the Food and Drug Administration for closure of PFO. Such devices can only be used in the United States through participation in a randomized trial or by application to an institutional review board exemption under circumstances that make anticoagulation undesirable and/or hazardous.

Pulmonary Arteriovenous Malformations

Pulmonary arteriovenous malformations may occur in isolation, in association with liver or congenital heart disease, or as a manifestation of hereditary hemorrhagic telangiectasia (192). These vascular structures may serve as transpulmonary conduits for venous-source emboli. Indeed, in a series of patients referred for endovascular occlusion of these vascular lesions, cerebral infarction was documented in 32% of patients with single malformations and in 60% of patients with multiple ones (193). There are no randomized data to guide optimal management of these vascular abnormalities, but transcatheter embolotherapy is favored for pulmonary arteriovenous malformations ≥3 mm in diameter, especially following documented cerebral ischemia (193).

Spontaneous Echo Contrast

Spontaneous echo contrast (SEC), also known as "smoke," is visualized by echocardiography as swirling echodensities in cardiac chambers or vessels. SEC reflects formation of rouleaux by red-blood cells as a consequence of stasis of blood flow, increased fibrinogen concentration, or high hematocrit (194). It is most commonly detected in the left atrium and left atrial appendage in the setting of AF or mitral stenosis, but is also described in patients with prosthetic heart valves and severe ventricular dysfunction (195–197). TEE is the primary clinical modality used to visualize the left atrial appendage and to detect SEC (198,199).

An early study examined the relationship of left atrial appendage function to SEC and thrombus in 12 patients with rheumatic AF, 29 patients with nonrheumatic AF, and 30 patients in normal sinus rhythm (59). This investigation reported different flow-velocity and contraction patterns in these three groups of patients. Patients with rheumatic AF were found to have minimal visible fibrillatory contractions of the appendage with flow velocities <25 cm/s (low-flow profile). In turn, patients with nonrheumatic AF had either low-flow profiles or visible fibrillatory contractions of the appendage wall with velocities ≥25 cm/s (high-flow profiles). Finally, discrete appendage contraction, with flow velocities >50 cm/s, was observed in patients with normal sinus rhythm. SEC was not detected in any of the patients in sinus rhythm, but was observed in 5% of patients with nonrheumatic AF and high-flow profile, 80% of patients with nonrheumatic AF and low-flow profile, and 92% of patients with rheumatic AF. Overall, this study showed that SEC is closely related to reduced contractility of the left atrial appendage.

Studies have showed that SEC is associated with thrombus formation and thromboembolic events (200,201). In the SPAF III study (113), SEC was associated with decreased left atrial appendage emptying velocity. SEC was detected in 75% of patients with emptying velocity of ≤20 cm/s compared to 58% of patients with a higher velocity (P <0.001). In addition, the prevalence of thrombus was 17% and 5% in these two groups, respectively (P <0.001). The study also reported that SEC density was related to thrombus formation, since 24% of patients with dense smoke had thrombus in the left atrial appendage, as compared with 10% of those with faint smoke, and 3% without smoke (P <0.001). Peak left atrial appendage flow velocity was inversely related to the rate of thromboembolism in this study. The relative risk of ischemic stroke in study subjects was 2.6 for patients with flow velocity ≤20 cm/s compared to patients with flow velocity >20 cm/s (P = 0.02). Patients with dense smoke randomized to receive combination therapy of low-dose warfarin and aspirin had an annual thromboembolic event rate of 18.2%, which corresponded to a relative risk of 2.7 compared to subjects without dense contrast ($P = 0.06$). This risk was decreased to 4.5% per year in those subjects assigned to adjusted-dose warfarin (with target INR 2–3), although this difference was not statistically significant ($P = 0.09$).

Cardioversion leading to left atrial appendage stunning and dysfunction has also been associated with new or worsening SEC. This phenomenon has been described in direct-current external cardioversion (202,203), spontaneous cardioversion (204), pharmacologic cardioversion (205), and low-energy internal atrial defibrillation (206). Although the pathophysiologic nature of left atrial appendage stunning is unclear, these studies support the hypothesis that the conversion to normal sinus rhythm itself, instead of the method of cardioversion, leads to myocardial stunning.

SEC represents a prethrombotic condition. Since it has been shown to be a marker of thromboembolic risk in AF, mitral stenosis and mitral valve replacement (197), use of systemic anticoagulation should be considered in patients with cryptogenic stroke in sinus rhythm in whom SEC is detected.

Mitral Valve Prolapse

Several early studies reported an association between mitral valve prolapse (MVP) and stroke (207–209). For example, a case-control study detected MVP in 40% of 60 patients less than 45-years-old with prior TIA or strokes, compared to 6.8% of age-matched control subjects ($P <0.001$). These early studies, however, applied M-mode and 2-dimensional echocardiography criteria that did not account for the 3-dimensional shape of the mitral annulus (210). Diagnostic criteria for MVP were subsequently revised, leading to greater specificity and, accordingly, decreased prevalence (<2.5%) of MVP in population studies (211). More recent investigations using the newer diagnostic criteria have not shown a significant association between MVP and stroke (13,211,212). These studies are of relatively modest sample size, however, and cannot exclude a moderately strong relationship between MVP and stroke. The extent to which MVP predisposes to ischemic stroke requires further investigation.

Current guidelines recommend against antithrombotic therapy in patients with MVP who do not have history of systemic embolism, unexplained TIA, or

ischemic stroke (3,65). For patients with stroke or TIA with associated MVP, there is consensus across professional societies for antiplatelet drugs as the treatment of choice unless AF or left atrial thrombus is also detected (2,65,213), although one group recommends anticoagulation therapy in the presence of mitral regurgitation or mitral leaflet thickening (213). In terms of choice of antiplatelet therapy for secondary stroke prevention in the setting of MVP, the combination of aspirin and extended release dipyridamole or clopidogrel may be preferable over aspirin alone, as judged from clinical trials in noncardioembolic stroke (191).

Valvular Calcification

Mitral Annular Calcification

Mitral annular calcification (MAC) is a chronic, degenerative process of the fibrous skeleton of the mitral valve (214). It is identified by the presence of bright echoes at the base of the mitral leaflets by 2-dimensional TTE or TEE, and is graded on a semiquantitative scale based on the extent of annular calcific deposits. The relationship between MAC and incident stroke was detailed in a large population-based study, wherein an association between the thickness of calcium deposition and stroke risk was documented (215). Other studies have since confirmed that MAC is an independent predictor of stroke (12,216), but the mechanism underlying this relationship is not well delineated. It is accepted that MAC serves as a marker of overall atherosclerotic burden, with several studies showing an association of MAC with coronary artery disease (217–219), carotid artery disease (220–222), aortic arch atheroma (223–225), and peripheral vascular disease (226). However, there is evidence that MAC can act as a direct emboligenic substrate, provided by reports of MAC-associated thrombotic (227), vegetative (228), or mobile calcific debris (229), and of such material detected in the cerebral circulation at necropsy (230). Current guidelines do not recommend anticoagulation therapy unless patients have recurrent systemic embolic events, ischemic strokes, or TIAs (2,65). Besides antiplatelet therapy, standard secondary prevention of atherosclerosis with lifestyle modification and lipid-lowering therapy is essential.

Aortic Valve Sclerosis

Aortic valve sclerosis is characterized by calcium and lipid deposition in the leaflets of the aortic valve (231).

Like MAC, aortic valve calcification shares risk factors with atherosclerosis, and has been documented to be a predictor of cardiovascular events. An association between aortic valve calcification and stroke in particular, however, has only been documented in the setting of aortic stenosis (12,232–234). Although direct embolization of calcium fragments or thrombotic material has been proposed as the pathophysiologic basis for this relationship, supportive evidence is lacking. To the extent that aortic valve sclerosis predicts ischemic stroke, the relationship of aortic valve sclerosis with subclinical atherosclerotic disease, particularly in the proximal thoracic aorta and large cervical and cerebral arteries, is likely to be the predominant pathophysiologic basis. In the presence of stenosis, however, beyond greater severity of calcification, the resulting left ventricular hypertrophy and, with it, left atrial enlargement provide an additional arrhythmic and thrombogenic substrate that could drive a heightened stroke risk.

Use of antithrombotic therapy for primary stroke prevention in the setting of isolated aortic valve sclerosis (i.e., with no separate indication from known atherosclerotic disease or its risk factors) is controversial, although the presence of this condition might sway a decision to institute aspirin therapy in an individual with otherwise uncertain indications for such preventive treatment. Statin therapy for reducing progression of aortic valve calcification has been evaluated, but contrary to expectations, has not proven effective at influencing this process (235,236). For secondary prevention, guidelines are uniform in recommending antiplatelet therapy over anticoagulation for the patient with stroke and aortic valve calcification (2,65), and the same considerations regarding choice of antiplatelet agent mentioned earlier apply.

Valvular Strands

Strands of the cardiac valves were first described by Vilem Dusan Lambl in 1856 (237), in whose honor they are also known as Lambl's excrescences. These strands are thin, mobile, filiform structures that arise near the line of valvular closure. They most often occur on the native aortic and mitral valves, as well as on prosthetic valves, but are less common on the tricuspid and, especially, the pulmonic valve (238). Lambl's excrescences are typically 1 mm or less in width and 1 to 5 mm in length, but can attain lengths of 10 mm or greater. Echocardiographically, Lambl's excrescences are differentiated from vegetations and tumors by an upper width limit of 1 to 2 mm (14,239). Their composition includes a central, densely hyalinized, avascular core and a peripheral layer of connective tissue covered by a single layer of endothelial cells (239). The pathogenesis of valvular strands remains unclear. It is postulated, however, that endocardial microabrasions or tears secondary to shear stress and trauma can lead to fibrin deposition and an overgrowth of the endothelial layer (239). TEE is the primary imaging modality for detection of these structures. Using this imaging technique, the prevalence of valvular strands in a population-based sample was determined to be 5.5% (240).

Several similarities exist between valvular strands and papillary fibroelastomas, which leads to the proposition that these two may be part of the same continuum. In the literature, the terms "giant Lambl's excrescences" and papillary fibroelastoma are used interchangeably (239). Histopathologically, they both contain a core of elastic connective tissue. However, there are several differences between these lesions. Lambl's excrescences are typically covered by a single layer of endothelial cells, while fibroelastomas contain several areas of multiple endothelial layers. Lambl's excrescenses usually occur in areas of the valve under the highest mechanical stress, in particular the leaflet lines of closure. In contrast, fibroelastomas can be found on other parts of the valve and endocardium (237). In addition, fibroelastomas generally are attached to the valve by a stalk or pedestal and can exhibit frond-like projections, which are not seen on valvular strands. Finally, there is cytogenetic evidence to suggest that papillary fibroelastomas may be neoplastic (241).

Valvular strands have been associated with cerebral ischemia in several cross-sectional studies (242–245). It has been proposed that strands or portions of strands may break off and embolize, or that thrombi may form on the strands owing to trauma, tears, and microabrasions of the endothelium (246). Unlike cardiac myxomas, however, valvular strands have rarely been found in the affected arteries on pathology specimens (246). Moreover, three longitudinal studies have failed to show an association of valvular strands with incident cerebral ischemia (14,15,247). These observations, together with the frequent detection of valvular strands as incidental findings in stroke-free patients, call into question a meaningful causal relationship between Lambl's excrescences and stroke.

Available evidence does not support institution of antithrombotic therapy for primary stroke prevention in individuals with incidentally discovered valvular strands. With regard to secondary prevention, analyses of PICSS documented similar incidences of recurrent stroke or death among patients with valvular strands randomized to aspirin versus warfarin (247). Thus, professional-society guidelines recommend antiplatelet therapy for patients with stroke and valvular strands (3). Surgery is generally not recommended for the treatment of valvular strands, but should be a consideration in patients with recurrent and otherwise cryptogenic stroke on medical therapy who harbor giant Lambl's excrescences (246).

■ CONCLUSION

Familiarity with cardioaortic sources of embolism, and knowledge of the diagnostic approaches and therapeutic options available for individuals harboring such findings, is of paramount importance for the care of patients with ischemic stroke, especially when otherwise unexplained. Much remains uncertain concerning the management of individual cardioaortic sources, and their relevance in the setting of cerebral ischemia, but ongoing and future research efforts promise to enhance strategies for the evaluation and treatment of affected patients.

■ REFERENCES

1. Rosamond W, Flegal K, Furie K, et al. Heart disease and stroke statistics—2008 update: a report from the American Heart Association Statistics Committee and Stroke Statistics Subcommittee. *Circulation* 2008;117:e25–146.
2. Sacco RL, Adams R, Albers G, et al. Guidelines for prevention of stroke in patients with ischemic stroke or transient ischemic attack: a statement for healthcare professionals from the American Heart Association/American Stroke Association Council on Stroke: co-sponsored by the Council on Cardiovascular Radiology and Intervention: the American Academy of Neurology affirms the value of this guideline. *Stroke* 2006;37:577–617.
3. Albers GW, Amarenco P, Easton JD, Sacco RL, Teal P. Antithrombotic and thrombolytic therapy for ischemic stroke: American College of Chest Physicians Evidence-Based Clinical Practice Guidelines. (8th Ed.). *Chest* 2008;133: 630S–669S.
4. Kistler JP. Cerebral embolism. *Compr Ther* 1996;22:515–30.
5. Kittner SJ, Sharkness CM, Price TR, et al. Infarcts with a cardiac source of embolism in the NINCDS Stroke Data Bank: historical features. *Neurology* 1990;40:281–4.
6. Doufekias E, Segal AZ, Kizer JR. Cardiogenic and aortogenic brain embolism. *J Am Coll Cardiol* 2008;51:1049–59.
7. Arboix A, Oliveres M, Massons J, Pujades R, Garcia-Eroles L. Early differentiation of cardioembolic from atherothrombotic cerebral infarction: a multivariate analysis. *Eur J Neurol* 1999;6:677–83.
8. Adams HP, Jr., Bendixen BH, Kappelle LJ, et al. Classification of subtype of acute ischemic stroke. Definitions for use in a multicenter clinical trial. TOAST. Trial of Org 10172 in Acute Stroke Treatment. *Stroke* 1993;24:35–41.
9. Sacco RL, Ellenberg JH, Mohr JP, et al. Infarcts of undetermined cause: the NINCDS Stroke Data Bank. *Ann Neurol* 1989;25:382–90.
10. Kizer JR. Evaluation of the patient with unexplained stroke. *Coron Artery Dis* 2008;19:535–40.
11. Kizer JR, Silvestry FE, Kimmel SE, et al. Racial differences in the prevalence of cardiac sources of embolism in subjects with unexplained stroke or transient ischemic attack evaluated by transesophageal echocardiography. *Am J Cardiol* 2002;90:395–400.
12. Kizer JR, Wiebers DO, Whisnant JP, et al. Mitral annular calcification, aortic valve sclerosis, and incident stroke in adults free of clinical cardiovascular disease: the Strong Heart Study. *Stroke* 2005;36:2533–7.
13. Gilon D, Buonanno FS, Joffe MM, et al. Lack of evidence of an association between mitral-valve prolapse and stroke in young patients. *N Engl J Med* 1999;341:8–13.
14. Roldan CA, Shively BK, Crawford MH. Valve excrescences: prevalence, evolution and risk for cardioembolism. *J Am Coll Cardiol* 1997;30:1308–14.
15. Cohen A, Tzourio C, Chauvel C, et al. Mitral valve strands and the risk of ischemic stroke in elderly patients. The French Study of Aortic Plaques in Stroke (FAPS) Investigators. *Stroke* 1997;28:1574–8.
16. Warnes CA, Williams RG, Bashore TM, et al. ACC/AHA 2008 Guidelines for the Management of Adults with Congenital Heart Disease: a report of the American College of Cardiology/American Heart Association Task Force on Practice Guidelines (writing committee to develop guidelines on the management of adults with congenital heart disease). *Circulation* 2008;118:e714–833.
17. Bedard E, Shore DF, Gatzoulis MA. Adult congenital heart disease: a 2008 overview. *Br Med Bull* 2008;85:151–80.
18. Golledge J, Eagle KA. Acute aortic dissection. *Lancet* 2008;372:55–66.
19. Meltzer RS, Visser CA, Fuster V. Intracardiac thrombi and systemic embolization. *Ann Intern Med* 1986;104:689–98.
20. Koniaris LS, Goldhaber SZ. Anticoagulation in dilated cardiomyopathy. *J Am Coll Cardiol* 1998;31:745–8.
21. Cardiogenic brain embolism. The second report of the Cerebral Embolism Task Force. *Arch Neurol* 1989;46:727–43.
22. Weinreich DJ, Burke JF, Pauletto FJ. Left ventricular mural thrombi complicating acute myocardial infarction. Long-term follow-up with serial echocardiography. *Ann Intern Med* 1984;100:789–94.
23. Johannessen KA, Nordrehaug JE, von der Lippe G. Left ventricular thrombosis and cerebrovascular accident in acute myocardial infarction. *Br Heart J* 1984;51:553–6.

24. Mooe T, Eriksson P, Stegmayr B. Ischemic stroke after acute myocardial infarction. A population-based study. *Stroke* 1997;28:762–7.
25. Fuster V, Halperin JL. Left ventricular thrombi and cerebral embolism. *N Engl J Med* 1989;320:392–4.
26. Zielinska M, Kaczmarek K, Tylkowski M. Predictors of left ventricular thrombus formation in acute myocardial infarction treated with successful primary angioplasty with stenting. *Am J Med Sci* 2008;335:171–6.
27. van Dantzig JM, Delemarre BJ, Bot H, Visser CA. Left ventricular thrombus in acute myocardial infarction. *Eur Heart J* 1996;17:1640–5.
28. Asinger RW, Mikell FL, Elsperger J, Hodges M. Incidence of left-ventricular thrombosis after acute transmural myocardial infarction. Serial evaluation by two-dimensional echocardiography. *N Engl J Med* 1981;305:297–302.
29. Witt BJ, Brown RD, Jr., Jacobsen SJ, Weston SA, Yawn BP, Roger VL. A community-based study of stroke incidence after myocardial infarction. *Ann Intern Med* 2005;143:785–92.
30. Stratton JR, Resnick AD. Increased embolic risk in patients with left ventricular thrombi. *Circulation* 1987;75:1004–11.
31. Reeder GS, Lengyel M, Tajik AJ, Seward JB, Smith HC, Danielson GK. Mural thrombus in left ventricular aneurysm: incidence, role of angiography, and relation between anticoagulation and embolization. *Mayo Clin Proc* 1981;56:77–81.
32. Simpson MT, Oberman A, Kouchoukos NT, Rogers WJ. Prevalence of mural thrombi and systemic embolization with left ventricular aneurysm. Effect of anticoagulation therapy. *Chest* 1980;77:463–9.
33. Lapeyre AC 3rd, Steele PM, Kazmier FJ, Chesebro JH, Vlietstra RE, Fuster V. Systemic embolism in chronic left ventricular aneurysm: incidence and the role of anticoagulation. *J Am Coll Cardiol* 1985;6:534–8.
34. Witt BJ, Brown RD, Jr., Jacobsen SJ, et al. Ischemic stroke after heart failure: a community-based study. *Am Heart J* 2006;152:102–9.
35. Pullicino PM, Halperin JL, Thompson JL. Stroke in patients with heart failure and reduced left ventricular ejection fraction. *Neurology* 2000;54:288–94.
36. Freudenberger RS, Hellkamp AS, Halperin JL, et al. Risk of thromboembolism in heart failure: an analysis from the Sudden Cardiac Death in Heart Failure Trial (SCD-HeFT). *Circulation* 2007;115:2637–41.
37. Loh E, Sutton MS, Wun CC, et al. Ventricular dysfunction and the risk of stroke after myocardial infarction. *N Engl J Med* 1997;336:251–7.
38. Dries DL, Rosenberg YD, Waclawiw MA, Domanski MJ. Ejection fraction and risk of thromboembolic events in patients with systolic dysfunction and sinus rhythm: evidence for gender differences in the studies of left ventricular dysfunction trials. *J Am Coll Cardiol* 1997;29:1074–80.
39. Thanigaraj S, Schechtman KB, Perez JE. Improved echocardiographic delineation of left ventricular thrombus with the use of intravenous second-generation contrast image enhancement. *J Am Soc Echocardiogr* 1999;12:1022–6.
40. Mele D, Soukhomovskaia O, Pacchioni E, et al. Improved detection of left ventricular thrombi and spontaneous echocontrast by tissue harmonic imaging in patients with myocardial infarction. *J Am Soc Echocardiogr* 2006;19:1373–81.
41. Mansencal N, Nasr IA, Pilliere R, et al. Usefulness of contrast echocardiography for assessment of left ventricular thrombus after acute myocardial infarction. *Am J Cardiol* 2007;99:1667–70.
42. Weinsaft JW, Kim HW, Shah DJ, et al. Detection of left ventricular thrombus by delayed-enhancement cardiovascular magnetic resonance prevalence and markers in patients with systolic dysfunction. *J Am Coll Cardiol* 2008;52:148–57.
43. Srichai MB, Junor C, Rodriguez LL, et al. Clinical, imaging, and pathological characteristics of left ventricular thrombus: a comparison of contrast-enhanced magnetic resonance imaging, transthoracic echocardiography, and transesophageal echocardiography with surgical or pathological validation. *Am Heart J* 2006;152:75–84.
44. Antman EM, Anbe DT, Armstrong PW, et al. ACC/AHA guidelines for the management of patients with ST-elevation myocardial infarction—executive summary. A report of the American College of Cardiology/American Heart Association Task Force on Practice Guidelines (Writing Committee to revise the 1999 guidelines for the management of patients with acute myocardial infarction). *J Am Coll Cardiol* 2004;44:671–719.
45. Massie BM, Collins JF, Ammon SE, et al. Randomized trial of warfarin, aspirin, and clopidogrel in patients with chronic heart failure: the Warfarin and Antiplatelet Therapy in Chronic Heart Failure (WATCH) trial. *Circulation* 2009;119:1616–24.
46. Konstam MA. Antithrombotic therapy in heart failure: WATCHful wondering. *Circulation* 2009;119:1559–61.
47. Hart RG, Halperin JL. Atrial fibrillation and thromboembolism: a decade of progress in stroke prevention. *Ann Intern Med* 1999;131:688–95.
48. Hart RG, Halperin JL. Atrial fibrillation and stroke: concepts and controversies. *Stroke* 2001;32:803–8.
49. Wolf PA, Dawber TR, Thomas HE, Jr., Kannel WB. Epidemiologic assessment of chronic atrial fibrillation and risk of stroke: the Framingham study. *Neurology* 1978;28:973–7.
50. Wyse DG, Gersh BJ. Atrial fibrillation: a perspective: thinking inside and outside the box. *Circulation* 2004;109:3089–95.
51. Gage BF, Waterman AD, Shannon W, Boechler M, Rich MW, Radford MJ. Validation of clinical classification schemes for predicting stroke: results from the National Registry of Atrial Fibrillation. *JAMA* 2001;285:2864–70.
52. Singer DE, Albers GW, Dalen JE, et al. Antithrombotic therapy in atrial fibrillation: American College of Chest Physicians Evidence-Based Clinical Practice Guidelines (8th Ed.). *Chest* 2008;133:546S–592S.
53. Biblo LA, Yuan Z, Quan KJ, Mackall JA, Rimm AA. Risk of stroke in patients with atrial flutter. *Am J Cardiol* 2001;87:346–9, A9.
54. Greenspon AJ, Hart RG, Dawson D, et al. Predictors of stroke in patients paced for sick sinus syndrome. *J Am Coll Cardiol* 2004;43:1617–22.
55. Halligan SC, Gersh BJ, Brown RD, Jr., et al. The natural history of lone atrial flutter. *Ann Intern Med* 2004;140:265–8.
56. Sgarbossa EB, Pinski SL, Maloney JD, et al. Chronic atrial fibrillation and stroke in paced patients with sick sinus syndrome. Relevance of clinical characteristics and pacing modalities. *Circulation* 1993;88:1045–53.
57. Lanzarotti CJ, Olshansky B. Thromboembolism in chronic atrial flutter: is the risk underestimated? *J Am Coll Cardiol* 1997;30:1506–11.
58. Agmon Y, Khandheria BK, Gentile F, Seward JB. Clinical and echocardiographic characteristics of patients with left atrial

thrombus and sinus rhythm: experience in 20 643 consecutive transesophageal echocardiographic examinations. *Circulation* 2002;105:27–31.

59. Mugge A, Kuhn H, Nikutta P, Grote J, Lopez JA, Daniel WG. Assessment of left atrial appendage function by biplane transesophageal echocardiography in patients with non-rheumatic atrial fibrillation: identification of a subgroup of patients at increased embolic risk. *J Am Coll Cardiol* 1994;23:599–607.

60. Leung DY, Davidson PM, Cranney GB, Walsh WF. Thromboembolic risks of left atrial thrombus detected by transesophageal echocardiogram. *Am J Cardiol* 1997;79: 626–9.

61. Rahmatullah AF, Rahko PS, Stein JH. Transesophageal echocardiography for the evaluation and management of patients with cerebral ischemia. *Clin Cardiol* 1999;22:391–6.

62. de Bruijn SF, Agema WR, Lammers GJ, et al. Transesophageal echocardiography is superior to transthoracic echocardiography in management of patients of any age with transient ischemic attack or stroke. *Stroke* 2006;37:2531–4.

63. Feuchtner GM, Dichtl W, Bonatti JO, et al. Diagnostic accuracy of cardiac 64-slice computed tomography in detecting atrial thrombi. Comparative study with transesophageal echocardiography and cardiac surgery. *Invest Radiol* 2008;43:794–801.

64. Ohyama H, Hosomi N, Takahashi T, et al. Comparison of magnetic resonance imaging and transesophageal echocardiography in detection of thrombus in the left atrial appendage. *Stroke* 2003;34:2436–9.

65. Salem DN, O'Gara PT, Madias C, Pauker SG. Valvular and structural heart disease: American College of Chest Physicians Evidence-Based Clinical Practice Guidelines (8th Edition). *Chest* 2008;133:593S–629S.

66. Hart RG, Pearce LA, Aguilar MI. Meta-analysis: antithrombotic therapy to prevent stroke in patients who have nonvalvular atrial fibrillation. *Ann Intern Med* 2007;146:857–67.

67. Gage BF, van Walraven C, Pearce L, et al. Selecting patients with atrial fibrillation for anticoagulation: stroke risk stratification in patients taking aspirin. *Circulation* 2004;110:2287–92.

68. Fuster V, Ryden LE, Cannom DS, et al. ACC/AHA/ESC 2006 Guidelines for the Management of Patients with Atrial Fibrillation: a report of the American College of Cardiology/ American Heart Association Task Force on Practice Guidelines and the European Society of Cardiology Committee for Practice Guidelines (Writing Committee to Revise the 2001 Guidelines for the Management of Patients With Atrial Fibrillation): developed in collaboration with the European Heart Rhythm Association and the Heart Rhythm Society. *Circulation* 2006;114:e257–354.

69. Reynen K. Cardiac myxomas. *N Engl J Med* 1995; 333:1610–7.

70. Yoon DH, Roberts W. Sex distribution in cardiac myxomas. *Am J Cardiol* 2002;90:563–5.

71. Wilkes D, McDermott DA, Basson CT. Clinical phenotypes and molecular genetic mechanisms of Carney complex. *Lancet Oncol* 2005;6:501–8.

72. Hannah H 3rd, Eisemann G, Hiszcznskyj R, Winsky M, Cohen L. Invasive atrial myxoma: documentation of malignant potential of cardiac myxomas. *Am Heart J* 1982;104:881–3.

73. Read RC, White HJ, Murphy ML, Williams D, Sun CN, Flanagan WH. The malignant potentiality of left atrial myxoma. *J Thorac Cardiovasc Surg* 1974;68:857–68.

74. Markel ML, Armstrong WF, Waller BF, Mahomed Y. Left atrial myxoma with multicentric recurrence and evidence of metastases. *Am Heart J* 1986;111:409–13.

75. Diflo T, Cantelmo NL, Haudenschild CC, Watkins MT. Atrial myxoma with remote metastasis: case report and review of the literature. *Surgery* 1992;111:352–6.

76. Lee VH, Connolly HM, Brown RD, Jr. Central nervous system manifestations of cardiac myxoma. *Arch Neurol* 2007;64:1115–20.

77. Quinn TJ, Codini MA, Harris AA. Infected cardiac myxoma. *Am J Cardiol* 1984;53:381–2.

78. Tunick PA, Fox AC, Culliford A, Levy R, Kronzon I. The echocardiographic recognition of an atrial myxoma vegetation. *Am Heart J* 1990;119:679–80.

79. Perez de Isla L, de Castro R, Zamorano JL, et al. Diagnosis and treatment of cardiac myxomas by transesophageal echocardiography. *Am J Cardiol* 2002;90:1419–21.

80. Tatli S, Lipton MJ. CT for intracardiac thrombi and tumors. *Int J Cardiovasc Imaging* 2005;21:115–31.

81. Rustemli A, Bhatti TK, Wolff SD. Evaluating cardiac sources of embolic stroke with MRI. *Echocardiography* 2007;24:301–8; discussion 308.

82. Gowda RM, Khan IA, Nair CK, Mehta NJ, Vasavada BC, Sacchi TJ. Cardiac papillary fibroelastoma: a comprehensive analysis of 725 cases. *Am Heart J* 2003;146:404–10.

83. Khair T, Mazidi P, Laos LF. Cardiac Papillary Fibroelastoma: Case report and review of the literature. *Int J Cardiol* 2008.

84. McFadden PM, Lacy JR. Intracardiac papillary fibroelastoma: an occult cause of embolic neurologic deficit. *Ann Thorac Surg* 1987;43:667–669.

85. Israel DH, Sherman W, Ambrose JA, Sharma S, Harpaz N, Robbins M. Dynamic coronary ostial obstruction due to papillary fibroelastoma leading to myocardial ischemia and infarction. *Am J Cardiol* 1991;67:104–105.

86. Waltenberger J, Thelin S. Papillary fibroelastoma as an unusual source of repeated pulmonary embolism. *Circulation* 1994;89:24–33.

87. Sun JP, Asher CR, Yang XS, et al. Clinical and echocardiographic characteristics of papillary fibroelastomas. A retrospective and prospective study in 162 patients. *Circulation* 2001;103:2687–2693.

88. Muir KW, McNeish I, Grosset DG, Metcalfe M. Visualization of cardiac emboli from mitral valve papillary fibroelastoma. *Stroke* 1996;27:1133–1134.

89. McAllister HA, Jr., Hall RJ, Cooley DA. Tumors of the heart and pericardium. *Curr Probl Cardiol* 1999;24:57–116.

90. Hananouchi GI, Goff WB, 2nd. Cardiac lipoma: six-year follow-up with MRI characteristics, and a review of the literature. *Magn Reson Imaging* 1990;8:825–8.

91. Straus R, Merliss R. Primary tumor of the heart. Arch pathol 1945;39:74–8.

92. Reardon MJ, Malaisrie SC, Walkes JC, et al. Cardiac autotransplantation for primary cardiac tumors. *Ann Thorac Surg* 2006;82:645–50.

93. Blackmon SH, Patel AR, Bruckner BA, et al. Cardiac autotransplantation for malignant or complex primary left-heart tumors. *Tex Heart Inst J* 2008;35:296–300.

94. Blackmon SH, Patel A, Reardon MJ. Management of primary cardiac sarcomas. *Expert Rev Cardiovasc Ther* 2008;6:1217–22.

95. Reardon MJ, Walkes JC, Benjamin R. Therapy insight: malignant primary cardiac tumors. *Nat Clin Pract Cardiovasc Med* 2006;3:548–53.

96. Dawson MA, Mariani J, Taylor A, Koulouris G, Avery S. The successful treatment of primary cardiac lymphoma with a dose-dense schedule of rituximab plus CHOP. *Ann Oncol* 2006;17:176–7.

97. Reynen K, Kockeritz U, Strasser RH. Metastases to the heart. *Ann Oncol* 2004;15:375–81.

98. Hoffmann U, Globits S, Schima W, et al. Usefulness of magnetic resonance imaging of cardiac and paracardiac masses. *Am J Cardiol* 2003;92:890–5.

99. Mylonakis E, Calderwood SB. Infective endocarditis in adults. *N Engl J Med* 2001;345:1318–30.

100. Cabell CH, Pond KK, Peterson GE, et al. The risk of stroke and death in patients with aortic and mitral valve endocarditis. *Am Heart J* 2001;142:75–80.

101. Di Salvo G, Habib G, Pergola V, et al. Echocardiography predicts embolic events in infective endocarditis. *J Am Coll Cardiol* 2001;37:1069–76.

102. Reisner SA, Brenner B, Haim N, Edoute Y, Markiewicz W. Echocardiography in nonbacterial thrombotic endocarditis: from autopsy to clinical entity. *J Am Soc Echocardiogr* 2000;13:876–81.

103. Edoute Y, Haim N, Rinkevich D, Brenner B, Reisner SA. Cardiac valvular vegetations in cancer patients: a prospective echocardiographic study of 200 patients. *Am J Med* 1997;102:252–8.

104. Dutta T, Karas MG, Segal AZ, Kizer JR. Yield of transesophageal echocardiography for nonbacterial thrombotic endocarditis and other cardiac sources of embolism in cancer patients with cerebral ischemia. *Am J Cardiol* 2006;97:894–8.

105. Reynolds HR, Jagen MA, Tunick PA, Kronzon I. Sensitivity of transthoracic versus transesophageal echocardiography for the detection of native valve vegetations in the modern era. *J Am Soc Echocardiogr* 2003;16:67–70.

106. Thamilarasan M, Griffin B. Choosing the most appropriate valve operation and prosthesis. *Cleve Clin J Med* 2002;69:688–90, 693–4, 696–8 passim.

107. Heras M, Chesebro JH, Fuster V, et al. High risk of thromboemboli early after bioprosthetic cardiac valve replacement. *J Am Coll Cardiol* 1995;25:1111–9.

108. Tunick PA, Perez JL, Kronzon I. Protruding atheromas in the thoracic aorta and systemic embolization. *Ann Intern Med* 1991;115:423–7.

109. Amarenco P, Duyckaerts C, Tzourio C, Henin D, Bousser MG, Hauw JJ. The prevalence of ulcerated plaques in the aortic arch in patients with stroke. *N Engl J Med* 1992;326:221–5.

110. Khatibzadeh M, Mitusch R, Stierle U, Gromoll B, Sheikhzadeh A. Aortic atherosclerotic plaques as a source of systemic embolism. *J Am Coll Cardiol* 1996;27:664–9.

111. Vaduganathan P, Ewton A, Nagueh SF, Weilbaecher DG, Safi HJ, Zoghbi WA. Pathologic correlates of aortic plaques, thrombi and mobile "aortic debris" imaged in vivo with transesophageal echocardiography. *J Am Coll Cardiol* 1997;30:357–63.

112. Atherosclerotic disease of the aortic arch as a risk factor for recurrent ischemic stroke. The French Study of Aortic Plaques in Stroke Group. *N Engl J Med* 1996;334:1216–21.

113. Transesophageal echocardiographic correlates of thromboembolism in high-risk patients with nonvalvular atrial fibrillation. The Stroke Prevention in Atrial Fibrillation Investigators Committee on Echocardiography. *Ann Intern Med* 1998;128:639–47.

114. Meissner I, Khandheria BK, Sheps SG, et al. Atherosclerosis of the aorta: risk factor, risk marker, or innocent bystander? A prospective population-based transesophageal echocardiography study. *J Am Coll Cardiol* 2004;44:1018–24.

115. Amarenco P, Cohen A, Tzourio C, et al. Atherosclerotic disease of the aortic arch and the risk of ischemic stroke. *N Engl J Med* 1994;331:1474–9.

116. Jones EF, Kalman JM, Calafiore P, Tonkin AM, Donnan GA. Proximal aortic atheroma. An independent risk factor for cerebral ischemia. *Stroke* 1995;26:218–24.

117. Weinberger J, Azhar S, Danisi F, Hayes R, Goldman M. A new noninvasive technique for imaging atherosclerotic plaque in the aortic arch of stroke patients by transcutaneous real-time B-mode ultrasonography: an initial report. *Stroke* 1998;29:673–6.

118. Katz ES, Konecky N, Tunick PA, Rosenzweig BP, Freedberg RS, Kronzon I. Visualization and identification of the left common carotid and left subclavian arteries: a transesophageal echocardiographic approach. *J Am Soc Echocardiogr* 1996;9:58–61.

119. Zaidat OO, Suarez JI, Hedrick D, et al. Reproducibility of transesophageal echocardiography in evaluating aortic atheroma in stroke patients. *Echocardiography* 2005;22:326–30.

120. Kutz SM, Lee VS, Tunick PA, Krinsky GA, Kronzon I. Atheromas of the thoracic aorta: A comparison of transesophageal echocardiography and breath-hold gadolinium-enhanced 3-dimensional magnetic resonance angiography. *J Am Soc Echocardiogr* 1999;12:853–8.

121. Fayad ZA, Nahar T, Fallon JT, et al. In vivo magnetic resonance evaluation of atherosclerotic plaques in the human thoracic aorta: a comparison with transesophageal echocardiography. *Circulation* 2000;101:2503–9.

122. Rutt BK, Clarke SE, Fayad ZA. Atherosclerotic plaque characterization by MR imaging. *Curr Drug Targets Cardiovasc Haematol Disord* 2004;4:147–59.

123. Kramer CM, Cerilli LA, Hagspiel K, DiMaria JM, Epstein FH, Kern JA. Magnetic resonance imaging identifies the fibrous cap in atherosclerotic abdominal aortic aneurysm. *Circulation* 2004;109:1016–21.

124. Kramer CM. Magnetic resonance imaging to identify the high-risk plaque. *Am J Cardiol* 2002;90:15L–17L.

125. Helft G, Worthley SG, Fuster V, et al. Progression and regression of atherosclerotic lesions: monitoring with serial noninvasive magnetic resonance imaging. *Circulation* 2002;105:993–8.

126. Bitar R, Moody AR, Leung G, et al. In vivo identification of complicated upper thoracic aorta and arch vessel plaque by MR direct thrombus imaging in patients investigated for cerebrovascular disease. *AJR Am J Roentgenol* 2006;187:228–34.

127. Harloff A, Handke M, Reinhard M, Geibel A, Hetzel A. Therapeutic strategies after examination by transesophageal echocardiography in 503 patients with ischemic stroke. *Stroke* 2006;37:859–64.

128. Tenenbaum A, Garniek A, Shemesh J, et al. Dual-helical CT for detecting aortic atheromas as a source of stroke: comparison with transesophageal echocardiography. *Radiology* 1998;208:153–8.

129. Tenenbaum A, Garniek A, Shemesh J, et al. Spiral computerized tomography (dual helical mode) as a detector of aortic atheromas in patients with stroke and systemic emboli: additional benefit of the contrast-enhanced technique. *Isr Med Assoc J* 2000;2:1–5.

130. Hussain SI, Gilkeson RC, Suarez JI, et al. Comparing multislice electrocardiogram-gated spiral computerized tomography and transesophageal echocardiography in evaluating aortic atheroma in patients with acute ischemic stroke. *J Stroke Cerebrovasc Dis* 2008;17:134–40.

131. Dressler FA, Craig WR, Castello R, Labovitz AJ. Mobile aortic atheroma and systemic emboli: efficacy of anticoagulation and influence of plaque morphology on recurrent stroke. *J Am Coll Cardiol* 1998;31:134–8.

132. Ferrari E, Vidal R, Chevallier T, Baudouy M. Atherosclerosis of the thoracic aorta and aortic debris as a marker of poor prognosis: benefit of oral anticoagulants. *J Am Coll Cardiol* 1999;33:1317–22.

133. Lewis SJ, Moye LA, Sacks FM, et al. Effect of pravastatin on cardiovascular events in older patients with myocardial infarction and cholesterol levels in the average range. Results of the Cholesterol and Recurrent Events (CARE) trial. *Ann Intern Med* 1998;129:681–9.

134. Baigent C, Keech A, Kearney PM, et al. Efficacy and safety of cholesterol-lowering treatment: prospective meta-analysis of data from 90,056 participants in 14 randomised trials of statins. *Lancet* 2005;366:1267–78.

135. Amarenco P, Bogousslavsky J, Callahan A, 3rd, et al. High-dose atorvastatin after stroke or transient ischemic attack. *N Engl J Med* 2006;355:549–59.

136. Tunick PA, Nayar AC, Goodkin GM, et al. Effect of treatment on the incidence of stroke and other emboli in 519 patients with severe thoracic aortic plaque. *Am J Cardiol* 2002;90:1320–5.

137. Lima JA, Desai MY, Steen H, Warren WP, Gautam S, Lai S. Statin-induced cholesterol lowering and plaque regression after 6 months of magnetic resonance imaging-monitored therapy. *Circulation* 2004;110:2336–41.

138. Corti R, Fuster V, Fayad ZA, et al. Effects of aggressive versus conventional lipid-lowering therapy by simvastatin on human atherosclerotic lesions: a prospective, randomized, double-blind trial with high-resolution magnetic resonance imaging. *J Am Coll Cardiol* 2005;46:106–12.

139. Yonemura A, Momiyama Y, Fayad ZA, et al. Effect of lipid-lowering therapy with atorvastatin on atherosclerotic aortic plaques detected by noninvasive magnetic resonance imaging. *J Am Coll Cardiol* 2005;45:733–42.

140. Hagen PT, Scholz DG, Edwards WD. Incidence and size of patent foramen ovale during the first 10 decades of life: an autopsy study of 965 normal hearts. *Mayo Clin Proc* 1984;59:17–20.

141. Patten B. The closure of the foramen ovale. Am J Anat 1931;48:19–44.

142. Kerut EK, Norfleet WT, Plotnick GD, Giles TD. Patent foramen ovale: a review of associated conditions and the impact of physiological size. *J Am Coll Cardiol* 2001;38:613–23.

143. Thaler DE, Saver JL. Cryptogenic stroke and patent foramen ovale. *Curr Opin Cardiol* 2008;23:537–44.

144. Di Tullio M, Sacco RL, Venketasubramanian N, Sherman D, Mohr JP, Homma S. Comparison of diagnostic techniques for the detection of a patent foramen ovale in stroke patients. *Stroke* 1993;24:1020–4.

145. Daniels C, Weytjens C, Cosyns B, et al. Second harmonic transthoracic echocardiography: the new reference screening method for the detection of patent foramen ovale. *Eur J Echocardiogr* 2004;5:449–52.

146. Ha JW, Shin MS, Kang S, et al. Enhanced detection of right-to-left shunt through patent foramen ovale by transthoracic contrast echocardiography using harmonic imaging. *Am J Cardiol* 2001;87:669–71, A11.

147. Souteyrand G, Motreff P, Lusson JR, et al. Comparison of transthoracic echocardiography using second harmonic imaging, transcranial Doppler and transesophageal echocardiography for the detection of patent foramen ovale in stroke patients. *Eur J Echocardiogr* 2006;7:147–54.

148. Mohrs OK, Petersen SE, Erkapic D, et al. Diagnosis of patent foramen ovale using contrast-enhanced dynamic MRI: a pilot study. *AJR Am J Roentgenol* 2005;184:234–40.

149. Kim YJ, Hur J, Shim CY, et al. Patent foramen ovale: diagnosis with multidetector CT—comparison with transesophageal echocardiography. *Radiology* 2009;250:61–7.

150. Williamson EE, Kirsch J, Araoz PA, et al. ECG-gated cardiac CT angiography using 64-MDCT for detection of patent foramen ovale. *AJR Am J Roentgenol* 2008;190:929–33.

151. Overell JR, Bone I, Lees KR. Interatrial septal abnormalities and stroke: a meta-analysis of case-control studies. *Neurology* 2000;55:1172–9.

152. Di Tullio MR, Sacco RL, Sciacca RR, Jin Z, Homma S. Patent foramen ovale and the risk of ischemic stroke in a multiethnic population. *J Am Coll Cardiol* 2007;49:797–802.

153. Meissner I, Khandheria BK, Heit JA, et al. Patent foramen ovale: innocent or guilty? Evidence from a prospective population-based study. *J Am Coll Cardiol* 2006;47:440–5.

154. Petty GW, Khandheria BK, Meissner I, et al. Population-based study of the relationship between patent foramen ovale and cerebrovascular ischemic events. *Mayo Clin Proc* 2006;81:602–8.

155. Loscalzo J. Paradoxical embolism: clinical presentation, diagnostic strategies, and therapeutic options. *Am Heart J* 1986;112:141–5.

156. Meacham RR 3rd, Headley AS, Bronze MS, Lewis JB, Rester MM. Impending paradoxical embolism. *Arch Intern Med* 1998;158:438–48.

157. Lechat P, Mas JL, Lascault G, et al. Prevalence of patent foramen ovale in patients with stroke. *N Engl J Med* 1988;318:1148–52.

158. Overell JR, Bone I, Less KR. Interatrial septal abnormalities and stroke. A meta-analysis of case-control studies. *Neurology* 2000;55:1172–1179.

159. Homma S, Sacco RL, Di Tullio MR, Sciacca RR, Mohr JP. Effect of medical treatment in stroke patients with patent foramen ovale: patent foramen ovale in Cryptogenic Stroke Study. *Circulation* 2002;105:2625–31.

160. Handke M, Harloff A, Olschewski M, Hetzel A, Geibel A. Patent foramen ovale and cryptogenic stroke in older patients. *N Engl J Med* 2007;357:2262–8.

161. Eggebrecht H, Naber CK, Plato C, Erbel R, Bartel T. Analysis of fossa ovalis membrane velocities by transesophageal

Doppler tissue echocardiography: a novel approach to functional assessment of patent foramen ovale. *J Am Soc Echocardiogr* 2004;17:1161–6.

162. Falk RH. PFO or UFO? The role of a patent foramen ovale in cryptogenic stroke. *Am Heart J* 1991;121:1264–6.

163. Kizer JR, Devereux RB. Clinical practice. Patent foramen ovale in young adults with unexplained stroke. *N Engl J Med* 2005;353:2361–72.

164. Stollberger C, Slany J, Schuster I, Leitner H, Winkler WB, Karnik R. The prevalence of deep venous thrombosis in patients with suspected paradoxical embolism. *Ann Intern Med* 1993;119:461–5.

165. Cramer SC, Rordorf G, Maki JH, et al. Increased pelvic vein thrombi in cryptogenic stroke: results of the Paradoxical Emboli from Large Veins in Ischemic Stroke (PELVIS) study. *Stroke* 2004;35:46–50.

166. Lock JE. Patent foramen ovale is indicted, but the case hasn't gone to trial. *Circulation* 2000;101:838.

167. Schuchlenz HW, Weihs W, Horner S, Quehenberger F. The association between the diameter of a patent foramen ovale and the risk of embolic cerebrovascular events. *Am J Med* 2000;109:456–62.

168. Steiner MM, Di Tullio MR, Rundek T, et al. Patent foramen ovale size and embolic brain imaging findings among patients with ischemic stroke. *Stroke* 1998;29:944–8.

169. Stone DA, Godard J, Corretti MC, et al. Patent foramen ovale: association between the degree of shunt by contrast transesophageal echocardiography and the risk of future ischemic neurologic events. *Am Heart J* 1996;131:158–61.

170. Bogousslavsky J, Garazi S, Jeanrenaud X, Aebischer N, Van Melle G. Stroke recurrence in patients with patent foramen ovale: the Lausanne Study. Lausanne Stroke with Paradoxal Embolism Study Group. *Neurology* 1996;46:1301–5.

171. Job FP, Ringelstein EB, Grafen Y, et al. Comparison of transcranial contrast Doppler sonography and transesophageal contrast echocardiography for the detection of patent foramen ovale in young stroke patients. *Am J Cardiol* 1994;74:381–4.

172. De Castro S, Cartoni D, Fiorelli M, et al. Morphological and functional characteristics of patent foramen ovale and their embolic implications. *Stroke* 2000;31:2407–13.

173. Mas JL, Arquizan C, Lamy C, et al. Recurrent cerebrovascular events associated with patent foramen ovale, atrial septal aneurysm, or both. *N Engl J Med* 2001;345:1740–6.

174. Homma S, Sacco RL, Di Tullio MR, Sciacca RR, Mohr JP. Atrial anatomy in non-cardioembolic stroke patients: effect of medical therapy. *J Am Coll Cardiol* 2003;42:1066–72.

175. Mas JL, Zuber M. Recurrent cerebrovascular events in patients with patent foramen ovale, atrial septal aneurysm, or both and cryptogenic stroke or transient ischemic attack. French Study Group on Patent Foramen Ovale and Atrial Septal Aneurysm. *Am Heart J* 1995;130:1083–8.

176. Hanley PC, Tajik AJ, Hynes JK, et al. Diagnosis and classification of atrial septal aneurysm by two-dimensional echocardiography: report of 80 consecutive cases. *J Am Coll Cardiol* 1985;6:1370–82.

177. Agmon Y, Khandheria BK, Meissner I, et al. Frequency of atrial septal aneurysms in patients with cerebral ischemic events. *Circulation* 1999;99:1942–4.

178. Silver MD, Dorsey JS. Aneurysms of the septum primum in adults. *Arch Pathol Lab Med* 1978;102:62–5.

179. Belkin RN, Hurwitz BJ, Kisslo J. Atrial septal aneurysm: association with cerebrovascular and peripheral embolic events. *Stroke* 1987;18:856–62.

180. Cabanes L, Mas JL, Cohen A, et al. Atrial septal aneurysm and patent foramen ovale as risk factors for cryptogenic stroke in patients less than 55 years of age. A study using transesophageal echocardiography. *Stroke* 1993;24:1865–73.

181. Marazanof M, Roudaut R, Cohen A, et al. Atrial septal aneurysm. Morphological characteristics in a large population: pathological associations. A French multicenter study on 259 patients investigated by transoesophageal echocardiography. *Int J Cardiol* 1995;52:59–65.

182. Mattioli AV, Aquilina M, Oldani A, Longhini C, Mattioli G. Atrial septal aneurysm as a cardioembolic source in adult patients with stroke and normal carotid arteries. A multicentre study. *Eur Heart J* 2001;22:261–8.

183. Mugge A, Daniel WG, Angermann C, et al. Atrial septal aneurysm in adult patients. A multicenter study using transthoracic and transesophageal echocardiography. *Circulation* 1995;91:2785–92.

184. Berthet K, Lavergne T, Cohen A, et al. Significant association of atrial vulnerability with atrial septal abnormalities in young patients with ischemic stroke of unknown cause. *Stroke* 2000;31:398–403.

185. Nendaz MR, Sarasin FP, Junod AF, Bogousslavsky J. Preventing stroke recurrence in patients with patent foramen ovale: antithrombotic therapy, foramen closure, or therapeutic abstention? A decision analytic perspective. *Am Heart J* 1998;135:532–41.

186. Dearani JA, Ugurlu BS, Danielson GK, et al. Surgical patent foramen ovale closure for prevention of paradoxical embolism-related cerebrovascular ischemic events. *Circulation* 1999;100:II171–5.

187. Devuyst G, Bogousslavsky J, Ruchat P, et al. Prognosis after stroke followed by surgical closure of patent foramen ovale: a prospective follow-up study with brain MRI and simultaneous transesophageal and transcranial Doppler ultrasound. *Neurology* 1996;47:1162–6.

188. Homma S, Di Tullio MR, Sacco RL, Sciacca RR, Smith C, Mohr JP. Surgical closure of patent foramen ovale in cryptogenic stroke patients. *Stroke* 1997;28:2376–81.

189. Bridges ND, Hellenbrand W, Latson L, Filiano J, Newburger JW, Lock JE. Transcatheter closure of patent foramen ovale after presumed paradoxical embolism. *Circulation* 1992;86:1902–8.

190. Windecker S, Wahl A, Chatterjee T, et al. Percutaneous closure of patent foramen ovale in patients with paradoxical embolism: long-term risk of recurrent thromboembolic events. *Circulation* 2000;101:893–8.

191. Adams RJ, Albers G, Alberts MJ, et al. Update to the AHA/ASA recommendations for the prevention of stroke in patients with stroke and transient ischemic attack. *Stroke* 2008;39:1647–52.

192. Gossage JR, Kanj G. Pulmonary arteriovenous malformations. A state of the art review. *Am J Respir Crit Care Med* 1998;158:643–61.

193. Moussouttas M, Fayad P, Rosenblatt M, et al. Pulmonary arteriovenous malformations: cerebral ischemia and neurologic manifestations. *Neurology* 2000;55:959–64.

194. Rastegar R, Harnick DJ, Weidemann P, et al. Spontaneous echo contrast videodensity is flow-related and is dependent on

the relative concentrations of fibrinogen and red blood cells. *J Am Coll Cardiol* 2003;41:603–10.

195. Black IW, Hopkins AP, Lee LC, Walsh WF. Left atrial spontaneous echo contrast: a clinical and echocardiographic analysis. *J Am Coll Cardiol* 1991;18:398–404.

196. Handke M, Harloff A, Hetzel A, Olschewski M, Bode C, Geibel A. Predictors of left atrial spontaneous echocardiographic contrast or thrombus formation in stroke patients with sinus rhythm and reduced left ventricular function. *Am J Cardiol* 2005;96:1342–4.

197. Daniel WG, Nellessen U, Schroder E, et al. Left atrial spontaneous echo contrast in mitral valve disease: an indicator for an increased thromboembolic risk. *J Am Coll Cardiol* 1988;11:1204–11.

198. Chan SK, Kannam JP, Douglas PS, Manning WJ. Multiplane transesophageal echocardiographic assessment of left atrial appendage anatomy and function. *Am J Cardiol* 1995;76:528–30.

199. Seward JB, Khandheria BK, Edwards WD, Oh JK, Freeman WK, Tajik AJ. Biplanar transesophageal echocardiography: anatomic correlations, image orientation, and clinical applications. *Mayo Clin Proc* 1990;65:1193–213.

200. Li YH, Hwang JJ, Lin JL, Tseng YZ, Lien WP. Importance of left atrial appendage function as a risk factor for systemic thromboembolism in patients with rheumatic mitral valve disease. *Am J Cardiol* 1996;78:844–7.

201. Shively BK, Gelgand EA, Crawford MH. Regional left atrial stasis during atrial fibrillation and flutter: determinants and relation to stroke. *J Am Coll Cardiol* 1996;27:1722–9.

202. Fatkin D, Kuchar DL, Thorburn CW, Feneley MP. Transesophageal echocardiography before and during direct current cardioversion of atrial fibrillation: evidence for "atrial stunning" as a mechanism of thromboembolic complications. *J Am Coll Cardiol* 1994;23:307–16.

203. Grimm RA, Stewart WJ, Maloney JD, et al. Impact of electrical cardioversion for atrial fibrillation on left atrial appendage function and spontaneous echo contrast: characterization by simultaneous transesophageal echocardiography. *J Am Coll Cardiol* 1993;22:1359–66.

204. Grimm RA, Leung DY, Black IW, Stewart WJ, Thomas JD, Klein AL. Left atrial appendage "stunning" after spontaneous conversion of atrial fibrillation demonstrated by transesophageal Doppler echocardiography. *Am Heart J* 1995;130:174–6.

205. Falcone RA, Morady F, Armstrong WF. Transesophageal echocardiographic evaluation of left atrial appendage function and spontaneous contrast formation after chemical or electrical cardioversion of atrial fibrillation. *Am J Cardiol* 1996;78:435–9.

206. Omran H, Jung W, Rabahieh R, et al. Left atrial chamber and appendage function after internal atrial defibrillation: a prospective and serial transesophageal echocardiographic study. *J Am Coll Cardiol* 1997;29:131–8.

207. Wilson LA, Keeling PW, Malcolm AD, Russel RW, Webb-Peploe MM. Visual complications of mitral leaflet prolapse. *Br Med J* 1977;2:86–8.

208. Barnett HJ, Boughner DR, Taylor DW, Cooper PE, Kostuk WJ, Nichol PM. Further evidence relating mitral-valve prolapse to cerebral ischemic events. *N Engl J Med* 1980;302:139–44.

209. de Bono DP, Warlow CP. Potential sources of emboli in patients with presumed transient cerebral or retinal ischaemia. *Lancet* 1981;1:343–6.

210. Levine RA, Stathogiannis E, Newell JB, Harrigan P, Weyman AE. Reconsideration of echocardiographic standards for mitral valve prolapse: lack of association between leaflet displacement isolated to the apical four chamber view and independent echocardiographic evidence of abnormality. *J Am Coll Cardiol* 1988;11:1010–9.

211. Freed LA, Levy D, Levine RA, et al. Prevalence and clinical outcome of mitral-valve prolapse. *N Engl J Med* 1999;341:1–7.

212. Orencia AJ, Petty GW, Khandheria BK, et al. Risk of stroke with mitral valve prolapse in population-based cohort study. *Stroke* 1995;26:7–13.

213. Bonow RO, Carabello BA, Chatterjee K, et al. ACC/AHA 2006 guidelines for the management of patients with valvular heart disease: a report of the American College of Cardiology/American Heart Association Task Force on Practice Guidelines (writing Committee to Revise the 1998 guidelines for the management of patients with valvular heart disease) developed in collaboration with the Society of Cardiovascular Anesthesiologists endorsed by the Society for Cardiovascular Angiography and Interventions and the Society of Thoracic Surgeons. *J Am Coll Cardiol* 2006;48:e1–148.

214. Fulkerson PK, Beaver BM, Auseon JC, Graber HL. Calcification of the mitral annulus: etiology, clinical associations, complications and therapy. *Am J Med* 1979;66:967–77.

215. Benjamin EJ, Plehn JF, D'Agostino RB, et al. Mitral annular calcification and the risk of stroke in an elderly cohort. *N Engl J Med* 1992;327:374–9.

216. Aronow WS, Ahn C, Kronzon I, Gutstein H. Association of mitral annular calcium with new thromboembolic stroke at 44-month follow-up of 2,148 persons, mean age 81 years. *Am J Cardiol* 1998;81:105–6.

217. Atar S, Jeon DS, Luo H, Siegel RJ. Mitral annular calcification: a marker of severe coronary artery disease in patients under 65 years old. *Heart* 2003;89:161–4.

218. Adler Y, Herz I, Vaturi M, et al. Mitral annular calcium detected by transthoracic echocardiography is a marker for high prevalence and severity of coronary artery disease in patients undergoing coronary angiography. *Am J Cardiol* 1998;82:1183–6.

219. Aronow WS, Ahn C, Kronzon I. Association of mitral annular calcium and of aortic cuspal calcium with coronary artery disease in older patients. *Am J Cardiol* 1999;84:1084–5, A9.

220. Aronow WS, Schoenfeld MR, Gutstein H. Frequency of thromboembolic stroke in persons greater than or equal to 60 years of age with extracranial carotid arterial disease and/or mitral annular calcium. *Am J Cardiol* 1992;70:123–4.

221. Adler Y, Koren A, Fink N, et al. Association between mitral annulus calcification and carotid atherosclerotic disease. *Stroke* 1998;29:1833–7.

222. Demopoulos LA, Tunick PA, Bernstein NE, Perez JL, Kronzon I. Protruding atheromas of the aortic arch in symptomatic patients with carotid artery disease. *Am Heart J* 1995;129:40–4.

223. Adler Y, Shohat-Zabarski R, Vaturi M, et al. Association between mitral annular calcium and aortic atheroma as detected by transesophageal echocardiographic study. *Am J Cardiol* 1998;81:784–6.

224. Adler Y, Vaturi M, Fink N, et al. Association between mitral annulus calcification and aortic atheroma: a prospective transesophageal echocardiographic study. *Atherosclerosis* 2000;152:451–6.

225. Karas MG, Francescone S, Segal AZ, et al. Relation between mitral annular calcium and complex aortic atheroma in patients with cerebral ischemia referred for transesophageal echocardiography. *Am J Cardiol* 2007;99:1306–11.

226. Aronow WS, Ahn C, Kronzon I. Association of mitral annular calcium with symptomatic peripheral arterial disease in older persons. *Am J Cardiol* 2001;88:333–4.

227. Eicher JC, Soto FX, DeNadai L, et al. Possible association of thrombotic, nonbacterial vegetations of the mitral ring-mitral annular calcium and stroke. *Am J Cardiol* 1997;79:1712–5.

228. Burnside JW, Desanctis RW. Bacterial endocarditis on calcification of the mitral anulus fibrosus. *Ann Intern Med* 1972;76:615–8.

229. Shohat-Zabarski R, Paz R, Adler Y, Vaturi M, Jortner R, Sagie A. Mitral annulus calcification with a mobile component as a possible source of embolism. *Am J Geriatr Cardiol* 2001;10:196–8.

230. Ridolfi RL, Hutchins GM. Spontaneous calcific emboli from calcific mitral annulus fibrosus. *Arch Pathol Lab Med* 1976;100:117–20.

231. Sell S, Scully RE. Aging changes in the aortic and mitral valves. Histologic and histochemical studies, with observations on the pathogenesis of calcific aortic stenosis and calcification of the mitral annulus. *Am J Pathol* 1965;46:345–65.

232. Boon A, Lodder J, Cheriex E, Kessels F. Risk of stroke in a cohort of 815 patients with calcification of the aortic valve with or without stenosis. *Stroke* 1996;27:847–51.

233. Otto CM, Lind BK, Kitzman DW, Gersh BJ, Siscovick DS. Association of aortic-valve sclerosis with cardiovascular mortality and morbidity in the elderly. *N Engl J Med* 1999;341:142–7.

234. Petty GW, Khandheria BK, Whisnant JP, Sicks JD, O'Fallon WM, Wiebers DO. Predictors of cerebrovascular events and death among patients with valvular heart disease: A population-based study. *Stroke* 2000;31:2628–35.

235. Antonini-Canterin F, Hirsu M, Popescu BA, et al. Stage-related effect of statin treatment on the progression of aortic valve sclerosis and stenosis. *Am J Cardiol* 2008;102:738–42.

236. Liebe V, Brueckmann M, Borggrefe M, Kaden JJ. Statin therapy of calcific aortic stenosis: hype or hope? *Eur Heart J* 2006;27:773–8.

237. Jaffe W, Figueredo VM. An example of Lambl's excrescences by transesophageal echocardiogram: a commonly misinterpreted lesion. *Echocardiography* 2007;24:1086–9.

238. Hort W, Horstkotte D. Fibrolelastoma and Lambl's excrescences: localization, morphology and pathogenesis, differential diagnosis and infection. *J Heart Valve Dis* 2006;15:591–3.

239. Voros S, Nanda NC, Thakur AC, Winokur TS, Samal AK. Lambl's Excrescences (Valvular Strands). *Echocardiography* 1999;16:399–414.

240. Meissner I, Whisnant JP, Khandheria BK, et al. Prevalence of potential risk factors for stroke assessed by transesophageal echocardiography and carotid ultrasonography: the SPARC study. Stroke Prevention: Assessment of Risk in a Community. *Mayo Clin Proc* 1999;74:862–9.

241. Speights VO, Jr., Dobin SM, Truss LM. A cytogenetic study of a cardiac papillary fibroelastoma. *Cancer Genet Cytogenet* 1998;103:167–9.

242. Freedberg RS, Goodkin GM, Perez JL, Tunick PA, Kronzon I. Valve strands are strongly associated with systemic embolization: a transesophageal echocardiographic study. *J Am Coll Cardiol* 1995;26:1709–12.

243. Tice FD, Slivka AP, Walz ET, Orsinelli DA, Pearson AC. Mitral valve strands in patients with focal cerebral ischemia. *Stroke* 1996;27:1183–6.

244. Orsinelli DA, Pearson AC. Detection of prosthetic valve strands by transesophageal echocardiography: clinical significance in patients with suspected cardiac source of embolism. *J Am Coll Cardiol* 1995;26:1713–8.

245. Roberts JK, Omarali I, Di Tullio MR, Sciacca RR, Sacco RL, Homma S. Valvular strands and cerebral ischemia. Effect of demographics and strand characteristics. *Stroke* 1997;28:2185–8.

246. Wolf RC, Spiess J, Vasic N, Huber R. Valvular strands and ischemic stroke. *Eur Neurol* 2007;57:227–31.

247. Homma S, Di Tullio MR, Sciacca RR, Sacco RL, Mohr JP. Effect of aspirin and warfarin therapy in stroke patients with valvular strands. *Stroke* 2004;35:1436–42.

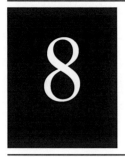

8 Cardiovascular Manifestations of Systemic Lupus Erythematosus

MARY J. ROMAN

OUTLINE

Vascular Disease   141

Myocardial Disease   145

Valvular Disease   146

Pericardial Disease   147

Arrhythmias and Conduction System
     Disease   147

Pulmonary Hypertension   147

Antiphospholipid Antibody Syndrome
     in SLE   148

Conclusions   148

References   149

Systemic lupus erythematosus (SLE) is a chronic, systemic, autoimmune disease. Its diagnosis (Table 8.1) is based on demonstration of multisystem clinical and laboratory manifestations (1). The population prevalence is about 1:2,500 with a marked (approximately 90%) female predominance; black women and men have substantially higher rates of disease and more severe disease manifestations than white women and men do (2,3). Although the cause of SLE is unknown, its expression is modulated by interactions among genetic, environmental, hormonal, and immunologic factors (4).

Valvular disease associated with Libman-Sacks lesions, pericardial disease due to serositis, and thromboses associated with the presence of antiphospholipid antibodies are well-established cardiovascular manifestations of SLE. However, newer manifestations of cardiovascular disease, particularly premature atherosclerosis, have emerged as important causes of morbidity and mortality in SLE as a consequence of (a) therapeutic advances in treatment of lupus nephritis resulting in longer life expectancy, (b) the ability to detect subclinical disease using sophisticated noninvasive cardiac and vascular diagnostic technology, and (c) a growing understanding of the pivotal roles of inflammation and the immune system in the initiation and progression of atherosclerosis.

This chapter will review cardiovascular manifestations of SLE with an emphasis on recent clinical research. Cardiovascular diseases will be categorized as vascular (accelerated atherosclerosis, arterial stiffness, endothelial dysfunction), myocardial (myositis, abnormalities of structure and function), valvular, pericardial, arrhythmias, conduction system, and pulmonary hypertension, for ease of reference. The influence of the presence of antiphospholipid antibodies on cardiovascular disease manifestations in SLE will also be discussed.

■ VASCULAR DISEASE

Accelerated Atherosclerosis

The premature development of atherosclerotic coronary artery disease in SLE was initially highlighted by an autopsy study published in 1975 that was designed to contrast the evolution in pathologic findings in SLE attributable to the advent of corticosteroid therapy (5). Of 36 autopsied patients, eight had significant atherosclerotic epicardial coronary artery disease, all of whom had received corticosteroid therapy for more than one year. Their average age at death was 35 years, and myocardial infarction was present in five of the eight patients.

■ **Table 8.1** Diagnostic criteria for systemic lupus erythematosus.[a]	
Criterion	**Description**
Malar rash	Fixed erythema, flat or raised, over the malar eminences, tending to spare the nasolabial folds
Discoid rash	Erythematosus raised patches with adherent keratotic scaling and follicular plugging; atrophic scarring may occur in older lesions
Photosensitivity	Skin rash as a result of unusual reaction to sunlight
Oral ulcers	Oral or nasopharyngeal ulcerations, usually painless
Arthritis	Nonerosive arthritis involving two or more peripheral joints, characterized by swelling or effusion
Serositis	Pleuritis: convincing history of pleuritic pain, or rub heard by physician, or evidence of pleural effusion Pericarditis: documented by EKG, or rub, or evidence of pericardial effusion
Renal disorder	Persistent proteinuria: ≥0.5 gm/day, or >3+, if quantification not performed Cellular casts: may be red, granular, tubular, or mixed
Neurologic disorder	Seizures: in the absence of offending drugs or known metabolic derangements Psychosis: in the absence of offending drugs or known metabolic derangements
Hematologic disorder	Anemia with reticulocytosis Leukopenia: <4,000/mL total on two or more occasions Lymphopenia: <1,500/mL on two or more occasions Thrombocytopenia: <100,000/mL in the absence of offending drugs
Immunologic disorder	Anti-DNA: antibody to native DNA in abnormal titer Anti-Sm: presence of antibody to Sm nuclear antigen. Positive test for APLA including: 1) abnormal serum IgG or IgM ACLA, 2) (+) test for LA, 3) false (+) test for syphillis known to be (+) for at least 6 months and confirmed by Treponema pallidum immoblization of fluorescent treponemal antibody absorption test.
Antinuclear antibody	Abnormal titer of ANA by IF or an equivalent assay at any point in time in the absence of drugs known to be associated with drug-induced lupus syndrome

[a]The 1982 revised criteria for the classification of systemic lupus erythematosus: four criteria must be present to qualify for a definite diagnosis.

Source: From Ref. 1, with permission.

This observation was subsequently reinforced by a mortality study that described a bimodal death pattern in a prospectively-studied Canadian cohort (6). Half of the deaths occurred within the first year of diagnosis in the setting of active disease and were attributable to acute nephritis or sepsis, whereas late deaths (an average of 8.6 years following diagnosis) were attributable to myocardial infarction rather than active disease and occurred in the setting of chronic corticosteroid therapy. Population-based, observational studies subsequently documented higher than expected rates of myocardial infarction (7–9), most notably in premenopausal women (8).

Although initial speculation centered on the importance of corticosteroid therapy in causing premature atherosclerosis (5,6), subsequent reports documented an excess of traditional risk factors that might predispose to coronary artery disease (10–13). Among 265 patients in the Hopkins Lupus Cohort, 53% had at least 3 traditional risk factors for coronary artery disease, even in the absence of prednisone therapy (14). Coincident with the recognition of the importance of inflammation in all aspects of the atherosclerotic process (15), evidence mounted that the risk of myocardial infarction was, at least in part, independent of traditional risk factors and therapy (16–18), suggesting that disease-related chronic inflammation might be atherogenic. SLE-related factors reported to be associated with clinical manifestations of coronary artery disease include older age at diagnosis (8,11), longer duration of SLE (8,11,19), higher damage score (a quantitative measure of cumulative organ damage attributable to SLE or its treatment) (19), and higher levels of oxidized low-density lipoprotein (LDL) cholesterol and homocysteine (20).

The independence of premature atherosclerosis in SLE from traditional risk factors and its direct relation to chronic inflammation was definitively documented in two case-control studies reported in 2003 (21,22). Both subclinical carotid atherosclerosis (21) and coronary artery calcification (22) were increased in lupus patients independent of traditional risk factors and unrelated to corticosteroid therapy (Figure 8.1) (21). Imaging studies indicate the underlying pathophysiology is primarily atherosclerosis rather than in situ thrombosis associated with antiphospholipid antibodies (12,21–23). Importantly, intimal-medial thickness, a less direct measure of atherosclerosis than focal plaque, is not abnormal in large cohorts of patients with SLE (12,21,24). Aspects of SLE associated with the presence of subclinical atherosclerosis include older age at diagnosis (21), longer duration of disease (21,25), longer duration of steroid therapy (12), less aggressive immunosuppressive therapy (21), higher damage score (21), and higher homocysteine concentrations (25). Subclinical atherosclerosis progresses at twice the rate seen in non-SLE populations (Figure 8.2) (27,28); the rate of progression is directly related to duration of disease and homocysteine levels (27) and to serum complement and use of immunosuppressive agents at baseline (28).

In addition to the overall proinflammatory and pro-oxidative milieu present in SLE, several additional specific mechanisms have been postulated as contributing to the development of premature atherosclerosis. Antibodies to monomeric C-reactive protein are found in a substantial percentage of SLE patients (29,30), possibly as a consequence of inadequate clearance of

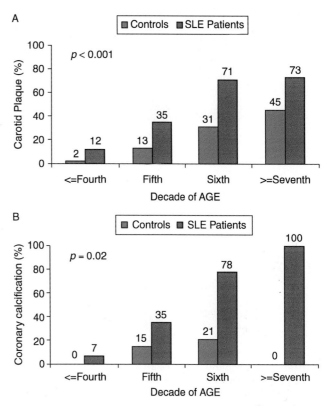

FIGURE 8.1 Prevalences of carotid atherosclerosis (A) and coronary artery calcification (B) in groups of control subjects and patients with systemic lupus erythematosus. (From Refs. 21, 22, with permission.)

apoptotic cells (31). These antibodies are associated with active disease, particularly nephritis (30,32), and may bind to antigen in vessels walls (33). Apoptotic endothelial cells (34) and antibodies to endothelial cells are increased in SLE patients and are also directly related to disease activity (35). In addition, circulating endothelial progenitor cells, important in vasculogenesis, have been reported to be either decreased (36,37) or dysfunctional (38) in SLE patients. Finally, proinflammatory high-density lipoprotein (HDL) (39) and antibodies to HDL (40), both of which have been detected in patients with SLE, may interfere with the atheroprotective effects of HDL cholesterol.

Intervention studies to limit development and progression of atherosclerosis in SLE have not been reported; however, the observation that more aggressive immunosuppressive and anti-inflammatory therapy is associated with a lesser prevalence of atherosclerosis (21) suggests that strategies to limit inflammation may be effective, provided toxicities can be minimized. In view

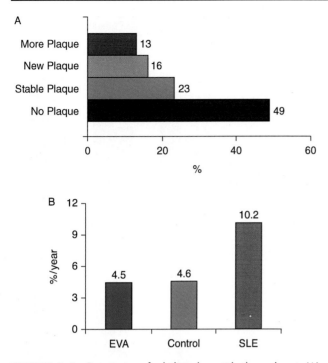

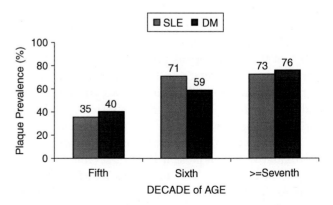

FIGURE 8.2 Progression of subclinical carotid atherosclerosis (A) in SLE patients during 3.4 years of observation. Annual rates of progression of atherosclerosis (B) in SLE patients and two control populations (EVA refers to the Aging Vascular Study reported in *Arterioscler Thromb Vasc Biol* 2000; 20:1622–9). (From Ref. 27, with permission.)

Guidelines for atherosclerosis screening in SLE do not exist. Stress testing is of limited value since flow-limiting coronary disease is uncommon, whereas false positive results are common (26). Although carotid ultrasonography to detect nonobstructive atherosclerosis or computed tomography to detect coronary calcium may yield age-adjusted abnormal results, a negative screening study does not preclude development of atherosclerosis in the short-term future (27,28). Thus, since both cardiovascular disease prevention efforts and control of disease activity should be aggressive, the presence or absence of subclinical atherosclerosis might arguably not alter overall management.

Arterial Stiffness

Arterial stiffness and central blood pressure, which can be accurately quantified using noninvasive techniques, are increasingly recognized as important independent risk factors for adverse cardiovascular outcomes in population-based studies (45–47). In view of the observation that arterial stiffening is associated with inflammatory markers in the general population (48), it is not surprising that arterial stiffness is increased in SLE (49–52), even in the absence of atherosclerosis (49). Arterial stiffening is related to disease duration, circulating levels of C-reactive protein and interleukin-6 (49), disease activity (50,52), and the organ damage index (50,51). Although preliminary studies in patients with rheumatoid arthritis suggest that antitumor necrosis factor therapy (53) and statin use (54) may favorably impact arterial stiffening, similar intervention studies have not been reported in SLE.

of the heightened risk of premature atherosclerosis in SLE, strict adherence to primary prevention guidelines is mandatory. Since the prevalence of carotid atherosclerosis in SLE is at least as high as in diabetes mellitus (Figure 8.3) (41), a coronary heart disease equivalent and indication for secondary prevention targets even in the absence of clinical cardiovascular disease, it is reasonable to consider application of more stringent (42) or secondary prevention guidelines in SLE patients (43,44). From a practical standpoint, a lower target for LDL cholesterol (< 70–100 mg/dL) and aspirin therapy would be the main differences in treatment. Secondary prevention measures should certainly be applied in the setting of established cardiovascular disease. Caution should be exercised in the consideration of percutaneous revascularization of coronary artery disease as SLE patients have worse outcomes following such procedures than non-SLE patients (102). The extent to which this observation is attributable to concomitant antiphospholipid antibody syndrome has not been systematically evaluated.

FIGURE 8.3 Comparison of prevalences of carotid atherosclerosis based on decade of age in SLE patients and 1,574 diabetic participants in the Strong Heart Study. (From Ref. 21, with permission.)

Endothelial Dysfunction

Endothelial function, assessed noninvasively by flow-mediated dilation in the brachial artery, is reduced in women with SLE compared to healthy control women matched with respect to age but not blood pressure (55,56). In contrast, endothelium-independent dilation (in response to sublingual nitroglycerin) is unaffected. Coronary flow reserve, measured noninvasively by transthoracic Doppler interrogation of the left anterior descending artery, was also found to be reduced in women with SLE compared to healthy women (57). In addition, endothelial function measured by plethysmography of the index finger in response to brachial artery occlusion was found to be reduced in SLE patients and was directly related to a reduction in endothelial progenitor cells (34). A randomized trial of ω-3 polyunsaturated fatty acids in 60 SLE patients reduced both disease activity and flow-mediated dilation of the brachial artery (58). Given the nonspecificity and variable nature of vascular reactivity, particularly in the setting of excess cardiovascular disease risk factors, the clinical relevance of these findings is uncertain.

■ MYOCARDIAL DISEASE

Myocarditis

Active myocarditis (focal infiltration of lymphocytes and plasma cells) is rarely diagnosed clinically or detected at autopsy in SLE patients in the current treatment era (5,59–61). It is most commonly associated with myositis and serositis (59). Systolic dysfunction and segmental wall motion abnormalities associated with lupus myocarditis are reversible by aggressive immunosuppressive therapy (60).

Abnormalities of Left Ventricular Structure and Function

Excess left ventricular (LV) hypertrophy has been reported in patients with SLE (52,62–65); however, these studies have been either observational or confounded by the presence of concomitant valvular, cardiovascular, or renal disease. In fact, several studies have attributed LV hypertrophy in SLE to the additional presence of hypertension (66–69). In a case-control study that excluded SLE patients with any of these associated conditions, LV mass index was markedly increased in SLE patients

(70). Arterial stiffness, in addition to traditional stimuli such as body size, hypertension and diabetes, was independently related to LV mass, suggesting that inflammation-related arterial stiffening (49) contributes to LV hypertrophy in SLE. This study convincingly demonstrated that hypertension is not the primary cause of LV hypertrophy in SLE, and is based on comparable prevalences of hypertension in the patient and control groups and on subgroup analyses in normotensive and hypertensive subjects demonstrating that the presence of both SLE and hypertension results in the greatest degree of LV hypertrophy (70). In fact, LV mass in normotensive SLE patients is comparable to that in hypertensive control subjects (Figure 8.4). Occult myocarditis is unlikely to be the cause of LV hypertrophy since it is so rare and, when present, is associated with heart failure and depressed ejection fraction (60,61). Insofar as hypertrophied myocardium provides an arrhythmogenic substrate and potentiates the magnitude of ischemia for a given stimulus, the observation of excess LV hypertrophy in SLE may be of considerable clinical importance, especially in the setting of premature atherosclerosis.

Similarly, LV systolic dysfunction has been reported in SLE (52,61). However, in the absence of concomitant disease, both LV ejection fraction (70) and fractional shortening (71) were reported to be not only preserved, but actually higher in SLE patients, likely due to the Starling phenomenon (higher end-diastolic and comparable end-systolic dimensions) (70). Although small studies have suggested a relation between LV systolic

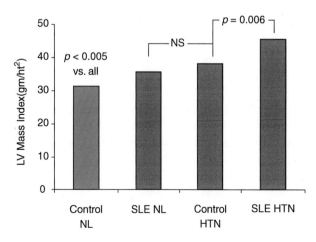

FIGURE 8.4 Comparisons of left ventricular mass index in normotensive and hypertensive control subjects and SLE patients. (LV, left ventricular; NL, normotensive; HTN, hypertensive.) (From Ref. 70, with permission.)

dysfunction and the presence of antiphospholipid antibodies (65,72), we did not detect such an association in a much larger population (23).

Abnormalities of diastolic filling have been reported in several small (n = 14–58) studies (52,71,73–76). Although these studies have mainly used older, load-dependent methods of assessment of diastolic function (71,73–76), disease activity has been associated with more abnormal diastolic relaxation both among (74–76) and within (73) patients. A more recent study using tissue Doppler methods in 32 young patients reported reductions in both diastolic and systolic myocardial velocities (52). Among 131 SLE patients without clinical cardiovascular disease in our study, deceleration time was prolonged in only 17 of them and isovolumic relaxation time was prolonged in only two (70). There are no data to suggest that isolated abnormalities of diastolic filling are of clinical relevance.

■ VALVULAR DISEASE

Libman-Sacks lesions ("atypical verrucous endocarditis") have been described in the majority of patients with SLE at autopsy (5,77,78). The verrucae have a variable morphology and distribution, but most commonly are the "flat spreading type," may occur diffusely on the valve (ring, commissures and both leaflet surfaces), and may extend onto the atrial and ventricular endocardium (78). Both gross and histopathologic changes to distinguish SLE-related endocardial disease from rheumatic disease have been proposed (78). The atrioventricular valves were more commonly involved than the semilunar valves, and both right- and left-sided valves were equally involved in hearts autopsied before the steroid treatment era (78). In contrast, widespread use of corticosteroid therapy has resulted in a reduction in the size and number of lesions, which now predominate on left-sided valves, particularly the left ventricular surface of the posterior mitral valve leaflet (5).

Although valvular lesions are frequently detected at autopsy, clinical disease solely attributable to valvular involvement appears to be much less common (<10%) (63,79–82). Prevalences of valvular abnormalities detected by echocardiography have been extremely variable, most likely due to frequent inclusion of nonspecific valvular thickening (separate from the presence of a vegetation or nodule) and valvular regurgitation (which may be mild and/or potentially due to other causes) as being representative of SLE-related involvement. In addition, echocardiographic studies vary with regard to the frequency of vegetations or nodules detected on the mitral (7–15%) and aortic (3–19%) valves (23,79,82,83). Significant (≥ moderate) valvular regurgitation occurs in less than 20% of relatively unselected patients undergoing Doppler echocardiography (23,63,83,84). Similar to more recent autopsy studies, the presence of echocardiographic evidence of valvular lesions is inversely related to corticosteroid therapy (82). The development of severe valvular regurgitation may be related to high levels of IgG anticardiolipin antibodies (84). Although valvular lesions (thickening and masses) and significant regurgitation were more commonly detected in 54 SLE patients undergoing transesophageal echocardiography (85), the extent to which selection bias or other comorbidities might influence these results is uncertain. A longitudinal echocardiographic study indicated that valvular vegetations may persist, resolve, or develop anew over time, independent of disease activity or therapy (81). This observation may also contribute to variations in prevalences of vegetations encountered in the echocardiographic literature.

An understanding of the impact of antiphospholipid antibodies on valvular involvement in SLE is confounded by differences in the literature in the definitions of valvular disease (thickening, nodules, presence of regurgitation) and of antiphospholipid antibody presence (method and titer used to define positivity, and presence or absence of antiphospholipid syndrome). Nevertheless, large transthoracic echocardiographic studies of relatively unselected patients document an association between higher anticardiolipin titers, valvular nodules, and significant regurgitation, particularly involving the mitral valve (23,63,72,84,86), whereas smaller (n <40) studies (64,87) using less stringent criteria for antibody positivity (85) have failed to demonstrate such an association. In fact, valvular disease is now considered an integral component of antiphospholipid antibody syndrome (*vide infra*).

Specific guidelines for antibiotic prophylaxis for SLE-related valvular disease do not exist. The presence of significant regurgitation, even in the absence of nodules, may heighten the risk of bacterial endocarditis, particularly in the setting of jet lesions; however, antibiotic prophylaxis is no longer recommended for valvular regurgitation per se in the absence of previous infective endocarditis (88). Nevertheless, it seems prudent to individualize consideration of antibiotic prophylaxis, particularly in the setting of long-standing immunosuppressant use. Indications for pharmacologic or surgical interventions for valvular heart disease do not differ from those applied in the general population. Major added risks in SLE patients include perioperative anticoagulation and the potential for thrombotic complications if antiphospholipid antibody syndrome coexists (89). In addition, wound healing may be impaired and infection risk may be increased in the setting of chronic and/or perioperative stress doses of corticosteroid therapy. Cerebrovascular and valvular disease may coexist, particularly when antiphospholipid antibodies are present (90). The extent to which in situ thrombosis (91), as opposed to valvular emboli, causes cerebrovascular disease may be impossible to clarify; hence the recommendation for valve replacement, as opposed to chronic anticoagulation, in such patients may be difficult to justify, particularly given the heightened risks of surgery.

■ PERICARDIAL DISEASE

Pericardial disease, a manifestation of serositis, is a diagnostic feature of SLE and is the most common clinical cardiovascular manifestation. Clinical features of pericarditis, with or without pericardial effusion, occur in 20% to 50% of patients in relatively large series (62,63,66,72,79,83). Pericardial effusions most commonly occur in the setting of acute flares (62,63,83), but may be asymptomatic (63). The effusions are usually small, although moderate-large pericardial effusions were detected in 5 of 70 (7%) patients in one series (63). Mild pericardial effusions associated with lupus pericarditis are usually not associated with typical electrocardiographic changes (63,66,79); the explanation for this observation is uncertain. Major complications (cardiac tamponade or constrictive pericarditis) of lupus pericarditis are very uncommon in the absence of renal failure. Treatment of symptomatic pericarditis and pericardial effusions includes high-dose aspirin, nonsteroidal anti-inflammatory drugs, or corticosteroid therapy, particularly if prednisone is required for management of other manifestations of active disease. In the rare instance of cardiac tamponade or constrictive pericarditis, treatment is not specific to SLE.

■ ARRHYTHMIAS AND CONDUCTION SYSTEM DISEASE

Arrhythmias and conduction system disease in SLE patients most commonly occur as a consequence of other disease manifestations such as pericarditis, coronary artery disease, significant valvular disease, or the rare case of myocarditis. In contrast, congenital heart block in offspring of women with SLE appears to be due to placental transfer of specific maternal autoantibodies. Antibodies to anti-SS-A/Ro were found in 100% of 54 women with SLE whose infants had congenital heart block, as opposed to 47% of 152 women with SLE whose infants did not have heart block (92). Corresponding prevalences anti-SS-B/La antibodies were 76% and 15%, respectively. (The presence of these maternal autoantibodies also increases the risk of neonatal lupus.) Heart block is usually complete and associated with an increased likelihood of intrauterine or neonatal death; permanent pacing is frequently required. Whether other conduction abnormalities such as first-degree heart block and QT prolongation are associated with the presence of maternal anti-SS-A/Ro is debated (93).

■ PULMONARY HYPERTENSION

Pulmonary hypertension occurs much less commonly in SLE than other rheumatologic disorders such as systemic sclerosis. Pulmonary hypertension not due to secondary causes such as systemic hypertension, significant mitral or aortic valvular disease, pulmonary embolism, or LV dysfunction caused by coronary heart disease may be multifactorial, as a consequence of vasoconstriction, vasculitis, or in situ thrombosis. Pulmonary hypertension was detected in about 6% of 786 SLE patients evaluated at a single center based on Doppler echocardiography or right heart catheterization, with comparable prevalences of primary and secondary hypertension (94). Raynaud's phenomenon was frequently present (35%) in patients with pulmonary hypertension and was associated with higher levels of pulmonary artery systolic pressure (94). In another large series, 6.2% of 194 SLE patients had pulmonary hypertension, especially in association with a systemic sclerosis overlap syndrome (95). Patients with unexplained pulmonary hypertension improved with immunosuppressive therapy with either corticosteroids or cyclophosphamide (95). Based on Doppler echocardiography, we detected pulmonary hypertension in 17% of 200 unselected SLE patients; however pulmonary hypertension was mild in over 90% of affected patients (23). In a small series of 28 SLE patients studied twice over a five-year period, pulmonary hypertension (defined as a pulmonary artery systolic pressure of >30 mm Hg) was initially present in 14% and subsequently in 43% of the patients (96). In all instances, the pulmonary hypertension was mild (≤ 38 mm Hg); however, no information was provided with regard to coexistent systemic hypertension, left ventricular dysfunction or valvular disease. Of note, Raynaud's phenomenon was almost twice as common (75% versus 40%) in those with pulmonary hypertension compared to those without it.

■ ANTIPHOSPHOLIPID ANTIBODY SYNDROME IN SLE

Antiphospholipid antibodies are a family of autoantibodies that recognize various combinations of phospholipids and phospholipid-binding proteins (97). Although these antibodies are present in a small percentage of the general population, they occur more commonly in patients with connective tissue disorders such as SLE (98). Persistent presence of these antibodies is strongly associated with recurrent fetal loss and arterial or venous thrombosis (antiphospholipid antibody syndrome). The primary antiphospholipid syndrome (absence of SLE or other connective tissue disorder) has also been associated with cardiac abnormalities. Indeed, in the most recent consensus conference, valvular heart disease was accepted as an integral part of the syndrome (99). As mentioned above (Valvular Disease), the presence of antiphospholipid antibodies in patients with SLE is strongly associated with valvular lesions and significant regurgitation or stenosis, particularly of the mitral valve (23,63,72,84,86).

In contrast, whether other cardiovascular manifestations are attributable to the presence of antiphospholipid antibodies in SLE has been controversial. Although SLE is associated with premature atherosclerosis, it is important to clarify whether myocardial infarction in the setting of antiphospholipid antibodies is attributable to unstable plaque rupture or progressive occlusive disease (atherosclerosis), as opposed to in situ

thrombosis due to endothelial cell activation, independent of underlying atherosclerotic plaque (100). In our study of 200 SLE patients, carotid atherosclerosis was comparably present in those with and without antiphospholipid antibodies (32% versus 37%, respectively, $P = 0.55$) (21,23), arguing against a significant atherogenic role for these antibodies. These findings have been confirmed in subsequent studies (22,101).

Similar considerations apply to cerebrovascular disease in SLE and antiphospholipid antibody syndrome wherein in situ thrombosis may be more important than atherosclerosis in causing ischemia. Pathological examination of brain lesions in patients with antiphospholipid antibodies (both primary and associated with SLE) show recanalized thrombi, fibrous and cellular occlusions, and fibrous webs which are suggestive of chronic recurring intravascular thrombosis not found in the cerebral arteries of patients without antiphospholipid antibodies (91).

Antiphospholipid antibodies have been suggested as potential causes of myocardial dysfunction (65) and pulmonary hypertension (91) in SLE. Our study, the largest to date to systematically examine these issues, does not support a role for antiphospholipid antibodies in myocardial disease (23). Left ventricular structure and function were comparable between 158 SLE patients without and 42 SLE patients with antiphospholipid antibodies. Similarly, prevalences of pulmonary hypertension (18% and 17%, respectively) were comparable. In addition, there were no differences in Raynaud's phenomenon or measures of vascular stiffness (Table 8.2).

■ CONCLUSIONS

SLE results in premature development of subclinical atherosclerosis as well as myocardial infarction as a direct consequence of chronic inflammation. Chronic inflammation is likewise responsible for premature arterial stiffening in SLE. Excess LV hypertrophy develops in SLE due to inflammation-related arterial stiffening and may potentiate the impact of premature atherosclerosis. LV systolic dysfunction is not a feature of SLE in the absence of concomitant disease. Although LV diastolic dysfunction and endothelium-dependent vasodilation appear to be impaired in SLE, the clinical relevance of these findings is uncertain. Clinically significant

■ **Table 8.2** Relationship of cardiovascular manifestations in SLE patients to the presence or absence of antiphospholipid antibodies

	Antibodies Absent ($n = 158$)	Antibodies Present ($n = 42$)	P Value
Mitral valve nodules (%)	4.4	14.3	0.32
Mitral regurgitation[a]	4.4	14.3	0.02
Aortic nodules (%)	6.3	2.4	0.32
Aortic regurgitation[b]	10.8	11.9	0.88
Carotid IMT (mm)	0.61 ± 0.15	0.62 ± 0.13	0.51
Carotid plaque (%)	36.7	31.7	0.55
LV mass (gm)	144.5 ± 46.1	151.2 ± 42.4	0.39
LV ejection fraction (%)	70 ± 6	70 ± 6	0.56
Raynaud's phenomenon (%)	51.2	40.0	0.19
Pulmonary hypertension (%)	17.7	16.7	0.87
Arterial stiffness index (β)	3.1 ± 1.5	2.8 ± 1.2	0.58

[a]Moderate or severe.

[b]Mild or moderate.

IMT, intimal-medial thickness; LV, left ventricular.

Source: Adapted from Ref. 23, with permission.

valvular disease develops in a minority of SLE patients and is influenced by the presence of antiphospholipid antibodies. Pericardial disease, a diagnostic feature, is common in SLE but is rarely associated with significant morbidity. Cardiac arrhythmias are usually secondary to other cardiovascular manifestations of SLE, whereas autoantibody-induced conduction system disease primarily affects the offspring of women with SLE. Pulmonary hypertension occurs in a minority of patients with SLE and is rarely severe. Antiphospholipid antibodies are associated with valvular disease, as well as arterial and venous thromboses in SLE, but not with atherosclerosis or myocardial disease. Effective treatment strategies need to be developed to retard the development and progression of novel manifestations of cardiovascular disease in SLE, particularly atherosclerosis, to reduce premature cardiovascular morbidity and mortality in this prototypic chronic inflammatory disease.

■ REFERENCES

1. Tan EM, Cohen AS, Fries JF, et al. The 1982 revised criteria for the classification of systemic lupus erythematosus. *Arthritis Rheum* 1982; 25:1271–77.
2. Lawrence RC, Helmick CG, Arnett FC, et al. Estimates of the prevalence of arthritis and selected musculoskeletal disorders in the United States. *Arthritis Rheum* 1998; 41:778–99.
3. Johnson AE, Gordon C, Palmer RG, Bacon PA. The prevalence and incidence of systemic lupus erythematosus in Birmingham, England: relationship to ethnicity and country of birth. *Arthritis Rheum* 1995; 38:551–58.
4. Rahman A, Isenberg DA. Mechanisms of disease: systemic lupus erythematosus. *N Engl J Med* 2008; 358:929–39.
5. Bulkley BH, Roberts WC. The heart in systemic lupus erythematosus and the changes induced in it by corticosteroid therapy: a study of 36 necropsy patients. *Am J Med* 1975; 58:243–64.
6. Urowitz MB, Bookman AA, Koehler BE, Gordon DA, Smythe HA, Ogryzlo, MA. The bimodal mortality pattern of SLE. *Am J Med* 1976; 60:221–5.
7. Björnådal L, Yin L, Granath F, Klareskog L, Ekbom A. Cardiovascular disease a hazard despite improved prognosis in patients with systemic lupus erythematosus: results from a

Swedish population based study 1964–95. *J Rheumatol* 2004; 31:713–19.

8. Manzi S, Meilahn EN, Rairie JE, et al. Age-specific incidence rates of myocardial infarction and angina in women with systemic lupus erythematosus—comparison with the Framingham study. *Am J Epidemiol* 1997; 145:408–15.

9. Fischer LM, Schlienger RG, Matter C, Jick H, Meier CR. Effect of rheumatoid arthritis or systemic lupus erythematosus on the risk of first-time acute myocardial infarction. *Am J Cardiol* 2004; 93:198–200.

10. Haider YS, Roberts WC. Coronary arterial disease in systemic lupus erythematosus. Quantification of degrees of narrowing in 22 necropsy patients (22 women) aged 16 to 37 years. *Am J Med* 1981; 70:775–81.

11. Petri M, Perz-Gutthan S, Spence D, Hochberg MC. Risk factors for coronary artery disease in patients with systemic lupus erythematosus. *Am J Med* 1992; 93:513–19.

12. Manzi S, Selzer F, Sutton-Tyrrell K, et al. Prevalence and risk factors of carotid plaque in women with systemic lupus erythematosus. *Arthritis Rheum* 1999; 42:51–60.

13. Selzer F, Sutton-Tyrrell K, Fitzgerald SG, et al. Comparison of risk factors for vascular disease in the carotid artery and aorta in women with systemic lupus erythematosus. *Arthritis Rheum* 2004; 50:151–9.

14. Petri M, Spence D, Bone LE, Hochberg MC. Coronary artery disease risk factors in the Johns Hopkins Lupus Cohort: prevalence, recognition by patients, and preventive practices. *Medicine* 1992; 71:291–302.

15. Ross R. Atherosclerosis--an inflammatory disease. *N Engl J Med* 1999; 34:115–26.

16. Esdaile JM, Abrahamowicz M, Grodzicky T, et al. Traditional Framingham risk factors fail to fully account for accelerated atherosclerosis in systemic lupus erythematosus. *Arthritis Rheum* 2001; 44:2331–37.

17. Rahman P, Urowitz M, Gladman DD, Bruce IN, Genest J Jr. Contribution of traditional risk factors to coronary artery disease in patients with systemic lupus erythematosus. *J Rheumatol* 1999:26:2363–68.

18. Fischer LM, Schlienger RG, Matter C, Jick H, Meier CR. Effect of rheumatoid arthritis or systemic lupus erythematosus on the risk of first-time acute myocardial infarction. *Am J Cardiol* 2004; 93:198–200.

19. de Leeuw K, Freire B, Smit AJ, Bootsma H, Kallenberg CG, Bijl M. Traditional and non-traditional risk factors contribute to the development of accelerated atherosclerosis in patients with systemic lupus erythematosus. *Lupus* 2006; 15:675–82.

20. Svenungsson E, Jensen-Urstad K, Heimbhrger M, et al. Risk factors for cardiovascular disease in systemic lupus erythematosus. *Circulation* 2001; 104:1887–93.

21. Roman MJ, Shanker B-A, Davis A, et al. Prevalence and correlates of accelerated atherosclerosis in systemic lupus erythematosus. *N Engl J Med* 2003; 349:2399–406.

22. Azanuma Y, Oeser A, Shintani AK, et al. Premature coronary-artery atherosclerosis in systemic lupus erythematosus. *N Engl J Med* 2003; 349:2407–15.

23. Farzaneh-Far A, Roman MJ, Lockshin MD, et al. Relationship of antiphospholipid antibodies to cardiovascular manifestations of systemic lupus erythematosus. *Arthritis Rheum* 2006; 54:3918–25.

24. de Leeuw K, Graaff R, de Vries R, et al. Accumulation of advanced glycation endproducts in patients with systemic lupus erythematosus. *Rheumatology* 2007; 46:1551–6.

25. Von Feldt JM, Scalzi LV, Cucchiara AJ, et al. Homocysteine levels and disease duration independently correlate with coronary artery calcification in patients with systemic lupus erythematosus. *Arthritis Rheum* 2006; 54:2220–7.

26. Sella EMC, Sato EI, Barbieri A. Coronary artery angiography in systemic lupus erythematosus patients with abnormal myocardial perfusion scintigraphy. *Arthritis Rheum* 2003; 48:3168–75.

27. Roman MJ, Crow MK, Lockshin MD, et al. Rate and determinants of progression of atherosclerosis in systemic lupus erythematosus. *Arthritis Rheum* 2007; 56:3412–19.

28. Thompson T, Sutton-Tyrrell K, Wildman RP, et al. Progression of carotid intima-media thickness and plaque in women with systemic lupus erythematosus. *Arthritis Rheum* 2008; 58:835–42.

29. Bell SA, Faust H, Schmid A, Meurer M. Autoantibodies to C-reactive protein (CRP) and other acute-phase proteins in systemic autoimmune diseases. *Clin Exp Immunol* 1998; 113: 327–32.

30. Figueredo MA, Rodriquez A, Ruiz-Yague M, et al. Autoantibodies against C-reactive protein: clinical associations in systemic lupus erythematosus and primary antiphospholipid syndrome. *J Rheumatol* 2006; 33:1980–86.

31. Hermann M, Voll RE, Zoller OM, Hagenhofer M, Ponner BB, Kalden JR. Impaired phagocytosis of apoptotic cell material by monocyte-derived macrophages from patients with systemic lupus erythematosus. *Arthritis Rheum* 1998; 41:1241–50.

32. Sjöwall C, Bengtsson AA, Stirfelt G, Skogh T. Serum levels of autoantibodies against monomeric C-reactive protein are correlated with disease activity in systemic lupus erythematosus. *Arthritis Res Ther* 2004; 6:R87–94.

33. O'Neill SG, Isenberg DA, Rahman A. Could antibodies to C-reactive protein link inflammation and cardiovascular disease in patients with systemic lupus erythematosus? *Ann Rheum Dis* 2007; 66:989–91.

34. Rajagopalan S, Somers EC, Brook RD, et al. Endothelial cell apoptosis in systemic lupus erythematosus: a common pathway for abnormal vascular function and thrombosis propensity. *Blood* 2004; 103:3677–83.

35. Constans J, Duouy R, Blann AD, et al. Anti-endothelial cell autoantibodies and soluble markers of endothelial cell dysfunction in systemic lupus erythematosus. *J Rheumatol* 2003; 30:1963–66.

36. Lee PY, Li Y, Richards HB, et al. Type 1 interferon as a novel risk factor for endothelial progenitor cell depletion and endothelial cell dysfunction in systemic lupus erythematosus. *Arthritis Rheum* 2007; 56:3759–69.

37. Westerweel PE, Luitjen RKMAC, Hoefer IE, et al. Haematopoietic and endothelial progenitor cells are deficient in quiescent systemic lupus erythematosus. *Ann Rheum Dis* 2007; 66:865–70.

38. Grisar J, Steiner CW, Bonelli M, et al. Systemic lupus erythematosus patients exhibit functional deficiencies of endothelial progenitor cells. *Rheumatology* 2008; 47:1476–83.

39. Hahn BH, Grossman J, Ansell BJ, Skaggs BJ, McMahon M. Altered lipoprotein metabolism in chronic inflammatory states: proinflammatory high-density lipoprotein and accelerated atherosclerosis in systemic lupus erythematosus and rheumatoid arthritis. *Arthritis Res Ther* 2008; 10:213–25.

40. Batuca JR, Ames PRJ, Amaral M, Favas C, Isenberg DA, Alves JD. Anti-atherogenic and anti-inflammatory properties of high-density lipoprotein are affected by specific antibodies

in systemic lupus erythematosus. *Rheumatology* 2009; 48: 26–31.

41. Roman MJ, Moeller E, Davis A, et al. Preclinical carotid atherosclerosis in patients with rheumatoid arthritis: prevalence and associated factors. *Ann Intern Med* 2006; 144:249–56.

42. Kavey R-EW, Allada V, Daniels SR, et al. Cardiovascular risk reduction in high-risk pediatric patients: a statement from the American Heart Association expert panel on population and prevention science; the Councils on Cardiovascular Disease in the Young, Epidemiology and Prevention, Nutrition, Physical Activity and Metabolism, High Blood Pressure Research, Cardiovascular Nursing, and the Kidney in Heart Disease; and the Interdisciplinary Working Group on Quality of Care and Putcomes Research: Endorsed by the American Academy of Pediatrics. *Circulation* 2006; 114:2710–38.

43. Salmon JE, Roman MJ. Accelerated atherosclerosis in systemic lupus erythematosus: implications for patient management. *Curr Opin Rheumatol* 2001; 13:341–44.

44. Wajed J, Ahmed Y, Durrington PN, Bruce IN. Prevention of cardiovascular disease in systemic lupus erythematosus—proposed guidelines for risk factor management. *Rheumatology* 2004; 43:7–12.

45. Hansen TW, Staessen JA, Torp-Pedersen C, et al. Prognostic value of aortic pulse wave velocity as index of arterial stiffness in the general population. *Circulation* 2006; 113:664–70.

46. Mattace-Raso FUS, van der Cammen TJM, Hofman A, et al. Arterial stiffness and risk of coronary heart disease and stroke: The Rotterdam Study. *Circulation* 2006; 113:657–63.

47. Roman MJ, Devereux RB, Kizer JR, et al. Central pressure more strongly relates to vascular disease and outcome than does brachial pressure: The Strong Heart Study. *Hypertension* 2007; 50:197–203.

48. Yasmin, McEniery CM, Wallace S, et al. C-reactive protein is associated with arterial stiffness in apparently healthy individuals. *Arterioscler Thromb Vasc Biol* 2004; 24:969–74.

49. Roman MJ, Devereux RB, Schwartz JE, et al. Arterial stiffness in chronic inflammatory diseases. *Hypertension* 2005; 46:194–99.

50. Shang Q, Tam LS, Li EKM, Yip GWK, Yu CM. Increased arterial stiffness correlated with disease activity in systemic lupus erythematosus. *Lupus* 2007; 17:1096–102.

51. Selzer F, Sutton-Tyrrell K, Fitzgerald S, Tracy R, Kuller L, Manzi S. Vascular stiffness in women with systemic lupus erythematosus. *Hypertension* 2001; 37:1075–82.

52. Chow P-C, Ho MH-K, Lee T-L, Lau Y-L, Cheung Y-F. Relation of arterial stiffness to left ventricular structure and function in adolescents and young adults with pediatric-onset systemic lupus erythematosus. *J Rheumatol* 2007; 1345–52.

53. Mäki-Petäjä KM, Hall FC, Booth AD, et al. Rheumatoid arthritis is associated with increased aortic pulse-wave velocity, which is reduced by anti-tumor necrosis factor-ά therapy. *Circulation* 2006; 114:1185–92.

54. van Doornum S, McColl G, Wicks IP. Atorvastatin reduces arterial stiffness in patients with rheumatoid arthritis. *Ann Rheum Dis* 2004; 63:1571–75.

55. El-Magadmi M, Bodill H, Ahmad Y, et al. Systemic lupus erythematosus: an independent risk factor for endothelial dysfunction in women. *Circulation* 2004; 110:399–404.

56. Wright SA, O'Prey FM, Rea DJ, et al. Microcirculatory hemodynamics and endothelial dysfunction in systemic lupus erythematosus. *Arterioscler Thromb Vasc Biol* 2006; 26:2281–87.

57. Hirata K, Kadirvelu A, Kinjo M, et al. Altered coronary vasomotor function in young patients with systemic lupus erythematosus. *Arthritis Rheum* 2007; 56:1904–09.

58. Wright SA, O'Prey FM, McHenry MT, et al. A randomized interventional trial of ω–3-polyunsaturated fatty acids on endothelial function and disease activity in systemic lupus erythematosus. *Ann Rheum Dis* 2008; 67:841–48.

59. Borenstein DG, Fye WB, Arnett FC, Stevens MB. The myocarditis of systemic lupus erythematosus: association with myositis. *Ann Intern Med* 1978;89:619–24.

60. Law WG, Thong BY, Lian TY, Kong KO, Chng HH. Acute lupus myocarditis: clinical features and outcome of an oriental case series. *Lupus* 2005; 14:827–31.

61. Wijetunga M, Rockson S. Myocarditis in systemic lupus erythematosus. *Am J Med* 2002; 113:419–23.

62. Crozier IG, Li E, Milne MJ, Nicholls GM. Cardiac involvement in systemic lupus erythematosus detected by echocardiography. *Am J Cardiol* 1990; 65:1145–48.

63. Cervera R, Font J, Pare C, et al. Cardiac disease in systemic lupus erythematosus: prospective study of 70 patients. *Annals Rheum Dis* 1992; 51:156–59.

64. Omdal R, Lunde P, Rasmussen K, Mellgren SI, Husby G. Transesophageal and transthoracic echocardiography and Doppler-examinations in systemic lupus erythematosus. *Scand J Rheumatol* 2001; 30:275–81.

65. Leung WH, Wong KL, Lau CP, Wong CK, Liu HW. Association between antiphospholipid antibodies and cardiac abnormalities in patients with systemic lupus erythematosus. *Am J Med* 1990; 89:411–19.

66. Doherty NE, Feldman G, Maurer G, Siegel RJ. Echocadiographic findings in systemic lupus erythematosus. *Am J Cardiol* 1988; 61:1144.

67. Gentile R, Lagana B, Tubani L, Casato M, Ferri GM, Fedele F. Assessment of echocardiographic abnormalities in patients with systemic lupus erythematosus: correlation with levels of antiphospholipid antibodies. *Ital Heart J* 2000; 1:487–92.

68. Falcao CA, Alves IC, Chahade WH, Branco Pinto Duarte AL, Lucena-Silva N. Echocardiographic abnormalities and antiphospholipid antibodies in patients with systemic lupus erythematosus. *Arq Bras Cardiol* 2002; 79:285–91.

69. Winslow TM, Ossipov MA, Fazio GP, Foster E, Simonson JS, Schiller NB. The left ventricle in systemic lupus erythematosus: Initial observations and a five-year follow-up in a university medical center population. *Am Heart J* 1993; 125:1117–22.

70. Pieretti J, Roman MJ, Devereux RB, et al. Systemic lupus erythematosus predicts increased left ventricular mass. *Circulation* 2007; 116:419–26.

71. Fujimoto S, Kagoshima T, Nakajima T, Dohi K. Doppler echocardiographic assessment of left ventricular diastolic function in patients with systemic lupus erythematosus. *Cardiology* 1994; 85:267–72.

72. Nihoyannopoulos P, Gomez PM, Joshi J, Loizou S, Walport MJ, Oakley CM. Cardiac abnormalities in systemic lupus erythematosus: association with raised anticardiolipin antibodies. *Circulation* 1990; 82:369–75.

73. Murai K, Oku H, Takeuchi K, Kanayama Y, Inoue T, Takeda T. Alterations in myocardial systolic and diastolic function in patients with active systemic lupus erythematosus. *Am Heart J* 1987; 113:966–71.

74. Leung WH, Wong KL, Lau CH, Wong CK, Cheng CH, Tai YT. Doppler echocardiographic evaluation of left ventricular

diastolic function in patients with systemic lupus erythematosus. *Am Heart J* 1990; 120:82–7.

75. Sasson Z, Rasooly Y, Chow WC, Marshall S, Urowitz MB. Impairment of left ventricular diastolic function in systemic lupus erythematosus. *Am J Cardiol* 1992; 69:1629–34.

76. Kalke S, Balakrishanan C, Mangat G, Mittal G, Kumar N, Joshi VR. Echocardiography in systemic lupus erythematosus. *Lupus* 1998; 7:540–44.

77. Libman E, Sacks B. A hitherto undescribed form of valvular and mural endocarditis. *Arch Intern Med* 1924; 33:701–37.

78. Gross L. The cardiac lesions in Libman-Sacks disease with a consideration of its relationship to diffuse lupus erythematosus. *Am J Pathol* 1940; 16:375–408.

79. Klinkhoff AV, Thompson CR, Reid GD, Tomlinson CW. M-mode and two-dimensional echocardiographic abnormalities in systemic lupus erythematosus. *JAMA* 1985; 253:3273–77.

80. Straaton KV, Chatham WW, Reveille JD, Koopman WJ, Smith SH. Clinically significant valvular heart disease in systemic lupus erythematosus. *Am J Med* 1988; 85:645–50.

81. Roldan CA, Shively BK, Crawford MH. An echocardiographic study of valvular heart disease associated with systemic lupus erythematosus. *N Engl J Med* 1996; 335:1424–30.

82. Galve E, Candell-Riera J, Pigrau C, Permanyer-Miralda G, Garcia-Del-Castillo H, Soler-Soler J. Prevalence, morphologic types, and evolution of cardiac valvular disease in systemic lupus erythematosus. *N Engl J Med* 1988; 319:817–23.

83. Sturfelt G, Eskilsson J, Nived O, Truedsson L, Valind S. Cardiovascular disease in systemic lupus erythematosus: a study of 75 patients from a defined population. *Medicine* 1992; 71:216–23.

84. Perez-Villa F, Font J, Azqueta M, et al. Severe valvular regurgitation and antiphospholipid antibodies in systemic lupus erythematosus: a prospective, long-term, follow-up study. *Arthritis Rheum* 2005; 53:460–67.

85. Roldan CA, Shively BK, Lau CC, Gurule FT, Smith EA, Crawford MH. Systemic lupus erythematosus valve disease by transesophageal echocardiography and the role of antiphospholipid antibodies. *J Am Coll Cardiol* 1992; 20:1127–34.

86. Khamasta MA, Cervera R, Asherson RA, et al. Association of antibodies against phospholipids with heart valve disease in systemic lupus erythematosus. *Lancet* 1990; 335:1541–44.

87. Gabrielli F, Alcini E, Di Prima MA, Mazzacurati G, Masala C. Cardiac valve involvement in systemic lupus erythematosus and primary antiphospholipid syndrome: lack of correlation with antiphospholipid antibodies. *Int J Cardiol* 1995; 51:117–26.

88. Wilson W, Taubert KA, Gewitz M, et al. Prevention of Infective Endocarditis: Guidelines From the American Heart Association: A Guideline From the American Heart Association Rheumatic Fever, Endocarditis, and Kawasaki Disease Committee, Council on Cardiovascular Disease in the Young, and the Council on Clinical Cardiology, Council on Cardiovascular Surgery and Anesthesia, and the Quality of Care and Outcomes Research Interdisciplinary Working Group. *Circulation* 2007; 116:1736–54.

89. Erkan D, Leibowitz E, Berman J, Lockshin MD. Perioperative medical management of antiphospholipid syndrome: Hospital for Special Surgery experience, review of literature, and recommendations. *J Rheumatol* 2002; 29:843–49.

90. Roldan CA, Gelgand EA, Qualls CR, Sibbitt WL Jr. Valvular heart disease as a cause of cerebrovascular disease in patients with systemic lupus erythematosus. *Am J Cardiol* 2005; 95:1441–47.

91. Hughson MD, McCarty GA, Sholer CM, Brumback RA. Thrombotic cerebral arteriopathy in patients with the antiphospholipid syndrome. *Mod Pathol* 1993; 6:644–53.

92. Buyon JP, Winchester RJ, Slade SG, et al. Identification of mothers at risk for congenital heart block and other neonatal lupus syndromes in their children: comparison of enzyme-linked immunosorbent assay and immunoblot for measurement of anti-SS-A/Ro and anti-SS-B/La antibodies. *Arthritis Rheum* 1993; 36:1263–73.

93. Costedoat-Chalumeau N, Amoura Z, Villain E, Cohen L, Piette J-C. Anti-SSA/Ro antibodies in the heart: more than complete congenital heart block? A review of electrocardiographic and myocardial abnormalities and of treatment options. *Arthritis Res Ther* 2005; 7:69–73.

94. Pan TL-T, Thumboo J, Boey M-L. Primary and secondary pulmonary hypertension in systemic lupus erythematosus. *Lupus* 2000; 9:338–42.

95. Tanaka E, Harigai M, Tanaka M, Kawaguchi Y, Hara M, Kamatani N. Pulmonary hypertension in systemic lupus erythematosus: evaluation of clinical characteristics and response to immunosuppressive treatment. *J Rheumatol* 2002; 29:282–87.

96. Winslow TM, Ossipov MA, Fazio GP, Simonson JS, Redberg RF, Schiller NB. Five-year follow-up study of the prevalence and progression of pulmonary hypertension in systemic lupus erythematosus. *Am Heart J* 1995; 129:510–15.

97. Levine JS, Branch DW, Rauch J. The antiphospholipid syndrome. *N Engl J Med* 2002; 346:752–63.

98. Petri M. Epidemiology of the antiphospholipid antibody syndrome. *J Autoimmun* 2000; 15:145–51.

99. Miyakis S, Lockshin MD, Atsumi T, et al. International consensus statement on an update of the classification criteria for definite antiphospholipid syndrome (APS). *J Thromb Haemost* 2006; 4:295–306.

100. Pierangeli SS, Colden-Stanfield M, Liu X, Barker JH, Anderson GL, Harris N. Antiphospholipid antibodies from antiphospholipid syndrome patients activate endothelial cells in vitro and in vivo. *Circulation* 1999; 99:1997–2002.

101. Petri M. The lupus anticoagulant is a risk factor for myocardial infarction (but not atherosclerosis): Hopkins Lupus Cohort. *Thromb Res* 2004; 114:593–95.

102. Maksimowicz-McKinnon K, Selzer F, Manzi S, et al. Poor 1-year outcomes after percutaneous coronary interventions in systemic lupus erythematosus. *Circ Cardiovasc Intervent* 2008; 1:201–8.

9 Tetralogy of Fallot in the Adult Congenital Heart Disease Patient

KIRSTEN O. HEALY

GINA LaROCCA

OUTLINE

Anatomic Features of Tetralogy
of Fallot   153

Palliative Surgery and Surgical
Repair   155

Complications Following TOF
Surgery   156

Cardiac Imaging   158

Pulmonary Valve Replacement   161

Percutaneous Pulmonary Valve
Replacement   162

Other TOF Complications Requiring
Interventions   163

Cardiopulmonary Exercise Testing   163

Pregnancy and Contraception   165

Long-term Survival   165

Conclusion   165

References   166

Over the past two decades, major advancements have been made in the diagnosis and management of congenital heart disease (CHD). Substantial progress in surgical techniques for repairing complex congenital heart defects has resulted in an increasing number of patients surviving into adulthood. There are currently over one million adult patients with either corrected or uncorrected CHD in the United States, and the prevalence is estimated to be increasing at a rate of about five percent per year (1). Therefore, it is inevitable that cardiologists will play an intricate role in the cardiovascular care of adult patients with CHD.

In 1888 Etienne-Louis Arthur Fallot (2) described a malformation composed of four constant components: a ventricular septal defect, an aortic valve with overriding of the ventricular septum, subpulmonary infundibular stenosis, and right ventricular hypertrophy (Figure 9.1). However, there is a broad morphologic spectrum to tetralogy of Fallot (TOF), ranging from minimal overriding of the aorta and mild pulmonic stenosis to almost complete aortic override and pulmonary atresia (3).

TOF is the most common cyanotic heart defect with which patients survive into adulthood and it accounts for approximately 10% of all congenital cardiac defects (4). It occurs equally in males and females (5), and approximately 15% of patients with TOF have a deletion of chromosome 22q11 (6). This deletion usually is a denovo noninherited abnormality but can be transmitted in families.

■ ANATOMIC FEATURES OF TETRALOGY OF FALLOT

Anterocephalad deviation of the outlet septum and hypertrophy of the septoparietal trabeculations are key morphologic features that unify the diagnosis of TOF and result in its four salient features: (a) ventricular septal defect, (b) an overriding aorta, (c) right ventricular outflow tract (RVOT) obstruction (infundibular, valvular, supravalvular or a combination), and (d) right ventricular hypertrophy as a result of the RVOT obstruction.

The ventricular septal defect (VSD) in TOF is usually single, large, and almost always nonrestrictive. In

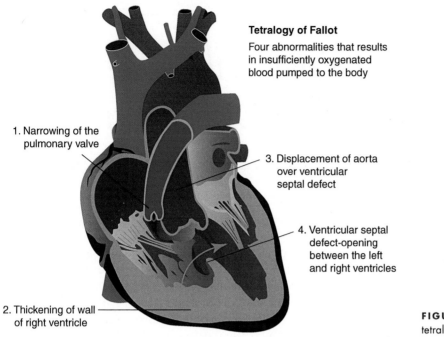

Tetralogy of Fallot
Four abnormalities that results
in insufficiently oxygenated
blood pumped to the body

1. Narrowing of the
   pulmonary valve

3. Displacement of aorta
   over ventricular
   septal defect

4. Ventricular septal
   defect-opening
   between the left
   and right ventricles

2. Thickening of wall
   of right ventricle

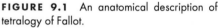

FIGURE 9.1 An anatomical description of tetralogy of Fallot.

the majority of cases, the VSD is perimembranous with the remainder having a muscular posteroinferior rim. However, the defect can be doubly committed juxta arterial, with the cephalad border being formed by the conjoined aortic and pulmonary valves. In this case some have argued whether the malformation should be referred to as TOF since there is an absence of the outlet septum (3).

In almost all cases, RVOT obstruction involves stenosis of the infundibulum. The main cause of the subvalvular obstruction is a result of the anterior and cephalad deviation of the outlet septum and/or hypertrophy of ventricular muscular bands. However, the pulmonic valve is typically abnormal and may be the cause of the RVOT obstruction. The annulus of the pulmonic valve is typically hypoplastic, and the pulmonic valve can be bicuspid and stenotic. In addition, it is not uncommon to have areas of supravalvar narrowing in the main pulmonary artery and the branch pulmonary arteries may be diffusely hypoplastic. Focal areas of pulmonic stenosis can occur from the bifurcation of the right and left pulmonary artery and their branches. In some cases, pulmonary atresia is present (3).

There is much variation in the degree of aortic override and this anatomy can overlap with that of double-outlet right ventricle, another congenital malformation.

The term double-outlet right ventricle (DORV) implies that more than 50% of each great artery arises from the right ventricle. In TOF, aortic override can vary from 5% to 95% of the valve being connected to the right ventricle. Therefore, when more than half of the aorta connects to the right ventricle, TOF coexists with double outlet right ventricle (3).

In addition to the salient features of TOF, there are a number of anatomic features that occur concomitantly. Clinical identification of these features in a given patient is important since it can impact surgical therapy. In about 25% of patients, a right aortic arch is present and needs to be noted prior to a palliative shunt surgery (7). Coronary artery anomalies occur in 9% of TOF patients, with the most common being a left anterior descending arising from the right coronary artery (8). Recognition of these abnormal coronaries is of therapeutic significance because their path can involve the right ventricular outflow tract. Therefore, surgical repair of TOF could inadvertently transect the anomalous coronary artery. An atrial septal defect (ASD) is present in 9% of patients with TOF, and this combination is referred to as pentology of Fallot (7). A patent foramen ovale and a second muscular inlet ventricular septal defect can also coexist with TOF (7).

■ PALLIATIVE SURGERY AND SURGICAL REPAIR

Prior to the era of open-heart surgery, the main treatment was surgical palliation via arterial shunts. Now with the widespread availability of cardiopulmonary bypass techniques, complete surgical repair has become the mainstay of treatment. This repair involves closure of the VSD and relief of the right ventricular outflow tract obstruction. Initially, total correction was carried out in late childhood, usually after an initial palliative shunt. However, total correction can now be offered during the first year of life, and in the majority of patients early shunt procedures can be avoided.

The first palliative shunt procedure for TOF was performed by Blalock and Taussig in 1945 (9). The Blalock-Taussig (B-T) shunt involved a subclavian artery anastamosis to the ipsilateral pulmonary artery resulting in increased pulmonary blood flow. This technique has been modified with the addition of a Gortex graft. The graft minimizes distortion of the pulmonary arteries and allows for easier elimination at the time of definitive repair. Although most patients initially undergo full anatomic repair, the B-T shunt remains an important palliative procedure for patients that are not initial or definitive candidates for intracardiac repair due to prematurity or hypoplastic pulmonary arteries. Central shunts—including the Waterson shunt, a side to side anastomosis of the ascending aorta and the right pulmonary artery, and the Potts shunt, a side to side anastomosis of the descending aorta and the left pulmonary artery—are two other palliative procedures. These central shunts have become obsolete due to complications relating to excessive pulmonary blood flow and possible pulmonary hypertension and pulmonary vascular obstructive disease. In addition, these shunts can also cause distortion of the pulmonary arterial branches at the site of the anastomosis, which may make it difficult for take down at the time of definitive repair. However, a number of TOF patients with these central shunts are now adults, and their consideration is important for the adult cardiologist.

In 1954, the first intracardiac repair of TOF was performed. It consisted of patch closure of the VSD and enlargement the right ventricular outflow tract (10). Since this time, this surgical technique has become the primary method of treatment for TOF patients. This procedure initially involved a right ventriculotomy, to expose the VSD and allow for resection and enlargement of the right ventricular outflow tract. More recently, a transatrial approach through the tricuspid valve was developed. This transatrial approach has been shown to be advantageous because it limits myocardial scar to the right ventricle and can limit ventricular arrhythmias later in life.

In the modern era, definitive TOF repair surgery is typically performed within the first few months of life, once the pulmonary arteries are large enough to support the increased right ventricular output (11). If there is significant pulmonic stenosis or the pulmonary artery size is inadequate, a palliative shunt can still be placed initially in order to augment growth of the pulmonary arteries until repair can be performed. Sometimes, augmentation of the pulmonary arteries via balloon dilatation, or a PA-plasty, is necessary to increase PA size during surgery.

Maintaining pulmonic valve competence during surgical repair is critical. This avoids progressive right ventricular dilatation, systolic and diastolic right ventricular (RV) failure and arrhythmias in the future. If the pulmonary annulus size is not adequate, a transannular patch can be applied across the valve in order to create unobstructed flow from the right ventricle into the pulmonary arteries. However, this transannular patch in the RVOT renders the pulmonary valve incompetent. Significant pulmonic insufficiency, therefore, is indefinitely present, and poses a threat to the right ventricular hemodynamics. As a result, surgical reintervention is required. Alternatively, a valved conduit (RV to PA conduit) from the right ventricle to the distal main pulmonary artery can be inserted in order to maintain pulmonary valve competence. This technique is particularly useful if pulmonary atresia is present. However, significant stenosis of the valved conduit can occur overtime, and replacement of the conduit is inevitable.

In one study by Stewart et al. (12), 80% of children who underwent full TOF repair had valve sparing procedures predominately through the transatrial and transpulmonary approach. Predictors of success in valve sparing surgery are a large pulmonary annulus, a trileaflet pulmonary valve, and a postoperative pressure ratio between the right and left ventricle of less than 70%. Only five patients with initial pulmonary valve-sparing operations required reoperation for residual stenosis. However, there are currently no guidelines to direct the size of the pulmonary annulus and the acceptable degree of residual outflow tract obstruction suitable for a valve sparing approach.

■ COMPLICATIONS FOLLOWING TOF SURGERY

It is unusual for unoperated TOF patients to present it in adulthood. Therefore, most adult cardiologists who encounter TOF will do so in individuals who have undergone some combination of palliative shunts and definitive repair. Adult cardiologists must be alert to the potential long-term complications of these procedures.

Pulmonary Regurgitation and Right Ventricular Dilatation

Pulmonary regurgitation (PR) is invariably present post-operatively when the transannular patch approach is used to repair TOF. In the majority of patients, mild to moderate pulmonary regurgitation is well tolerated and does not typically require reintervention. Such patients typically have normal pulmonary vascular resistance and no pulmonary arterial obstruction. However, over-time, severe PR leads to right ventricular (RV) dilation and both systolic and diastolic RV dysfunction.

For this reason, surgical management has focused on both pulmonic valve preservation when possible and limiting the amount of pulmonary regurgitation. In one series (13), 100 patients with repaired TOF underwent cardiac magnetic resonance imaging (CMR) at a median of 20 years postsurgery. There was a significantly greater pulmonary regurgitation fraction in patients with transannular patch repair compared to those patients with pulmonary atresia and subsequent surgical RV to PA conduit. In addition, the degree of right ventricular enlargement was more pronounced in those patients with transannular patch repair, as the median RV end-diastolic volume index was 122 mL/m^2 compared to 106 mL/m^2 with RV to PA conduit (13).

Inadequate myocardial preservation during surgery and the degree of residual right ventricular outflow tract obstruction may contribute to RV decompensation into adulthood. In addition, RV dilatation can lead to significant tricuspid regurgitation and beget worsening right ventricular failure. With the development of both pulmonic regurgitation and tricuspid regurgitation, it is difficult to determine the exact etiology of right ventricular decompensation. In such patients, pulmonary valve replacement and/or tricuspid repair has been shown to improve symptoms and right heart function (14). However, it is crucial to avoid the effects of longstanding volume overload to the right ventricle as

this can lead to irreversible right ventricle dysfunction. As discussed later in this chapter, the proper timing of pulmonary valve replacement is crucial in the repaired TOF adult patient.

Atrial Arrhythmias

Although ventricular arrhythmias are more important contributors to the morbidity and mortality of repaired TOF patients (15), the importance of atrial arrhythmias cannot be underestimated. Atrial tachyarrhythmias such as atrial fibrillation and atrial flutter are common after repair of TOF, with one study suggesting prevalence as high as 34% (16). The pathophysiology of atrial arrhythmias is multifactorial and includes increased atrial size, valvular regurgitation (mainly pulmonary) and ventricular dysfunction. Although surgical techniques have recently been optimized with this in mind, atrial arrhythmias complicate both former and newer surgical strategies. Previous surgical incisions can lead to progressive myocardial fibrosis and provide the substrate for reentrant rhythms that underlie atrial tachycardia (17).

The development of atrial tachyarrhythmias is more common in patients who have had long lasting systemic to pulmonary artery central shunts and in those who required early reoperations for residual hemodynamic lesions. However, even in the repaired patients, atrial arrhythmias are not uncommon. In one study of 793 patients with repaired TOF, 29 patients had new onset atrial fibrillation or flutter over a ten year follow-up. Older age at repair, and moderate to severe tricuspid and/or pulmonic regurgitation were found to be specific predictors of sustained atrial arrhythmias (18).

The presence of atrial arrhythmias contributes significantly to morbidity. Symptoms such as palpitations, near-syncope, and reduced exercise capacity are not uncommon in patients who develop atrial arrhythmias (15). In one retrospective cohort study of 242 patients with repaired TOF (19), 29 patients had sustained episodes of atrial tachycardia. Baseline characteristics and clinical outcomes were studied in this group and were compared to the other 213 repaired TOF patients who were arrhythmia free. The patients with atrial tachycardia were more likely to develop palpitations associated with presyncope, dyspnea or fatigue. The development of atrial tachycardias was also associated with substantial morbidity including congestive heart failure, need for reoperation, subsequent ventricular tachycardia, stroke and even death (19). Event-free survival after repair was approximately 10 years less in patients with atrial tachycardias.

Ventricular Arrhythmias and Sudden Cardiac Death

Ventricular tachyarrhythmias, including nonsustained and sustained ventricular tachycardia, and associated sudden cardiac death can occur early after surgery as well as years after intracardiac TOF repair. Nonsustained ventricular tachycardia (NSVT) can be seen in up to 60% of TOF patients (6). However, the prognostic significance of ventricular premature contractions (VPCs) and their frequency is unclear. Cullen et al. followed TOF patients prospectively for twelve years and neither the presence of frequent VPCs (>30 per hour) nor NSVT were significant predictors of sudden death (20). In addition, a 10-year multicenter cohort study showed no correlation between NSVT and sudden cardiac death or the subsequent development of clinical ventricular tachycardia (18). Therefore, there is currently no evidence for the initiation of antiarrhythmic therapy to suppress VPCs or NSVT.

In contrast to NSVT, sustained monomorphic ventricular tachycardia is less common and occurs in about 4% to 5% of patients (19). Sudden cardiac death occurring from ventricular arrhythmias, and less frequently atrial arrhythmias, has an incidence of almost 6%. The QRS duration, older age at repair, and significant pulmonary regurgitation are important predictors of late complications.

The most common mechanism for ventricular arrhythmias is reentry and the arrhythmic focus is usually near the previous infundibulectomy and right ventricular outflow tract. In less than 20% of patients, the reentry focus may involve the body of the right ventricle. Right ventricular dilatation and RV stretch slows intraventricular conduction and creates an electromechanical substrate for reentrant rhythms. Impaired hemodynamics from significant pulmonary regurgitation are thought to be responsible for sustaining the ventricular tachycardia once initiated (21).

Clinical predictors of ventricular arrhythmias and sudden cardiac death are important to identify in order to risk-stratify patients These include but are not limited to: the coexistence of other congenital cardiac defects, late repair of undetected TOF (22), transannular patching predisposing to free pulmonary regurgitation (18), and repair via a right ventriculotomy

rather than an atriotomy (23). Right ventricular dilatation with or without pulmonary stenosis is commonly seen in patients with sustained ventricular tachycardias with moderate to severe pulmonic regurgitation, and is associated with an increased likelihood of sudden cardiac death (24,25). Therefore, thorough hemodynamic assessment of these patients is required upon presentation, and one can consider restoring pulmonic valve competency in order to reduce this risk. Interestingly, right ventricular hypertension in isolation has not been shown to be predictive of sudden cardiac death or sustained ventricular arrhythmias (18).

Electrocardiographic wave (QRS) duration also correlates with the size of the right ventricle and is predictive of the development of sustained ventricular arrhythmias and sudden cardiac death (21). Typically a right bundle branch pattern (RBBB) is present on the electrocardiogram (ECG) of patients with repaired TOF. RBBB initially develops from damage to the bundle during repair, but progressive lengthening of the QRS complex is also caused by right ventricular dilatation (26). There is great variability in the QRS duration in repaired TOF patients. Gatzoulis et al., observed the QRS durations ranging from 70 to 240 msec (mean of 151 msec). A QRS duration ≥180 msec is both a sensitive and specific marker for ventricular tachycardia and sudden cardiac death (18).

Echocardiographic parameters have also been studied in attempts to risk stratify patients. The most convincingly implicated echocardiographic findings are pulmonic regurgitation, right ventricular dilatation, right ventricular dysfunction, and left ventricular dysfunction. In a retrospective analysis of 125 patients, moderate to severe left ventricular dysfunction was significantly more common in patients with sudden cardiac death (42% versus 9%; $P \leq 0.01$) with a positive predictive value of 29% (27). Left ventricular dysfunction was a marker of severe right-sided dysfunction, a phenomenon referred to as ventricular-ventricular interdependence (13).

In the current era, invasive electrophysiological (EP) testing is useful for diagnosis and treatment of underlying arrhythmias. EP testing is performed frequently in TOF patients in order to risk-stratify for tachyarrhythmias. In a recent multicenter cohort study of 252 patients who underwent an EP study at a mean of 12 years after surgical repair, monomorphic ventricular tachycardia and polymorphic ventricular tachycardia were inducible in 30% and 4.4% of the patients, respectively. Patients with inducible ventricular tachycardia had a significantly increased risk of clinical ventricular tachycardia and sudden cardiac death, and the sensitivity and specificity of sustained ventricular tachycardia on EP testing for subsequent episodes of subsequent ventricular tachycardia or sudden cardiac death were 77% and 80%, respectively (28). Event-free survival rates in noninducible patients were significantly higher when compared to inducible patients.

Only limited data are available regarding the utility of implantable cardioverter-defibrillators (ICD) in patients with TOF. In one series of 121 high-risk patients with TOF followed over a four-year period postimplantation, 30% of patients received at least one appropriate and effective ICD discharge and five patients died of sudden cardiac death (29). A higher left ventricular end diastolic pressure and the presence nonsustained ventricular tachycardia independently predicted appropriate ICD shocks. However, inappropriate shocks occurred in 6% of patients annually and 36% of patients experienced complications. ICD therapy for TOF patients is not specifically addressed in the recent ACC/AHA guidelines. However, ICD implantation is usually an adjuvant therapy for secondary prevention of sustained ventricular tachycardia and sudden cardiac death, following restoration of the residual hemodynamic problems. ICD therapy should be considered for high-risk patients when ventricular dysfunction is present, and no target hemodynamic lesions for either catheter and/or surgical intervention are found (6,29).

■ CARDIAC IMAGING

Cardiac imaging has become the cornerstone in adult TOF management. During the third postoperative decade, mortality more than triples to 0.94% per year (30). As described below, close observation of the adult TOF patient by echocardiography and cardiac magnetic resonance imaging (CMR) to closely monitor the adult TOF patient is required. Echo provides valuable estimates of cardiac function and myocardial performance, while CMR quantifies pulmonary regurgitation (pulmonary regurgitant fraction), right and left ventricular volumes as well as ventricular dimensions, and mass and systolic ventricular function.

The importance of a comprehensive noninvasive evaluation combining these imaging modalities should

not be underestimated, since these tools are needed to determine clinical status as well as the proper timing for pulmonary valve replacement, a key issue in the proper management the adult TOF patient.

Echocardiography

Echocardiography has been used as the mainstay for imaging patients with congenital heart disease, mostly due to its ease of use and wide availability. Since many adult CHD patients may have pacemakers or defibrillators, echocardiography is presently the optimal imaging modality. However, because of the complex crescentic RV shape, there is no ideal geometric model to calculate RV volumes and derive accurate RVEF from standard views. However, Doppler-derived RV myocardial performance index (MPI) measurements correlate with MRI-derived RVEF, and offer a simple and reliable method for the evaluation of RVEF in adults with repaired TOF (31). The RV MPI in adult repaired TOF patients has been reported to be 0.21 ± 0.10 compared with the RV MPI in adults without cardiac disease of 0.28 ± 0.04. The decreased RV MPI in adult repaired TOF is not surprising since more than half of adult TOF patients have signs of restrictive physiology with high RV filling pressures, independent of RV systolic function (32). Similar to patients with left ventricular restriction, RV relaxation time is shortened.

Pulse Doppler tissue imaging (DTI) is a unique tool for measurement of the systolic and diastolic motion velocities of the tricuspid valve annulus with high spatial and temporal resolution, and is associated with RV function and performance. DTI evaluation of the lateral tricuspid annular motion has been correlated with RVEF in adult patients with heart failure (33), while DTI velocities have been associated with RV performance in congenital heart disease whether the RV supports the pulmonic or systemic circulation. Pulse DTI of the RV may be more sensitive than standard echocardiographic measurements for identifying patients with RV dysfunction. It has been well established that DTI indices of RV systolic and diastolic function correlate with radionuclide angiography measurements (34), and patients with repaired TOF have significantly lower RV DTI velocities when compared to control population (35).

Pulsed DTI of the RV is performed from the apical four-chamber view by placing a 5 mm sample volume at the tricuspid annulus (free wall). Peak myocardial velocities during systole (S′), early diastole (E′), atrial contraction (A′) and isovolumic contraction (IVV′), in addition to myocardial acceleration during isovolumic contraction (IVA′), are measured.

Apostolopoulou et al. (36) observed systolic and diastolic parameters derived from Doppler tissue imaging of tricuspid annular motion at rest and during dobutamine infusion as indices of RV function in adult repaired TOF patients. They concluded that DTI evaluation of the tricuspid annular motion with dP/dt and RV stroke volume index to BSA helps in assessing RV function.

DTI evaluation has been useful in characterizing adult repaired TOF patients' highly variable but mild to moderate impairment in exercise capacity. Salehian et al. (37) related DTI indices of RV function in TOF patients (Figure 9.2) to their exercise capacity as measured by maximal oxygen consumption (VO$_2$ max). They found that DTI peak RV systolic velocity obtained at the tricuspid valve annulus is an independent predictor of VO$_2$ max in adult patients with repaired TOF, and postulated that diminished RV DTI systolic velocities likely reflect RV systolic dysfunction and exercise capacity in these patients.

The combination of transthoracic 2-dimensional echocardiographic imaging, myocardial RV performance index (MPI), pulse Doppler tissue imaging (DTI) of the tricuspid valve annulus, and color Doppler and continuous Doppler of the pulmonary valve of the adult repaired TOF patient, provide an accurate assessment of RV systolic and diastolic function and degree of pulmonary regurgitation.

Cardiac MRI

Cardiac magnetic resonance imaging (CMR) is the gold standard in accurate assessing right ventricular size, function and degree of pulmonary regurgitation. CMR scans are performed most often today on a 1.5-T scanner using three plane localizing images; biventricular volume and function are assessed using a breath hold ECG gated steady state free precession sequence (FIESTA). Imaging is performed in the two and four chamber view planes followed by 12 contiguous short axis slices perpendicular to the long-axis of the ventricles extending from the plane of the atrioventricular valve to the apex. Left and right ventricular end-diastolic and end-systolic volumes, mass and ejection fraction are measured. The end-diastolic (RVEDVi, LVEDVi) and end-systolic

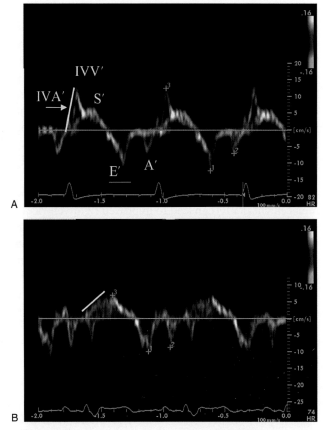

FIGURE 9.2 Doppler tissue imaging (DTI) recording from tricuspid annulus in control subject (A) and patient with repaired TOF (B) showing different parameters measured. A′, Late diastolic velocity (2); E′, early diastolic velocity (1); IVA′, acceleration during isovolumic contraction; IVV′, isovolumic contraction velocity; S′ (3), systolic velocity. (From Adult Congenital Echocardiography Laboratory, Weill Cornell Medical Center, 2008.)

volumes (RVESVi, LVESVi) and mass of the right and left ventricles (RV massi, LV massi) are indexed to body surface area. Gadolinium enhanced 3D (MRA) are performed in the sagittal or coronal planes.

Using such parameters, Tal Geva et al. (13) have demonstrated that moderate RV and LV systolic dysfunction is an important determinant of poor clinical status of long-term survivors of TOF repair. They showed that the combination of lower left ventricular ejection fraction (LVEF) and older age at TOF repair predicted a high sensitivity and a New York Heart Association (NYHA) functional class ≥III at a median of two decades after repair. The RV–LV interaction that is pivotal to understand the pathophysiology leading to clinical deterioration late after TOF repair, and demonstrated that the PR induced volume load leads to the ultimate failure of compensatory mechanisms with consequent biventricular dysfunction. Tal Geva et al. concluded that when using CMR to consider pulmonary valve replacement in an asymptomatic patient with repaired TOF, physicians should take into account not only the age of the TOF repair but also that all patients with RVESVi ≥95 mL/m² exhibited RV dysfunction, and all patients with LVESVi ≥50 mL/m² had LV systolic dysfunction. In addition, LVEF <50% or RVEF <35% predicts poor clinical status.

For the adult repaired TOF patient, pulmonary valve replacement (PVR) can lead to improved right ventricular (RV) volumes and function, improved functional status, stabilization of the QRS duration, and a reduction in both atrial and ventricular arrhythmias. However, the timing of PVR still remains controversial. In addition to RV and LV function, and degree of PR, CMR studies (38) have demonstrated that the presence of an akinetic or aneurysmal RV outflow tract wall segment diminishes RVEF late after TOF repair (Figure 9.3). RVOT aneurysm/akinesia, lack of systolic thickening, and inward motion of

the RVOT, are common in TOF patients regardless of whether they have undergone transannular patch repair, and they contribute to increased RV systolic volumes and decreased RVEF, irrespective of the degree of PR. Thus, other factors such as myectomy or infundibular resection and/or ischemic insult (due to coronal branch interruption) may be responsible for the formation of RVOT aneurysm/akinesia. (Figure 9.4) Therefore, measures to maintain or restore pulmonary valve function and to avoid RVOT aneurysm/akinesia are mandatory for preserving both RV and LV dysfunction late after TOF repair. Like echo, CMR also provides an estimate of RV systolic function as a powerful predictor of exercise capacity (40).

Sheehan et al. (39) have used three dimensional shape analysis to further analyze the RV in adult TOF patients. They observed that the RV undergoes a significant shape change and dilatation in repaired TOF patients: it broadens at the apex, bulges at the base, and widens in cross-section from crescentic to rectangular. The elevated eccentricity in such TOF patients

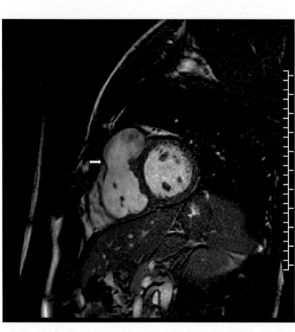

FIGURE 9.3 The right ventricular outflow tract (RVOT) after repair of TOF by CMR demonstrates RVOT aneurysms (arrow). Short axis images at end-diastole, at the RVOT level. Lack of systolic thickening and inward motion of the RVOT in a TOF patient with transannular patch repair is seen and RVOT akinesia. The PV is not seen. (From Weill Cornell Medical Center, 2008.)

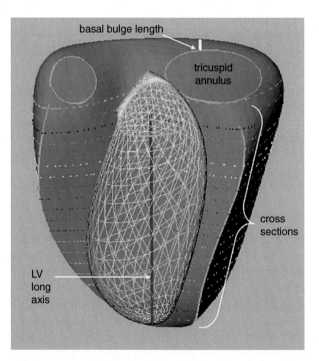

FIGURE 9.4 3-D CMR reconstruction of the RV. Twenty-one evenly spaced planes were constructed orthogonal to the long axis spanning the distance from the lowest point of the RV apex to the most apical point on the tricuspid annulus. The intersection of the RV surface with these planes produed 20 cross sections on which areas and perimeters were measured. Each area was normalized by the distance from the RV apex to tricuspid annulus. (From Ref. 39, with permission.)

corresponds to the septal flattening and free wall bulging seen in RV volume overload, and an "apex-forming right ventricle" is a well-known sign of RV overload. Such use of piecewise smooth subdivision surface 3-dimensional reconstruction gives a more accurate quantitative analysis of right ventricular shape to avoid underestimation of RV volume as seen by CMR without 3-dimensional reconstruction. The present study graphically confirms previous reports that abnormalities in RV shape may invalidate geometric models used to compute RV volume by 2-dimensional imaging. This study demonstrated that the right ventricle has greater than one pattern of remodeling its shape and perhaps all RV remodeling should be done using 3-dimensional.

There is broad consensus that the adult repaired TOF patient should be carefully followed by the two imaging modalities, echocardiography and CMR, and that multiple approaches should be made to maximize accurate assessment of RV end-diastolic and end-systolic size, RV systolic and diastolic function, presence of RVOT aneurysm/akinesia, degree of pulmonary regurgitation, and LVEF for ventricular-ventricular interaction. To this end, echocardiography offers pulse Doppler tissue imaging (DTI) with myocardial performance index (MPI). CMR with and without reconstruction offers accurate RV volumes and RVEF, and accurately determines the degree of pulmonary regurgitation by regurgitant fraction using phase contrast imaging and even using CMR 3-dimensional imaging. Together, echocardiography and CMR imaging provide an accurate assessment of cardiac structural function that can assist (along with cardiopulmonary exercise testing as described later in this chapter) in the timing of pulmonary valve replacement.

■ PULMONARY VALVE REPLACEMENT

Due to the increasing number of repaired adult TOF patients requiring an initial transannular patch in order to relieve outflow tract obstruction, significant right ventricular volume overload secondary PR is an increasingly common problem. Long-term effects of progressive RV volume overload can lead to the many complications discussed above: RV dysfunction, atrial and ventricular arrhythmias, and impaired exercise tolerance. The timing of pulmonary valve replacement (PVR) remains controversial. Whether all the consequences

of longstanding PR are reversible after intervention remains to be seen. However, beneficial effects of PVR can include improvement in functional class and exercise capacity, reduction of RV size (41), and a decrease in the QRS duration (42). Therrien et al. (42) showed that mean RV end-diastolic volume measured by CMR decreased significantly after PVR, but that mean global RVEF did not change significantly. In this study, no patients spontaneously remodeled to normal RV volume if operated on when RVEDV >170 mL/m² or RVESV >85 mL/m². Oosterhof et al. (43) observed similar RV volume effects; normalization of RV volumes tried to demonstrate the optimal time for PVR in adult repaired TOF patients. Normalization of RV volumes could be achieved when preoperative values are RVEDV <160 mL/m² or RVESV <82 mL/m². Therefore, these studies suggest RVEDV and RVESV values to guide PVR in the adult TOF patient (Figure 9.5).

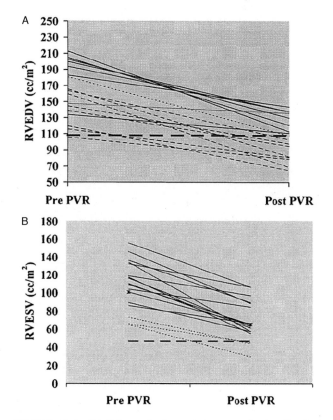

FIGURE 9.5 (A) This graph demonstrates normalization (hatched lines) of RV end-diastolic volume (RVEDV) in 9 of 17 patients (<108 mL/m²) post PVR. The solid lines demonstrate those who did not normalize. (B) This graph demonstrates normalization (hatched lines) of RV end-systolic volume (RVESV) in 3 of 17 patients (<47mL/m²) post PVR. The solid lines demonstrate those who did not normalize. (From Ref. 42, with permission.)

PVR in adults with moderate/severe pulmonary regurgitation after TOF repair can improve clinical outcomes without altering RVEF. Graham et al., (44) observed no surgical mortality with PVR and only 2% mortality within a year postoperation. At eleven years postoperation, approximately half of the prosthetic valves (mostly porcine) exhibited acceptable performance, and 59% of patients displayed improved ability in the Warnes-Somerville ability index. Importantly, this clinical improvement occurred in the setting of decreased RV size without improvement in RV systolic function. As in the two previous studies, RV size did decrease in the majority of patients, but the RV systolic function did not show consistent improvement. However, this study supports PVR

should be performed early to preserve systolic function. To further make our decision process for PVR more accurate, CMR and cardiopulmonary exercise testing (CPET) should be performed in all repaired adult TOF patients.

■ PERCUTANEOUS PULMONARY VALVE REPLACEMENT

Percutaneous pulmonary valve implantation (PPVI) was first introduced in the year 2000 as a nonsurgical treatment for patients with RV and RVOT dysfunction. PPVI can relieve both pulmonic stenosis (PS) and regurgitation (PR), and involves transcatheter placement of a

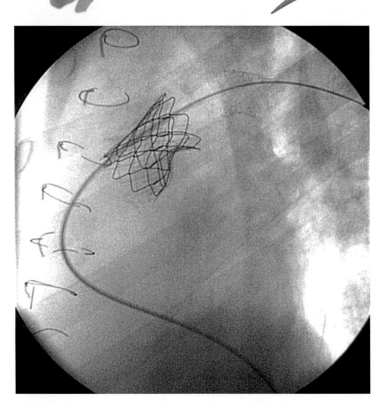

FIGURE 9.6 (A) Percutaneous pulmonary valve implantation device. (B) This fluoroscopy demonstrates proper PPVI at the level of the original pulmonary valve. (From Ref. 45, with permission.)

valved stent (Figure 9.6) within the existed degenerated valve or conduit and can be performed without cardiopulmonary bypass and without residual pulmonary regurgitation. In a recent publication in *Circulation* by Lurz et al. (45), 155 patients with either PS or PR underwent PPVI between September 2000 and February 2007 (Figure 9.6). In one series of pulmonic stenosis and PR patients with RV systolic pressures (RVSP) >2/3 systemic with symptoms, or RVSP >3/4 without symptoms, moderate or severe PR and symptoms; or patients with severe RV dysfunction or severe RV dilatation or impaired exercise tolerance <65% of predicted, as well as appropriately sized RVOT (between 14 × 14 mm to 22 × 22 mm), RV systolic pressure decreased significantly post PPVI (45) (Table 9.1). No patient had more than mild PR on angiography post-PPVI. The availability of this minimally invasive approach can facilitate decision making for the clinician who may have been hesitant to have early surgical valve replacement, and earlier intervention may prevent further RV dysfunction in adult TOF patients.

However, evaluation of RVOT morphology is necessary following the repair of congenital heart disease and has an important implication for PPVI patient selection to ensure device stability (46). The current available device is bovine-jugular venous valve sutured into a balloon-expandable platinum-iridium stent. It has an unexpanded length of 35 mm and can be deployed to a maximum diameter of 22 mm.

Schievano et al. (46) have used CMR with 3-dimensional reconstruction to describe five types of RVOT morphology in adult CHD patients. The type I morphology, a pyramidal shape occurred in 49% of the patients and was associated with the transannular patch repair; this type of morphology may be unsuitable for PPVI. Thus, CMR provides key anatomic information for the pre-PPVI evaluation. The development of larger devices and new device designs that permit downsizing of dilated outflow tracts to the size of biologically available valves is underway and will increase the number patients who are able to undergo PPVI.

■ OTHER TOF COMPLICATIONS REQUIRING INTERVENTIONS

In addition to PR, other complications in TOF patients can lead to the need for surgical reintervention. Although mild right ventricular outflow obstruction is well tolerated, significant obstruction may require a surgical revision in the adult patient. Residual pulmonary stenosis with right ventricular pressure two-thirds or greater than systemic pressure should warrant reintervention (3). Residual VSD, patent arterial shunts, significant aortic regurgitation associated with symptoms and/or progressive deterioration of left ventricular function, and progressive aortic root enlargement with aortic regurgitation should all be intervened upon early in the adult TOF patient. Residual right ventricular outflow tract obstruction, hypertrophy of subvalvular muscle, annular hypoplasia, pulmonary valve stenosis, or branch pulmonary artery stenosis can occur as a consequence of TOF repair and will warrant further surgical corrections (47).

■ CARDIOPULMONARY EXERCISE TESTING

In addition to ECG and arrhythmia assessment, and echocardiography and CMR, cardiopulmonary exercise testing (CPET) is valuable for risk stratification in the TOF patient. Approximately 50% of TOF patients will develop ventricular ectopy during exercise. Ventricular arrhythmias are more commonly induced during stress in those patients who are older at the time of their repair, and in those with the longest period of follow-up between repair and stress (48). In addition, a high right ventricular systolic pressure (>60 mm Hg) has also been shown to be associated with exercise-induced arrhythmias (49). However, a direct correlation between stress-induced ectopy and the risk of sudden cardiac death has not been shown (50).

In CPET, a reduced value of peak oxygen uptake (peak VO_2) during peak exercise and an enhanced ventilator response have been shown to be adverse prognostic markers. In a large cohort of adult patients with surgically repaired TOF, peak oxygen uptake (peak VO_2), the slope of ventilation per unit of carbon dioxide production (VCO_2), and New York Heart Association functional class (NYHA) were independent predictors of death and/or hospitalization. In addition, patients with peak VO_2 ≤36% of predicted and those with VE/VCO2 slope ≥39 were at greater risk for cardiac related death and cardiac hospitalizations (5 year mortality of 48% versus 0%, *P* <0.0001, and 31% versus 0%, *P* <0.0001), respectively (51). Echocardiographically

TABLE 9.1 RV systolic pressure and RVOT gradient after PPVI

Parameter	Total Population (n = 151)			Predominantly Stenosis (n = 61)			Predominantly Regurgitant (n = 46)			Combined Lesions (n = 44)		
	Pre	Post	P	Pre	Post	P	Pre	Post	P	Pre	Post	P
RV systolic pressure, mm Hg	63 ± 18	45 ± 13	<0.001	72 ± 16	46 ± 13	<0.001	48 ± 13	43 ± 12	0.002	62 ± 15	46 ± 12	<0.001
RV end diastolic pressure, mm Hg	12 ± 4	10 ± 5	<0.001	12 ± 4	9 ± 4	<0.001	11 ± 5	10 ± 5	0.016	11 ± 4	11 ± 5	0.507
PA systolic pressure, mm Hg	27 ± 11	29 ± 12	0.056	25 ± 11	26 ± 9	0.373	31 ± 10	31 ± 9	0.917	25 ± 9	29 ± 13	0.027
PA diastolic pressure, mm Hg	10 ± 4	14 ± 9	<0.001	10 ± 4	12 ± 4	0.003	11 ± 5	15 ± 6	<0.001	9 ± 4	13 ± 6	<0.001
RV-tp-PA gradient, mm Hg	37 ± 20	17 ± 10	<0.001	48 ± 18	19 ± 12	<0.001	20 ± 13	13 ± 9	<0.001	37 ± 18	17 ± 8	<0.001
Aortic systolic pressure, mm Hg	94 ± 15	101 ± 16	<0.001	95 ± 15	98 ± 14	0.004	94 ± 14	102 ± 16	0.002	94 ± 17	105 ± 17	0.001
Aortic diastolic pressure, mm Hg	54 ± 10	58 ± 10	<0.001	54 ± 9	57 ± 10	0.021	55 ± 9	58 ± 8	0.01	53 ± 11	59 ± 11	0.004
RV-to-systemic pressure, %	69 ± 19	45 ± 14	<0.001	81 ± 16	47 ± 12	<0.001	52 ± 15	42 ± 11	<0.001	67 ± 11	44 ± 15	<0.001

This table demonstrates RV systolic pressure and RVOT gradient after PPVI, as well as PA diastolic pressures. After successful valve implantation, RV systolic pressure (63 ± 18 to 45 ± 13 mm Hg, $P < 0.001$) and RVOT gradient (37 ± 20 to 17 ± 10 mm Hg, $P < 0.001$) fell significantly.

PA, pulmonary artery; RV, right ventricular; RVOT, right ventricular outflow tract.

Source: From Ref. 45, with permission.

assessed high right ventricular MPI and left ventricular MPI values, representing impaired ventricular function, are associated with diminished peak VO_2 (52).

■ PREGNANCY AND CONTRACEPTION

Pregnancy in the unoperated patient with TOF poses significant risk of maternal and fetal complications with a high mortality rate. This risk appears to be inversely proportional to the oxygen saturation with a significant increase in risk when the arterial oxygen saturation is less than 85%. Preexisting cyanosis can be exacerbated by increased right to left shunting as a result of hypotension and peripheral dilation that accompanies labor and delivery (6).

In the repaired patient, the risk of pregnancy is related directly to the hemodynamic status. In patients with relatively normal hemodynamics, the risk of complications from pregnancy is close to the general population. The increased volume load of pregnancy can lead to right heart failure and arrhythmias, especially in patients with either RVOT residual obstruction or significant pulmonary regurgitation. In one report, arrhythmias (the majority being supraventricular) and clinically significant right heart failure occurred in 6.4% and 2.4% of completed pregnancies, respectively. There were no cases of myocardial infarction, stroke, or cardiovascular mortality in this patient group (53). Veldtman et al. studied patients with repaired and unrepaired TOF. Pregnancy outcomes in women who had undergone intracardiac repair were generally similar to those in the general obstetric population. However, patients who had severe RV dilatation and/or RV dysfunction, RV outflow tract obstruction, and/or pulmonary hypertension were more likely to have significant cardiovascular complications. In addition, unrepaired TOF and morphologic pulmonary artery abnormality were independently predictive of infant birth rate (54).

Fertility is preserved in women with TOF and appears to be similar to that in age matched controls (55). It is recommended that all patients with TOF have cardiology counseling prior to conception and close follow-up during pregnancy. Approximately 15% of patients with TOF have the chromosome 22q11.2 microdeletion, and preconception genetic counseling is recommended. There are presently no guidelines for pregnancy termination in the unoperated TOF and each case should be individualized.

■ LONG-TERM SURVIVAL

Without surgical intervention, the majority of patients die in childhood. Survival rate is 66% at one year of age, 40% at three years of age, 11% at 20 years and 3% at 40 years of age (56). Morbidity in these patients is high and relates to progressive cyanosis, exercise intolerance, and atrial and ventricular arrhythmias. The few patients that survive into the fourth decade of life usually have profound congestive heart failure secondary to right ventricular hypertension.

Long-term survival in patients with TOF who undergo complete operative repair is excellent. Nollert and colleagues (30) reported 10-, 20-, and 30-year survival rates of about 97%, 94%, and 89%, respectively. Bertranou et al. (56) estimated survival was 92% at 10 years and 76% at 40 years. The major cause of death in these patients was sudden cardiac death. Heart failure and sudden cardiac death are the most common causes of death. Major risk factors for impaired survival included operation prior to 1970, preoperative polycythemia, and use of a right ventricular outflow patch (30). TOF patients with transient complete heart block that persisted beyond the third postoperative day have a lower long-term survival rate (56) and a less favorable long-term functional status.

■ CONCLUSION

Tetralogy of Fallot (TOF) is the most common cyanotic heart defect in infancy, and major advancements in the diagnosis and management of this disease have resulted in increasing numbers of patients surviving to adulthood. The vast majority of patients undergo corrective surgery within the first two years of life. Although the long-term outcome is relatively good, survival in adult repaired TOF patients is not the same as for age and sex-matched controls. Recent studies on large cohorts of survivors of TOF repair have shown that the risk of complications or death increases during the third postoperative decade since chronic pulmonic regurgitation can lead to right ventricular failure, as well as subsequent atrial and ventricular arrhythmias. Therefore, risk assessment of these patients by clinical parameters, electrocardiogram, echocardiogram, CPET, and CMR is essential. It is also imperative to identify TOF patients where surgical replacement of the pulmonic valve or percutaneous pulmonary valve implantation is feasible, although the optimal time for these procedures remains to be clearly defined.

■ REFERENCES

1. Moddie DS. Adult congenital heart disease. *Curr Opin Cardiol* 1994; 9,137–42.
2. Hoffman JI. Incidence of congenital heart disease: I. Postnatal incidence. *Pediat Cardiol* 1995; 16(3),103–13..
3. Perloff JK, Rosove MH, Sietsema KE, et al. Cyanotic Congenital Heart Disease: a multisystem disorder. In: Perloff JK, Childs JS, eds. *Congenital heart disease in adults* 2nd ed. Philadelphia: WB Sanders, 1998, 199–226.
4. Goldmuntz E, Clark BJ, Mitchell LE, et al. Frequency of 22q11 deletions in patients with conotruncal defects. *Pediat Cardiol* 1998; 32(2):492–8.
5. Acierno LJ. Etienne-Louis Fallot: is it his tetralogy? Profiles in Cardiology. *Clin Cardiol* 1999; 22:176–82.
6. Gatzoulis MA, Webb GD, Daubeney P. Tetralogy of Fallot. In: Gatzoulis MA, Webb GD, Daubeney PEF, eds. *Diagnosis and Management of adult congenital heart disease*. Churchill Livingstone, 2003, 315–27.
7. Rao BN, Anderson RC, Edwards JE. Anatomic variations in the tetrology of Fallot. *American Heart Journal* 1971; 81:361–71.
8. Dabizzi RP, Teodori G, Barletta GA, et al. Associated coronary and cardiac abnormalities in the tetrology of Fallot: an angiographic study. *Eur Heart J* 1990; 11:692–704.
9. Blalock A, Taussig HB. Surgical treatment of malformations of the heart. *American Journal of Medicine* 1945; 128(3):189–202.
10. Lillehei CW, Cohen M, Warden HE, et al. The direct vision intracardiac correction of congenital anomalies by controlled cross circulation; results in thirty-two patients with ventricular septal defects, tetralogy of fallot, and atrioventricularis communis defects. *Surgery* 1955; 38(1):11–29.
11. Reddy, VM, Liddicoat, JR, McElhinney DB, et al. Routine primary repair of tetralogy of Fallot in neonates and infants less than three months of age. *Ann Thorac Surg* 1995; 60(6 Suppl):S592–6.
12. Stewart RD, Backer CL, Young L, et al. Tetralogy of Fallot: results of a pulmonary valve sparing strategy. *Ann Thorac Surg* 2005; 80(4):1431–8.
13. Geva T, Sandweiss, BM, Gauvreau K, et al. Factors associated with impaired clinical status in long term survivors of tetralogyt of Fallot repair evaluated by magnetic resonance imaging. *J Am Coll Cardiol* 2004; 43(6):1068–74.
14. Gersony W, Rosenbaum M. *Tetralogy of Fallot. Congenital Heart Disease in the Adult*. NY: McGraw-Hill, 2002, 145–67.
15. Roos-Hesselink J, Perlroth MG, McGhie J, et al. Atrial arrhythmias in adults after repair of tetralogy of Fallot. *Circulation* 1995; 91:2214–9.
16. Meijboom F, Szatmari A, Deckers JW, et al. Cardiac status and health-related quality of life in the long term after surgical repair of tetralogy of Fallot in infancy and childhood. *J Thorac Cardiovasc Surg* 1955; 110:883–91.
17. Kalman JM, VanHare GF, Olgin JE, et al. Ablation of "incisional" reentrant atrial tachycardia complicating surgery for congenital heart disease. Use of entrainment to define a critical isthmus of conduction. *Circulation* 1996; 93:502–12.
18. Gatzoulis MA, Balaji S, Weber SA, et al. Risk factors for arrhythmia and sudden death in repaired tetralogy of Fallot: a multi-centre study. *Lancet* 2000; 356:975–81.
19. Harrison DA, Siu SC, Hussain F, et al. Sustained atrial arrhythmias in adults late after repair of tetralogy of Fallot. *Am J Cardiol* 2001; 87(5):584–8.
20. Cullen S, Celermajer DS, Franklin RC, et al. Prognostic significance of ventricular arrhythmia after repair of tetralogy of Fallot: a 12-year prospective study. *J Am Coll Cardiol* 1994; 23:1151–5.
21. Gatzoulis M, Till JA, Redington AN. Depolarisation-repolarisation inhomogeneity after repair of tetralogy of Fallot. *Circulation* 1997; 95:401–4.
22. Murphy JG, Gersh BJ, Mair DD, et al. Long-term outcome in patients undergoing surgical repair of tetralogy of Fallot. *N Engl J Med* 1993; 329:593–9.
23. Dietl CA, Cazzaniga ME, Dubner SJ, et al. Life-threatening arrhythmias and RV dysfunction after surgical repair of tetrology of Fallot. Comparison between transventricular and transatrial approaches. *Circulation* 1994; 90:II7–II12.
24. Harrison DA, Harris L, Siu SC, et al. Sustained ventricular tachycardia in adult patients late after repair of tetrology of Fallot. *J Am Coll Cardiol* 1997; 30:1368–73.
25. Garson A, Randall DC, Gillette PC. Prevention of sudden death after repair of tetrology of Fallot: treatment of ventricular arrhythmias. *J Am Coll Cardiol* 1985; 6:221–7.
26. Norgard G, Gatzoulid M, Moraes F, et al. The relationship between type of outflow tract repair and postoperative right ventricular diastolic physiology in tetralogy of Fallot: implications for long term outcome. *Circulation* 1996; 94:3276–81.
27. Ghai A, Silversides C, Harris L. Left ventricular dysfunction is a risk factor for sudden cardiac death in adults late after repair of tetrology of Fallot. *J Am Coll Cardiol* 2002; 40:1675–80.
28. Khairy P, Landzberg MJ, Gatzoulis MA, et al. Value of programmed ventricular stimulation after tetralogy of Fallot repair: a multicenter study. *Circulation* 2004; 109(16):1994–2000.
29. Khairy P, Harris L, Landzberg MJ, et al. Implantable cardioverter-defibrillators in tetralogy of Fallot. *Circulation* 2008; 117(3):363–70.
30. Nollert G, Fischlein T, Bouterwek S, et al. Long term survival in patients with repair of tetrology of Fallot: 36-year follow-up of 490 survivors of the first year after surgical repair. *J Am Coll Cardiol* 1997; 30(5):1374–83.
31. Schwerzmann M, Samman A, Salehian O, et al. Comparison of Echocardiographic and Cardiac Magnetic Resonance Imaging for Assessing Right Ventricular Function in Adults with Repaired Tetralogy of Fallot. *Am J Cardiol* 2007; 99:1593–7.

32. Gatzoulis MA, Clark AL, Cullen S, et al. Right ventricular diastolic function 15 to 35 years after repair of tetrology of Fallot. Restrictive physiology predicts superior exercise performance. *Circulation* 1995; 91(6):1775–81.

33. Meluzin J, Spinarova L, Bakala J, et al. Pulsed Doppler tissue imaging of the velocity of tricuspid annular systolic motion; a new, rapid, and non-invasive method of evaluating right ventricular systolic function. *Eur Heart J* 2001; 22(4):340–8.

34. Ueti OM, Camargo EE, Ueti AA, et al. Assessment of right ventricular function with Doppler echocardiographic indices derived from tricuspid annular motion:comparison with radionuclide angiography. *Heart* 2002; 88(3):244–8.

35. Brili S, Alexopoulos N, Latsios G, et al. *J Am Soc Echocardiog* 2005; 18(11):1149–54.

36. Apostolopoulou AC, Laskari CV, Tsoutsinos A, et al. Doppler tissue imaging evaluation of right ventricular function at rest and during dobutamine infusion in patients after the repair of tetrology of Fallot. *Int J Cardiovasc Imag* 2007; 23(1):25–31.

37. Salehian O, Burwash IG, Chan KL, et al. Tricuspid annular systolic velocity predicts maximal oxygen consumption during exercise in adult patients with repaired tetralogy of Fallot. *J Am Soc Echocardiog* 2008; 21(4):342–6.

38. Davlouros P, Kilner P, Hornung T, et al. Right ventricular function in adults with repaired tetrology of Fallot assessed with cardiovascular magnetic resonance imaging: Detrimental role of right ventricular outflow aneurysms or akinesia and adverse right-to-left ventricular interaction. *J Am Coll Cardiol* 2002; 40(11):2044–52.

39. Sheehan FH, GE S, Vick GW, et al. Three dimentional shape analysis of right ventricular remodeling in repaired tetrology of Fallot. *Am J Cardiol* 2008; 101(1):107–13.

40. Meadows J, Powell AJ, Geva T, et al. Cardiac magnetic resonance imaging correlates of exercise capacity in patients with surgically repaired tetrology of Fallot. *Am J Cardiol* 2007; 100(9):1446–50.

41. Vliegen HW, van Straten A, de Roos A. Magnetic resonance imaging to assess the hemodynamic effects of pulmonary valve replacement in adults late after repair of tetrology of Fallot. *Circulation* 2002; 106(13):1703–7.

42. Therrien J, Provost Y, Merchant N, et al. Optimal timing for pulmonary valve replacement in adults after tetralogy of Fallot repair. *Am J Cardiol* 2005; 95:779–82.

43. Oosterhof T, van Straten A, Vliegen HW, et al. Preoperative thresholds for pulmonary valve replacement in patients with corrected tetralogy of Fallot using cardiovascular magnetic resonance. *Circulation* 2007; 116:545–51.

44. Graham TP, Bernard Y, Arbogast P, et al. Outcome of pulmonary valve replacements in adults after tetralogy repair: a multi-institutional study. *Congenit Heart Dis* 2008; 3(3):162–7.

45. Lurz P, Coats L, Khambadkone S, et al. Percutaneous pulmonary valve implantation: impact of evolving technology and learning curve on clinical outcome. *Circulation* 2008; 117:1964–72.

46. Schievano S, Coats L, Migliavacca F, et al. Variations in right ventricular outflow tract morphology following repair of congenital heart disease: implications for percutaneous pulmonary valve implantation. *J Cardiovasc Magn Reson* 2007; 9:687–95.

47. Hennein HA, Mosca RS, Urcelay G, et al. Intermediate results after complete repair of tetralogy of Fallot in neonates. *J Thor Cardiovasc Surg* 1995; 109(2):332–42.

48. Wessel H, Paul M. Exercise studies in tetralogy of Fallot: a review. *Pediat Cardiol* 1999; 20:39–47.

49. Garson A, Gillette P, Gutgesell H, et al. Stress induced ventricular arrhythmias after repair of tetralogy of Fallot. *Am J Cardiol* 1980; 46:1006–12.

50. Steeds RP, Oakley D. Predicting late sudden death from ventricular arrhythmia in adults following surgical repair of tetralogy of Fallot. *QJ Medicine* 2004; 97:7–13.

51. Giardini A, Specchia A, Tacy T. Usefulness of cardiopulmonary exercise to predict long-term prognosis in adults with repaired tetralogy of Fallot. *Am J Cardiol* 2007; 99:1462–7.

52. Samman A, Schwerzmann M, Balint OH. Exercise capacity and biventricular function in adult patients with repaired tetralogy of Fallot. *Am Heart J* 2008; 156:100–5.

53. Drenthen W, Pieper P, Hesselink R. Outcome of pregnancy in women with congenital heart disease. *Journal of the American College of Cardiology* 2007; 49:2304–11.

54. Veldtman GR, Connolly HM, Grogan M, et al. Outcomes of pregnancy in women with tetralogy of Fallot. *Journal of the American College of Cardiology* 2004; 44(1):174–80.

55. Engelfriet P, Boersma E, Oechslin E, et al. The spectrum of adult congenital heart disease in Europe: morbidity and mortality in a five year follow-up period. *Eur Heart J* 2005; 26(21):2325–33.

56. Bertranou EG, Blackstone EH, Hazelrig JB, et al. Life expectancy without surgery in tetralogy of Fallot. *Am J Cardiol* 1978; 43(3):458–66.

Index

AAA. *See* Abdominal aortic aneurysm (AAA)

ABCD trial. *See* Appropriate Blood Pressure Control in Diabetes (ABCD) trial

Abdominal aortic aneurysm (AAA), 106–107
  ultrasound for, 111

ABI. *See* Ankle-brachial index (ABI)

Abnormal repolarization, 51, 52, 56, 57, 58, 63

ACCORD. *See* Action to Control Cardiovascular Risk in Diabetes (ACCORD)

ACCURACY trial, for evaluating diagnostic test performance of CCTA, 8–9

ACS. *See* Acute coronary syndrome (ACS)

Action in Diabetes and Vascular Disease Study (ADVANCE), 75, 77

Action to Control Cardiovascular Risk in Diabetes (ACCORD), 75, 77

Acute coronary syndrome (ACS), 20, 59, 70
  diagnosis of, 9–10
  plaques associated with, 12

Acute mesenteric ischemia, 109, 110

ADVANCE. *See* Action in Diabetes and Vascular Disease Study (ADVANCE)

Advanced glycation end products (AGEs), 75, 82

Albuminuria, 75, 82

Amaurosis fugax, 102

Anatomic and functional imaging
  clinical applications, 21
  imaging concepts, 20–21

Anatomic coronary artery, CCTA technology for evaluating, 1–2

Angina, 11, 13, 15, 37, 42, 59

Angiotensin-converting enzyme (ACE) inhibitor, 75

Anithrombotic prophylaxis, 123

Ankle-brachial index (ABI), 89, 90
  indications for measurement, 93
  limitations of, 93–94
  measurement technique, 91
  prognostic utility of, 91–93

Antibiotic prophylaxis, 146

Anticoagulation therapy, 119, 125

Antihypertensive therapy, 61, 64

Antihypertensive treatment, 63

Anti-inflammatory drugs, 147

Antiphospholipid antibodies, 141, 146

Antiphospholipid antibody syndrome, 146, 147, 148

Antiplatelet therapy, 119, 125, 129, 130

Antithrombotic therapy, 29, 123, 125
  for primary stroke prevention, 131, 132

Aortic atheroma, 124, 125

Aortic atherosclerosis, 14

Aortic valve sclerosis, 130–131

Aortoiliac stenosis, 95

Apex-forming right ventricle, 161

Apoptotic endothelial cells, 143

Appropriate Blood Pressure Control in Diabetes (ABCD) trial, 75

Arrhythmias and conduction system disease, 147

Arterial duplex ultrasound
  abdominal aortic aneurysm, 106–107
  carotid duplex ultrasonography, 102–105
  carotid ultrasound and cardiovascular risk assessment, 105–106
  color Doppler, 100–101
  Doppler ultrasound, 97
  grayscale imaging, 99–100
  hemodynamics of blood flow, 96–97

mesenteric artery disease, 109–111
peripheral arterial ultrasonography, 101–102
renal artery duplex ultrasonography, 107–109
spectral Doppler analysis, 97–99

Arterial occlusive disease, 90, 96

Arterial stiffness, 144

Arterial thrombosis, 77

Arteriography, for evaluating patients with acute mesenteric ischemia, 110

ASA. *See* Atrial septal aneurysm (ASA)

ASD. *See* Atrial septal defect (ASD)

Aspirin, 78, 125, 130

Atherosclerosis, 102, 105, 107

Atherosclerotic occlusive disease, 89

Atherosclerotic plaque, 1

Atherothrombotic strokes, 117

Atrial arrhythmias, 156–157

Atrial fibrillation (AF), 59, 61, 117, 119

Atrial flutter, 120, 121

Atrial septal aneurysm (ASA), 127–128

Atrial septal defect (ASD), 154

Atrial tachyarrhythmias, 156

AUC. *See* Area under the receiver-operating curve (AUC)

Autonomic neuropathy, 72

BARI. *See* Bypass Angioplasty Revascularization Investigation (BARI)

Bayesian analysis, Diamond–Forrester model of, 7

Beta-blockers, 27, 39

Beyond obstructive *vs.* nonobstructive stenosis
  for identification of individuals with ischemia, 11

[Beyond obstructive *vs.*
nonobstructive stenosis]
for risk stratification, 11–12
Bioprosthetic heart valves, 123
"Black blood" imaging, 20
B-mode ultrasound, 105
Body habitus, 55
Brachiocephalic artery, 104
Bronx Longitudinal Aging Study, 59
Bruce protocol, 38, 42
Bypass Angioplasty Revascularization
Investigation (BARI), 78, 79

CABG. *See* Coronary artery bypass
graft surgery (CABG)
CAD. *See* Coronary artery disease
(CAD)
Calcific coronary atherosclerosis, 10
Calcium channel blocking drugs, 39
Candesartan in Heart Failure:
Assessment of Reduction in
Mortality and Morbidity
(CHARM), 59
Cardiac arrhythmias, 2, 149
Cardiac autotransplation, for treating
difficult tumors, 123
Cardiac death, ventricular
arrhythmias and, 157–158
Cardiac embolism, 117
Cardiac imaging
cardiac MRI, 159–161
echocardiography, 158–159
Cardiac magnetic resonance
(CMR), 156
in adult TOF management, 158
anatomic and functional imaging
clinical applications, 21
imaging concepts, 20–21
cardiac flow imaging
clinical applications, 22
imaging concepts, 21–22
emerging concepts for applications
of, 27–28
for post-MI risk stratification,
28–29
imaging principles of, 19–20
myocardial perfusion imaging
clinical applications, 22–23
imaging concepts, 22
pulse sequences for localizing
protons, 19
tissue characterization using, 20,
23–27

Cardiac MRI, 159–161
Cardiac myxomas. *See* Myxomas
Cardiac tumors
metastatic, 123
myxomas, 121–122
other benign cardiac tumors, 122
papillary fibroelastoma, 122
primary malignant tumors,
122–123
Cardioembolic strokes, diagnosis
of, 117
Cardiomyopathy, 80–81
left ventricular function, 81–82
left ventricular hypertrophy, 81
potential mechanisms, 82
Cardiopulmonary exercise testing
(CPET), 162, 163–165
Cardiovascular disease (CVD), 105
age-adjusted rates of, 69
Cardiovascular mortality, 29, 56, 89,
91, 92, 93
CARE trial. *See* Cholesterol and
Recurrent Events (CARE) trial
Carney Complex, 121, 122
Carotid artery stenosis, 102
Doppler criteria for, 103
Carotid duplex ultrasonography,
102–105
Carotid intima-media thickness
(C-IMT), 105
Carotid plaque, 105
CCA. *See* Common carotid artery
(CCA)
CCTA. *See* Coronary computed
tomographic angiography
(CCTA)
Celiac artery (CA), 107, 108, 110
Cell metabolism, 40
Cellular necrosis, 24
Cerebrovascular disease, 79–80
CHARM. *See* Candesartan in
Heart Failure: Assessment of
Reduction in Mortality and
Morbidity (CHARM)
CHD. *See* Congenital heart disease
(CHD)
Chemotherapy, for treatment of
lymphomas, 123
Chest pain syndromes, 15, 16
Chiari network, 127, 128
Cholesterol and Recurrent Events
(CARE) trial, 73
Chronic mesenteric ischemia, 109
C-IMT. *See* Carotid intima-media
thickness (C-IMT)

Clopidogrel, 130
CMR. *See* Cardiac magnetic
resonance (CMR)
Common carotid artery (CCA), 102
Comorbid disease, 62
"Complex" aortic atheromas (CAA),
clinical significance of, 124
Computed tomography (CT), 1, 21
Computerized tomographic
angiography (CTA), 90, 102
Congenital heart disease (CHD)
cardiac imaging, 158–161
cardiovascular care of adult patients
with, 153
diagnosis and management of, 153
long-term survival in patients with
TOF, 165
palliative surgery and surgical
repair, 155
percutaneous pulmonary valve
replacement, 162–163
pregnancy and contraception, 165
pulmonary valve replacement,
161–162
tetralogy of Fallot
anatomic features of, 153–154
complications following, 156–158
CORAL trial, 111
CORE 64 trial, for evaluating
diagnostic test performance of
CCTA, 8–9
Cornell voltage, 52, 59
Coronary artery bypass graft patency,
CCTA for evaluation of, 10
Coronary artery bypass graft surgery
(CABG), 78
Coronary artery disease (CAD), 1, 38,
69–70
management in diabetic patients, 78
Coronary artery stenosis, 8, 9, 11
Coronary artery stents, CCTA for
evaluation of, 10
Coronary atherosclerosis, 71
Coronary atherosclerotic lesions, 72
Coronary computed tomographic
angiography (CCTA)
ACCURACY and CORE 64 trial
for evaluating diagnostic test
performance of, 8–9
cost considerations for adoption of,
14–15
current indications and
appropriateness criteria for,
15–16
diagnostic accuracy of

[Coronary computed tomographic angiography (CCTA)]
  for acute coronary syndrome, 9–10
  for detecting and excluding obstructive coronary artery stenosis, 7–9
  for evaluation of coronary artery bypass graft patency, 10
  for evaluation of coronary artery stents, 10
  for intraluminal stenosis to detect perfusion defects, 9
  for evaluating coronary artery, 1–2, 5
  future directions of, 16
  methods of evaluation by, 4
  noninvasive method of plaque characterization by, 12–13
  practice of, 2–5
  predictive values of, 9
  prognostic value of
    for all-cause mortality, 13
    noncoronary findings by CCTA, 14
    plaque composition, 14
    plaque severity for adverse events, 13–14
    warranty period of normal CCTA, 14
  radiation considerations for, 15
  temporal resolution of, 2
Coronary heart disease (CHD), 71
  Kaplan–Meier plot of, 38
  MRFIT trial for, 43
Coronary revascularization, 44
Corticosteroid therapy, 141
Cox proportional hazards model, 43
Cox regression analysis, 62
CPET. See Cardiopulmonary exercise testing (CPET)
C-reactive protein, 144
Cryptogenic brain embolism, 129
Cryptogenic stroke, 126
CT. See Computed tomography (CT)
CTA. See Computerized tomographic angiography (CTA)
CVD. See Cardiovascular disease (CVD)

DCCT. See Diabetes Control and Complications Trial (DCCT)
Delayed enhancement CMR (DE-CMR)

  for post-MI risk stratification
    clinical applications, 29
    current evidence, 28–29
  for post-MI thrombus assessment
    clinical applications, 31
    current evidence, 29–31
    thrombus imaging, 29, 30
Detection of Ischemia in Asymptomatic Diabetics (DIAD-2), 72
Diabetes Control and Complications Trial (DCCT), 77
Diabetes mellitus (DM)
  cardiomyopathy, 80–81
    left ventricular function, 81–82
    left ventricular hypertrophy, 81
    potential mechanisms, 82
  cerebrovascular disease, 79–80
  coronary artery disease, 69–70
    management of, 78
    myocardial infarction, 70–71
    silent ischemia, 71–72
  pathophysiology/risk factors, 72–73
    cigarette smoking, obesity, and physical activity, 78
    coronary revascularization, 78–79
    dyslipidemia, 73–74
    hyperglycemia, 75–78
    hypertension, 74–75
    management of CAD, 78
    procoagulant state, 78
Diabetic cardiomyopathy, 81
Diabetic heart muscle disease, 70
Diabetic patients, 64–65
Diamond–Forrester model, of Bayesian analysis, 7
Diastolic dysfunction, 82
Digital subtraction aortogram (DSA), 107
Diltiazem Reinfarction Study Group, 59
Dipyridamole, 130
DM. See Diabetes mellitus (DM)
Doppler echocardiography, 146
Doppler tissue imaging (DTI), 158, 159, 161
Doppler ultrasound, 97
Doppler velocity waveform, 98
Double-outlet right ventricle (DORV), 154
Drug therapy, for LDL cholesterol reduction, 74
DSA. See Digital subtraction aortogram (DSA)

DTI. See Doppler tissue imaging (DTI)
Duke coronary artery jeopardy score, 11, 13
Duplex ultrasonography, 89
Duplex ultrasound surveillance, studies of grafts, 102
Dyslipidemia, 72, 73

EAST. See Emory Angioplasty Versus Surgery Trial (EAST)
EBCTA. See Electron beam computed tomographic angiography (EBCTA)
ECA. See External carotid artery (ECA)
ECG. See Exercise electrocardiography (ECG)
ECG strain
  development of, 63
  as predictor of CV mortality, 57
  prognostic value of, 57
Echocardiographic LV mass index, 63
Echocardiography, 21, 123, 126, 158–159
EDV. See End diastolic velocity (EDV)
Electrocardiographic LVH, 61
Electro-cardio-graphic wave, 157
Electrocardiography, evaluation of, 37
Electron beam computed tomographic angiography (EBCTA), 14
Emory Angioplasty Versus Surgery Trial (EAST), 79
End diastolic velocity (EDV), 97
Endocardial blood flow, 40
Endothelial dysfunction, 145
Eustachian valve, 125, 127, 128
Exercise electrocardiography (ECG)
  chronotropic response, 38–39
  detection of LVH
    additional factors affecting, 54–55
    characteristic ECG manifestations of LVH, 51–53
    Cornell voltage criteria for, 53
    criteria for identification of LVH for, 53
    multivariate analyses to improve accuracy of, 54
    and performance of voltage criteria, 53
    Perugia score and Cornell/strain index, 54

[Exercise electrocardiography (ECG)]
  prognostic implications for, 55–58
  signal averaged electrocardiography for, 54
  fundamental principles of, 37
  for identification of coronary obstruction, 38
  for identification of myocardial ischemia, 37
  LVH and CV morbidity
    atrial fibrillation, 59
    heart failure, 58–59
    stroke, 58
    sudden death, 59
  LVH in selected populations
    older patients, 59–60
    patients with acute MI/unstable angina, 59
    patients with heart failure, 59
  ST segment depression response to, 39
    anatomic and physiologic bases of, 40
    heart rate adjustment, 40–41
    regression-based ST segment/heart rate slope, 42
    ST segment/heart rate index, 42–43
Exercise-induced ischemia, 37
External carotid artery (ECA), 102

FACET. See Fosinopril versus Amlodipine Cardiovascular Events Randomized Trial (FACET)
Familial syndrome, 121
Fenofibrate Intervention and Event Lowering in Diabetes (FIELD), 73
FFR. See Fractional flow reserve (FFR)
Fibromas, 122
Fibromuscular dysplasia (FMD), 102, 107, 117
FIELD. See Fenofibrate Intervention and Event Lowering in Diabetes (FIELD)
FMD. See Fibromuscular dysplasia (FMD)
Fosinopril versus Amlodipine Cardiovascular Events Randomized Trial (FACET), 75

Fractional flow reserve (FFR), 11
Framingham cohort, 58
Framingham criteria, 52
Framingham Offspring Study, 38

Gene transfer, 21
Global Utilization of Strategies to Open Occluded Arteries (GUSTO) IV ACS trial, 59
Glucose intolerance, 72
Glucose metabolism, 74, 81
Gortex graft, 155
Gradient echo-echo planar hybrid, 22
Gradient echo (GRE), 22
Granular-cell tumors, 121
Grayscale imaging, 99–100
GRE. See Gradient echo (GRE)
Gubner–Ungerleider voltage criteria, 53
GUSTO IV ACS trial. See Global Utilization of Strategies to Open Occluded Arteries (GUSTO) IV ACS trial

Hazard ratio (HR), 13, 14, 74
HDL. See High-density lipoprotein (HDL)
HDL cholesterol. See High-density lipoprotein (HDL) cholesterol
Heart Outcomes Prevention Evaluation trial (HOPE), 55–56, 58, 60, 61, 75
Heart rate
  adjustment in postexercise recovery period
    quantitative rate-recovery loops, 46
    simple rate-recovery loop, 45
  recovery in postexercise period, 43–45
Heart rate recovery (HRR), 43–45
Heart tumors. See Cardiac tumors
Heart valves, mechanical and bioprosthetic, 123
High-density lipoprotein (HDL), 143
High-density lipoprotein (HDL) cholesterol, 39, 73
Histopathology, 23, 24, 25
HOPE. See Heart Outcomes Prevention Evaluation trial (HOPE)

HOT. See Hypertension Optimal Treatment (HOT)
HR. See Hazard ratio (HR)
HRR. See Heart rate recovery (HRR)
Hydrogen protons, 19
Hyperglycemia, 75–78
Hyperinsulinemia, 72
Hyperkalemia, 75
Hypertension, 74, 82, 120
Hypertension Detection and Follow-Up Program, 60
Hypertension Optimal Treatment (HOT), 74

ICA. See Internal carotid artery (ICA)
ICD. See Implantable cardioverter-defibrillators (ICD)
IMA. See Inferior mesenteric arteries (IMA)
Implantable cardioverter-defibrillators (ICD), 158
IMT. See Intima-media thickness (IMT)
Infective endocarditis, 123. See also Noninfective endocarditis
Inferior mesenteric arteries (IMA), 110
Inferior vena cava, 125
In-stent restenosis, 10
Interleukin-6, 144
Internal carotid artery (ICA), 98
Intima-media thickness (IMT), 105
Intracoronary vascular ultrasound (IVUS), 11, 12
Intraluminal stenosis, 9
Intravascular ultrasound, 3
Intravenous beta blockers, 2
Invasive angiograms, 9
Invasive coronary angiography, 2, 6
  anatomic evaluation by, 13
Ischemia
  beyond obstructive vs. nonobstructive stenosis for identification of, 11
  and detection of coronary atherosclerosis, 9
  methods for provoking, 37
  in patients with coronary artery disease, 38
Ischemic heart disease, 63, 69

Ischemic strokes, 79
  classification of, 117
  clinical relevance of PFO to, 126
  medical management for prevention
    of, 129
IVUS. *See* Intracoronary vascular
    ultrasound (IVUS)

Left ventricular ejection fraction
    (LVEF), 159
Left ventricular hypertrophy (LVH),
    51, 70, 81
  common electrocardiogram criteria
    for identifying, 52
  ECG detection of
    additional factors affecting,
      54–55
    characteristic ECG
      manifestations of LVH, 51–53
    Cornell voltage criteria for, 53
    criteria for identification, 53
    multivariate analyses to improve
      accuracy of, 54
    performance of voltage criteria,
      53–54
    Perugia score and Cornell/strain
      index, 54
    prognostic implications and, 55–58
    signal averaged
      electrocardiography, 54
  regression of ECG
    antihypertensive therapy, 60
    for improving outcome, 61–64
    special considerations for, 64–65
Libman–Sacks lesions, 141, 146
Lifetime attributable risk (LAR), of
    cancer incidence, 15
LIFE trial. *See* Losartan Intervention
    for Reduction in Endpoints
    (LIFE) trial
Long-term survival, in patients with
    TOF, 165
Losartan-based therapy, 61
Losartan Intervention for Reduction in
    Endpoints (LIFE) trial, 57, 60
Low-density lipoprotein (LDL), 143
Low-density lipoprotein (LDL)
    cholesterol, 73
Lown's arrhythmia score, 59
Lumenography, 11
Luminal stenosis, 3
Lupus nephritis, 141
Lupus pericarditis, 147

LVEF. *See* Left ventricular ejection
    fraction (LVEF)
LVH. *See* Left ventricular
    hypertrophy (LVH)
LV mass index (LVMI), 52
LV strain pattern, 51
Lymphangiomas, 121
Lymphomas, 123

MAC. *See* Mitral annular calcification
    (MAC)
MACE. *See* Major adverse cardiac
    events (MACE)
Magnetic resonance angiography
    (MRA), 90
Magnetic resonance imaging (MRI),
    119, 159
  advantages of, 125
Major adverse cardiac events
    (MACE), 13, 14
Mechanical heart valves, 123
Medicare category III transaction
    codes, 15
Mesenchymal cells, 121
Mesenteric artery disease,
    109–111
Metabolic syndrome, 78
Metastatic tumors, 123
MI. *See* Myocardial infarction (MI)
Microvascular obstruction (MVO),
    25, 27
Minnesota code, 52, 60
Mitral annular calcification
    (MAC), 130
Mitral valve prolapse (MVP), 130
MPI. *See* Myocardial performance
    index (MPI)
MPS. *See* Myocardial perfusion
    scintigraphy (MPS)
MRA. *See* Magnetic resonance
    angiography (MRA)
MRFIT. *See* Multiple Risk Factor
    Intervention Trial (MRFIT)
MRI. *See* Magnetic resonance
    imaging (MRI)
Multiple Risk Factor Intervention
    Trial (MRFIT), 43,
    60, 73
Muscle cells, 77
MVO. *See* Microvascular obstruction
    (MVO)
MVP. *See* Mitral valve prolapse
    (MVP)

Myocardial disease
  abnormalities of left ventricular
    structure and function, 145–146
  myocarditis, 145
Myocardial infarction (MI), 20, 63
Myocardial ischemia, 11, 22, 71
  exercise electrocardiography for
    identification of, 37
Myocardial oxygen demand, 38, 40
Myocardial performance index (MPI),
    158, 161
Myocardial perfusion imaging
  clinical applications, 22–23
  imaging concepts, 22
Myocardial perfusion scintigraphy
    (MPS), 9, 15
Myocarditis, 145
Myxomas, 121–122

National Cholesterol Education
    Program (Adult Treatment
    Panel III) guidelines, 74
Neurofibromas, 121
Neuropeptide Y, 46
Nicotinic acid, 74
Nonbacterial thrombotic (marantic)
    endocarditis, 123
Noncardioembolic stroke, 130. *See
    also* Stroke
Noncoronary cardiac anatomy, 3
Noninfective endocarditis, 123. *See
    also* Infective endocarditis
Noninvasive imaging test, usefulness
    of, 5–7
Nonischemic cardiomyopathy, 30
Nonsustained ventricular tachycardia
    (NSVT), 59, 157
Norepinephrine, 46
NSVT. *See* Nonsustained ventricular
    tachycardia (NSVT)
Nyquist limit, 100

Obstructive coronary artery disease, 39
Obstructive coronary stenoses, 1
Oral beta blockers, 2

Painless ischemia, 72
Palliative surgery, and surgical
    repair, 155

Papillary fibroelastomas, 122, 131
Patent Foramen Ovale in Cryptogenic Stroke Study (PICSS), 128, 132
Patent foramen ovale (PFO), 125–127, 128–129
Patients
    with acute MI/unstable angina, 59
    with cryptogenic stroke, 126
    with heart failure, 59
    with ischemic limb symptoms, 90
Peak systolic velocity (PSV), 98, 108
Percutaneous coronary angioplasty (PTCA), 78
Percutaneous pulmonary valve implantation (PPVI), 162
Percutaneous transluminal angioplasty (PTA), 101
Pericardial disease, 147
Peripheral arterial disease (PAD)
    ankle-brachial index for diagnosis of
        indications for measurement, 93
        limitations of, 93–94
        measurement technique, 91
        prognostic utility of, 91–93
    arterial duplex ultrasound
        abdominal aortic aneurysm, 106–107
        carotid duplex ultrasonography, 102–105
        carotid ultrasound and cardiovascular risk assessment, 105–106
        color Doppler, 100–101
        Doppler ultrasound, 97
        gray scale imaging, 99–100
        hemodynamics of blood flow, 96–97
        mesenteric artery disease, 109–111
        peripheral arterial ultrasonography, 101–102
        renal artery duplex ultrasonography, 107–109
        spectral Doppler analysis, 97–99
    lower extremity, 89–90
    physiologic testing for
        peripheral arterial ultrasonography, 101–102
        pulse volume recordings, 95
        segmental pressure measurements, 94–95
        toe-brachial index, 95
        treadmill exercise testing, 95–96
Peripheral arterial ultrasonography, 101–102
Perugia index, 52, 54

Perugia score, 58
PFO. *See* Patent foramen ovale (PFO)
Phase velocity encoded imaging, 22
"Phase velocity encoded" pulse sequences, 21–22
Phospholipid-binding proteins, 148
PICSS. *See* Patent Foramen Ovale in Cryptogenic Stroke Study (PICSS)
Plaque
    characteristics in stable and unstable coronary syndromes, 12–13
    composition, 12
    obstructive coronary artery, 40
    remodeling, 12
    severity for adverse events, 13–14
    volume, 12
PPVI. *See* Percutaneous pulmonary valve implantation (PPVI)
Prednisone therapy, 143
Pregnancy, and contraception, 165
Prospective Pioglitazone Clinical Trial in Macro Vascular Events (PROACTIVE), 77
Prosthetic valves, 123–124
PSV. *See* Peak systolic velocity (PSV)
PTA. *See* Percutaneous transluminal angioplasty (PTA)
PTCA. *See* Percutaneous coronary angioplasty (PTCA)
Pulmonary arteriovenous malformations, 129
Pulmonary hypertension, 147–148
Pulmonary regurgitation (PR), 156
Pulmonary valve replacement (PVR), 160, 161–162
Pulse volume recordings (PVRs), 95

QCA. *See* Quantitative coronary angiography (QCA)
QRS complex voltage amplitude, 51
QRS prolongation, and delayed ventricular activation, 51–53
Quantitative coronary angiography (QCA), 9

Radiation dose, 15
Radionuclide angiography, 158
RAS. *See* Renin-angiotensin system (RAS)

Receiver operating characteristics (ROC) analysis, 28
Refractory hypertension, 107
Renal artery
    duplex ultrasonography, 107–109
    resistive index, 109
    revascularization, 109
    stenosis, 111
        clinical predictors of, 107
Renal parenchymal disease, 109
Renin-angiotensin-aldosterone system inhibitors, 74
Renin-angiotensin system (RAS), 60
Renovascular disease, types of, 107
Rhabdomyomas, 122
Rheumatoid arthritis, 144
Right bundle branch pattern (RBBB), 157
Right ventricular outflow tract (RVOT), 153, 154, 155
ROC analysis. *See* Receiver operating characteristics (ROC) analysis
Romhilt–Estes point score, 52, 53, 56
ROMICAT trial, 16
Rouleaux, formation by red-blood cells, 129
RVOT. *See* Right ventricular outflow tract (RVOT)
RV systolic pressures (RVSP), 163

SAECG. *See* Signal-averaged electrocardiogram (SAECG)
SANDS. *See* Stop Atherosclerosis in Native Diabetics Study (SANDS)
SCD. *See* Sudden cardiac death (SCD)
SEC. *See* Spontaneous echo contrast (SEC)
Sick sinus syndrome, 120, 121
Signal-averaged electrocardiogram (SAECG), 54
Signal-to-noise ratio, 106
    of cardiac potentials, 54
Silent ischemia, 71–72
Single-photon emission computed tomography (SPECT), 21, 28
SLE. *See* Systemic lupus erythematosus (SLE)
SMA. *See* Superior mesenteric artery (SMA)
Smoke. *See* Spontaneous echo contrast (SEC)

Sokolow–Lyon voltage criteria, 52, 53, 54, 55, 56, 58

SPECT. *See* Single-photon emission computed tomography (SPECT)

Sphygmomanometric cuffs, 94

Spontaneous echo contrast (SEC), 129–130

SSFP. *See* Steady-state free precession (SSFP)

Statin therapy, for reducing progression of aortic valve calcification, 131

STD. *See* ST-segment depression (STD)

Steady-state free precession (SSFP), 20, 21, 22

ST-elevation myocardial infarction (STEMI), 119

Stem cell transfer, 21

STEMI. *See* ST-elevation myocardial infarction (STEMI)

Stepped-care (SC) antihypertensive therapy, 60

Stop Atherosclerosis in Native Diabetics Study (SANDS), 75
  baseline and follow-up carotid and cardiac measures in, 76

Stress-recovery index, 46

Stroke
  high-risk cardioembolic sources of
    cardiac tumors, 121–123
    complex aortic atheroma, 124–125
    left atrial thrombus, 120–121
    left ventricular thrombus, 118–119
    prosthetic valves, 123–124
    valvular vegetations, 123
  medium or uncertain risk cardioembolic sources of, 118
    interatrial septal abnormalities, 125–129
    mitral valve prolapse, 130
    pulmonary arteriovenous malformations, 129
    spontaneous echo contrast, 129–130
    valvular calcification, 130–131
  nature of, 117

Stroke Prevention: Assessment of Risk in a Community (SPARC) study, 124

Stroke Prevention in Atrial Fibrillation (SPAF) III study, 124

ST-segment depression (STD), 57

Sudden cardiac death (SCD), 59, 61

Superficial femoral artery (SFA) stenosis, 95

Superior mesenteric artery (SMA), 110

Symptom-limited treadmill thallium testing, 39

Syndrome X, 78

Systemic lupus erythematosus (SLE)
  antiphospholipid antibody syndrome, 148
  arrhythmias and conduction system disease, 147
  diagnostic criteria for, 142
  myocardial disease
    abnormalities of left ventricular structure and function, 145–146
    myocarditis, 145
  pericardial disease, 147
  pulmonary hypertension, 147–148
  relationship of cardiovascular manifestations in, 149
  valvular disease, 146–147
  vascular disease
    accelerated atherosclerosis, 141–144
    arterial stiffness, 144
    endothelial dysfunction, 145

Systolic dysfunction, 31

TEI. *See* Transmural extent of infarction (TEI)

Tetralogy of Fallot (TOF)
  anatomic features of, 153–154
  complications following
    atrial arrhythmias, 156–157
    pulmonary regurgitation and right ventricular dilatation, 156
    ventricular arrhythmias and sudden cardiac death, 157–158
  coronary artery anomalies, 154
  intracardiac repair of, 155
  long-term survival in patients with, 165
  other complications requiring interventions, 163
  palliative shunt procedure for, 155
  ventricular septal defect in, 153

Thrombus imaging, 29

TIA. *See* Transient ischemic attack (TIA)

Tissue characterization, using delayed enhancement CMR
  clinical applications of
    assessment of mechanical complications, 27
    guidance of medical therapy, 27
    guidance of revascularization, 25–27
  pathophysiologic basis of, 23–25

Toe-brachial indices, 93, 95

TOF. *See* Tetralogy of Fallot (TOF)

TOMHS. *See* Treatment of Mild Hypertension Study (TOMHS)

Transesophageal echocardiograms (TTE), 120

Transient ischemic attack (TIA), 121

Transmural extent of infarction (TEI), 25, 26

Transthoracic echocardiography (TTE), 119

Treadmill exercise test, 38, 90, 95–96

Treatment of Mild Hypertension Study (TOMHS), 60

TTE. *See* Transesophageal echocardiograms (TTE); Transthoracic echocardiography (TTE)

UK Prospective Diabetes Study (UKPDS), 75, 77

Valvular calcification
  aortic valve sclerosis, 130–131
  mitral annular calcification, 130
  valvular strands, 131–132

Valvular disease, 141, 146–147, 149

Valvular heart disease, 51, 147, 148

Valvular regurgitation, 14, 19, 21, 146, 156

Valvular strands, 118, 131–132

Valvular vegetations, 123

Vascular disease
  accelerated atherosclerosis, 141–144
  arterial stiffness, 144
  endothelial dysfunction, 145

Vascular ultrasonography, 97
Venography, conventional and
  MRI, 127
Venous thrombosis, 127
Ventricular arrhythmias, and sudden
  cardiac death, 157–158
Ventricular ectopy, 59

Ventricular premature contractions
  (VPCs), 157
Ventricular tachyarrhythmias, 28
Vertebral artery
  stenosis, 104
Very low-density lipoprotein (VLDL)
  triglycerides, 73

VPCs. *See* Ventricular premature
  contractions (VPCs)

Warnes–Somerville ability index, 162
Waterson shunt, 155